This book is dedicated to my mother,
Lillian P. Stanley, forever a nurse!

Advanced Practice Nursing:
Emphasizing Common Roles

Edition 2

Joan M. Stanley, PhD, RN, CRNP
Director of Education Policy
American Association of Colleges of Nursing
Washington, DC

 F.A. Davis Company • Philadelphia

F. A. Davis Company
1915 Arch Street
Philadelphia, PA 19103
www.fadavis.com

Printed in the United States of America

Last digit indicates print number: 10 9 8 7 6 5 4 3 2 1

Acquisitions Editor: Joanne Patzek DaCunha, RN, MSN
Developmental Editor: Kristin L. Kern
Design Manager: Joan Wendt

As new scientific information becomes available through basic and clinical research, recommended treatments and drug therapies undergo changes. The author(s) and publisher have done everything possible to make this book accurate, up to date, and in accord with accepted standards at the time of publication. The author(s), editors, and publisher are not responsible for errors or omissions or for consequences from application of the book, and make no warranty, expressed or implied, in regard to the contents of the book. Any practice described in this book should be applied by the reader in accordance with professional standards of care used in regard to the unique circumstances that may apply in each situation. The reader is advised always to check product information (package inserts) for changes and new information regarding dose and contraindications before administering any drug. Caution is especially urged when using new or infrequently ordered drugs.

Library of Congress Cataloging-in-Publication Data

Advanced practice nursing : emphasizing common roles / [edited by] Joan M. Stanley.—2nd ed.
  p. ; cm.
  Includes bibliographical references and index.
  ISBN 0-8036-1229-X (hardcover : alk. paper)
  1. Nurse practitioners. 2. Midwives. 3. Nurse anesthetists.
  [DNLM: 1. Nurse Clinicians. 2. Nurse Practitioners. 3. Nurse Midwives. WY 128 A2445 2005] I. Stanley, Joan M.
  RT82.8.A37 2005
  610.73′06′92—dc22
                2004001938

Foreword

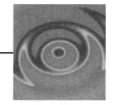

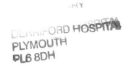

With information overload a challenge in all of our lives, why should anyone read this book? The answer is simple—this book is not only informative, covering the major issues facing advanced practices nurses (APNs), but it is also vital to understanding the past, present, and future of advanced practice. This effort weaves together historical views of APNs with present-day issues and trends. The contributors have masterfully analyzed the issues so that the reader will come to know both the larger policy issues facing APNs and how these issues translate into day-to-day care of patients.

The critical examination of financing, values, politics, and intraprofessional education and practice as well as interprofessional relationships combines to bring APNs into sharp focus. The evolution of APNs has been a major event in the history of nursing. While each of the four APN disciplines—clinical nurse specialist, nurse practitioner, certified nurse midwife, and nurse anesthetist—has a unique history and place within nursing, the commonalities have established a force within health care that has changed the way care is delivered and will continue to change the system. In fact, the commonalities provide a critical basis for forging an even more powerful coalition of APNs to tackle common challenges related to ensuring patients get the best care possible. The social contract that nurses have with the public is unique, and APNs have extended that contract to higher levels of service, decision-making, and accountability.

This book captures the vitality of advanced practice nursing as an aggregated entity. The label of APN is now widely used and recognized by policy makers and patients alike. This represents unprecedented progress in nursing, when few knew what a clinical specialist or nurse practitioner was. We are largely past the days of having to prove the viability, utility, and safety of APNs. We are now constructively examining practice issues in order to advance patient care, not defend the practice.

Each chapter presents perspectives that are useful resources unto themselves. A valuable part of each chapter is the suggested exercises. Readers will appreciate the challenge that these exercises afford them. Taking the time to think through the questions will give APNs and others a chance to explore issues they may not have thought to explore. Even though each chapter is a resource itself, the collection of chapters is so well orchestrated that the full picture is definitely greater than the parts.

Whether this book is used by students, practicing APNs, policy makers, or other health professionals, it will be an extraordinary resource.

Jean Johnson, PhD, FAAN
Senior Associate Dean and Professor
George Washington University Medical Center
Washington, DC

Acknowledgments

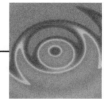

As an APN for the past 30 years, more years than I want to count, I have made many lasting and cherished friends among the APN community. A very heart-felt thanks goes out to all on whom I called and who allowed me to cajole them into contributing to this project. The collegiality of the APN community was truly demonstrated.

I also am deeply indebted to all my friends and colleagues who provided support throughout this endeavor. Several people were particularly helpful in providing guidance and wisdom. A special thanks goes to Christine Sheehy and Marilyn Edmunds, who shared their expertise and insight on editing a book. I also am indebted to my editor, Joanne DaCunha, for her patience and confidence through the many stages of learning and production.

Finally, loving thanks go to my husband, Jack, and my two boys, Jonny and Jeff, for their understanding, love, and support. And to my little sister, June, an FNP, who has always been there for me when I needed a listening ear or a laugh: thank you.

JMS

Contributors

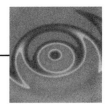

Janet Allan, PhD, RN, NP, FAAN
Dean
University of Maryland School of Nursing
Baltimore, Maryland

Geraldine "Polly" Bednash, PhD, RN, FAAN
Executive Director
American Association of Colleges of Nursing
Washington, DC

Debra Bergstrom, MS, RN, FNP
Nurse Practitioner
Neighborhood Family Practice, PC

Linda A. Bernhard, PhD, RN
Associate Professor and
Associate Dean of Academic Affairs
The Ohio State University
Columbus, Ohio

Pier Angeli Broadnax, PhD, RN
Assistant Professor
Howard University
Washington, DC

Vicki L. Buchda, MS, RN
Director, Patient Care Resources
Mayo Clinic
Scottsdale, Arizona

Christine E. Burke, PhD, CNM
Clinical Practice
The Denver Health Authority
Denver, Colorado

Linda Callahan, PhD, CRNA
Associate Professor
Department of Nursing
California State University
Long Beach, California

Dennis J. Cheek, PhD, RN, FAHA
Professor, Harris School of Nursing and
School of Anesthesia
Texas Christian University, Texas

Katherine Crabtree, DNSc, FAAN APRN, BC
Professor
Oregon Health and Science University
Portland, Oregon

Linda Lindsey Davis, PhD, RN
Professor, School of Nursing
Senior Scientist, Center for Aging
University of Alabama at Birmingham
Birmingham, Alabama

Julie Reed Erickson, PhD, RN, FAAN
Associate Professor
University of Arizona College of Nursing
Tucson, Arizona

Margaret Faut-Callahan, DNSc, CRNA, FAAN
Professor and Chair of Adult Health Nursing and
Director of the Nurse Anesthesia Program
Rush University College of Nursing
Chicago, Illinois

Linda Gibbs, BSN, RN, MBA
Assistant Professor of Clinical Nursing
Associate Dean for Practice Development
Columbia University School of Nursing
New York, New York

Catherine L. Gilliss, DNSc, RN, FAAN
Dean and Professor
Yale University
New Haven, Connecticut

Karol S. Harshaw-Ellis, MSN, RN, A/GNP, ACNP-CS
Consulting Clinical Associate
Durham Regional Hospital

Practicing Acute Care Nurse Practitioner
Durham, North Carolina

Judy Honig, EdD, CPNP
Associate Professor of Clinical Nursing
and Associate Dean, Student Services
Columbia University School of Nursing
New York, New York

Betty J. Horton, CRNA, DNS
Immediate Past Director
American Association of Nurse Anesthetists Accreditation Council
Chicago, Illinois

Anita Hunter, PhD, RN, CNS, CPNP
Associate Professor and PNP
University of San Diego
San Diego, California

Lucille A. Joel. EdD, RN, FAAN
Professor
Rutgers—The State University of New Jersey, College of Nursing
Newark, New Jersey

Jean Johnson, PhD, FAAN
Senior Associate Dean and Professor
George Washington
University Medical Center
Washington, DC

Suzanne Hall Johnson MN, RN,C, CNS
Director, Hall Johnson Consulting, Inc
Editor Emeritus, *Nurse Author & Editor* and *Dimensions of Critical Care Nursing*
Lakewood, Colorado

Mary Knudtson MSN, NP
Professor of Family Medicine
University of California,
Irvine, California

Pauline Komnenich, PhD, RN
Professor
Arizona State University College of Nursing
Tempe, Arizona

Michael J. Kremer, DNSc, CRNA, FAAN
Associate Professor of Adult Health Nursing and
Assistant Director of the Nursing Anesthesia Program
Rush University College of Nursing
Chicago, Illinois

Brenda L. Lyon, DNS, FAAN
Professor, Adult Health Nursing
Indiana University School of Nursing
Indianapolis, Indiana

Mary Jeannette Mannino, JD, CRNA
Director, Anesthesia and Ambulatory Surgery
The Mannino Group
Washington, D.C.

Eileen T. O'Grady, PhD, RN, NP
Adjunct Assistant Professor
George Washington University School of Medicine
and Health Sciences and
George Mason University College of Nursing
and Health Science
Fairfax, Virginia

Mary Ann Shah, CNM, MS, FACNM
President, American College of Nurse-Midwives
Editor Emeritus, *Journal of Midwifery & Women's Health*
White Plains, New York

Christine Sheehy, PhD, RN
Chief, Quality of Care and Program Monitoring for
Geriatrics and Extended Care in the Veterans Health Administration
Washington, DC

Michelle Walsh, PhD, RN, CPNP
Pediatric Nurse Practitioner
Columbus, Ohio

Marla J. Weston, MS, RN
Executive Director
Arizona Nurses' Association
Phoenix, Arizona

Consultants

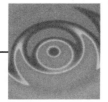

Lynne M. Dunphy, PhD, FNP, CS
Associate Professor
Florida Atlantic University
Boca Raton, Florida

Laurie Kennedy-Malone, PhD, RN, APRN-BC, GNP
Associate Professor
Director of the Adult/Gerontological Nurse Practitioner Program
School of Nursing
The University of North Carolina at Greensboro
Greensboro, North Carolina

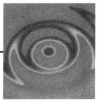

Contents

Introduction

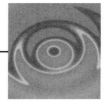

Joan M. Stanley, PhD, RN, CRNP

Joan Stanley, PhD, RN, CRNP, is currently Director of Education Policy at the American Association of Colleges of Nursing (AACN), a position she has held since 1994. She has served on many of the association's task forces and committees, including the Task Forces on Essentials of Master's Education for Advanced Practice Nursing, Essentials of Baccalaureate Education for Professional Nursing Practice, Hallmarks of Professional Nursing Practice, Quality Indicators for Research-Focused Doctoral Programs, and Education, Regulation and Practice II. She codirected the national project to develop consensus-based Primary Care Competencies for Adult, Family, Gerontology, Pediatric and Women's Health. She has also served as the association's representative to numerous advanced practice nursing projects, including the American Nurses Association's Task Force on the Scope and Standards for Advanced Practice Nursing, The National Council of State Boards of Nursing' Advisory Committee for the Family Nurse Practitioner Pharmacology Curriculum Project, and the first and second national task forces that developed the Criteria for Evaluation of Nurse Practitioner Programs. In addition, since 1991, Dr. Stanley has served as project director for a contract awarded to the AACN by the National Health Service Corps and served on the NHSC Technical Advisory Group on the Evaluation of the Effectiveness of the NHSC. She also maintains a practice as an adult nurse practitioner at the University of Maryland Hospital Faculty Practice Office. Before joining the AACN, Dr. Stanley was assistant professor at the School of Nursing at the University of Maryland and associate director of Primary Care Nursing Services at the University of Maryland Hospital. Dr. Stanley received her bachelor's of science degree in nursing from Duke University and her master's of science in nursing and her doctorate in higher education organization and policy from the University of Maryland.

One commonality undergirds all four advanced practice nursing roles–the discipline of nursing. At the same time, it is the unique combination of nursing knowledge, science, and practice that differentiates each of the advanced practice nursing roles from one another and from other health professional roles and practice. Now is an exciting time for advanced practice nurses (APNs). After many decades, cost-effectiveness and beneficial outcomes of advanced nursing practice are being widely recognized by policy makers, other health professionals, and the public. Despite or because of the increased recognition and advances made, APNs face many issues, some recurrent and others emerging, related to education, certification, regulation, and practice. Increasingly over the past 10 years, leaders in the APN community have recognized the need and benefit to collaborate in addressing these common concerns. Some of the most critical emerging and recurrent practice issues confronting APNs include attempts to limit scope of practice, rising costs of malpractice insurance premiums, establishing parity with other health professions, maintenance of ongoing competence, and standardized recognition for reimbursement, primary care status, and practice privileges. Current education issues facing the APN community include concern over subspecialization, maintenance of quality programs, and the exponential growth of scientific knowledge, technology, and role expectations, all of which have increased credit requirements and length of education programs. A comprehensive list of critical issues currently facing APNs could probably be developed. However, the nuances, importance of, and interaction of events affecting each of these issues are changing constantly. Just since beginning work on this text, changes in economic and health policies, funding sources, and even organizational policies are just of a few of the things that have significantly impacted, both positively and negatively, APN practice and education. An overall and ongoing awareness of these issues, and of others not yet evident, is what is imperative for each APN in order to navigate the current and future health care environment successfully.

Four nursing leaders, each recognized for leadership and expertise in one of the APN specialties, were asked to identify and briefly discuss the critical issues facing their APN specialty, now and in the near future. These perspectives represent the individual's opinion and personal thoughts and are presented here as a basis for reflection and discussion.

THE CERTIFIED REGISTERED NURSE ANESTHETIST ISSUES TODAY AND TOMORROW

Betty J. Horton, CRNA, DNSc
Immediate Past Director

American Association of Nurse Anesthetists (AANA)
Accreditation Council

Nurses were chosen by surgeons to administer anesthesia in the United States shortly after the discovery of ether in the middle of the 19th century. In 1893, Isabel Robb documented the education of nurses as anesthetists by including a chapter on the administration of anesthesia in her nursing textbook. She indicated that nurses needed the information because they were often asked to give anesthesia to alleviate the pain and suffering of patients. Thus, Robb identified nurses as the first professional group to provide anesthesia in the United States prior to the establishment of anesthesiology as a specialty option for physicians following World War II.

In the early 20th century, court decisions established that nurse anesthetists were not practicing medicine but rather practicing nursing when they administered anesthesia. These legal opinions paved the way for a current population of approximately 30,000 certified registered nurse anesthetists (CRNAs) to administer more than 65 percent of the 26 million anesthetics given annually in 50 states and Puerto Rico. CRNAs practice in all types of practice settings, from large urban centers to more than two-thirds of rural hospitals where they are the sole anesthesia providers. Fifty-eight percent of CRNAs are women, and 42 percent are men.[i]

There are many important education and practice issues facing CRNAs in the early 21st century. Key issues in education include approval of schools, certification, academic degrees, and continuing education. Key practice issues are changes in the work environment, equitable reimbursement for services, continuing education, maintaining a full scope of practice, and staffing shortages.

Education Issues

Nurse anesthetists recognized education as a top priority at the first meeting of the National Association of Nurse Anesthetists (later renamed the American Association of Nurse Anesthetists [AANA]) in 1931. This focus on education was maintained throughout the 20th century with the establishment of educational standards, accreditation of schools, certification of nurse anesthetists for entry into practice, and a recertification process requiring mandatory continuing education. Civilian and military employers, insurers, and governments soon recognized the value of the accreditation, certification, and recertification requirements as established prerequisites for nurses as anesthetists to provide safe care to patients. The maintenance of strong accreditation, certification, recertification, and continuing education programs will continue to hold value and high priority for CRNAs.

Support of graduate education for nurse anesthetists has also been a key issue. Following the move of all certificate nurse anesthesia programs into graduate education to comply with a 1998 deadline set by the Council on Accreditation of Nurse Anesthesia Education Programs, it is projected that every practicing CRNA will possess a minimum of a master's degree sometime in the first half of the 21st century. Continued support for graduate education will undoubtedly increase knowledge from research on education and practice.

Another key issue is the education of adequate numbers of students to meet the increasing demands for anesthesia services. Nurse anesthesia programs have been admitting more students as resources permit to meet a national need for increased staffing. However, the recruitment and retention of more qualified faculty are vital to meeting anesthesia personnel needs. Success in obtaining government funding for education and payment for patient care services provided by CRNA clinical instructors will affect the availability of adequate resources necessary to continue educating enough anesthetists in the future.

Practice Issues

Providing safe hands-on care to one patient at a time is the hallmark of nurse anesthesia care. Close patient contact is provided in an environment where major health care reform has redefined how and where anesthesia care is to be provided, with significant reduction in the amount of time nurse anesthetists can spend with patients. Changes in the practice environment have also included a tremendous expansion of knowledge and technology in recent decades. This requires that nurse anesthetists use a great deal of technology in all kinds of practice settings whether part of an anesthesia team or not. Complex services must be provided that require a full scope of practice with a wide variety of anesthesia techniques, drugs, and equipment. The need to keep abreast of changes within the field will continue to commit CRNAs to continuing education and evidence-based practice throughout their careers.

The AANA and state nurse anesthesia organizations have made concerted efforts to avoid reimbursement disincentives for the use of CRNAs. Although opposed vigorously by anesthesiologists, nurse anesthetists were the first nurses to initiate a successful lobbying effort resulting in direct reimbursement from Medicare in 1989. Today, nurse anesthesia services are additionally reimbursed by various states and federal programs plus some commercial insurance carriers. A proposal to eliminate physician supervision as a condition of Medicare reimbursement was deemed to be each state's prerogative rather than a federal policy, which had been strongly supported by nursing. A number of states have opted out of the requirement that tied reimbursement for CRNAs to physician supervision. Lobbying for equitable reimbursement for services of civilian CRNAs and financial incentives for military CRNAs will be ongoing. Contributions to political campaigns are an important part of organized lobbying efforts. In 2002, the national political action committee, CRNA PAC, ranked 107 out of approximately 3,000 federal PACs.

In addition to equitable reimbursement for CRNAs, other critical practice issues include the availability and affordability of liability insurance; the regulation of clinical practice at the institutional, state, and federal levels; the maintenance of a full scope of practice; and strained relationships between anesthesiologists and nurse anesthetists at the national and state levels. Undoubtedly, lobbying, public relations, and liaisons with other APN groups will continue to be at the forefront in attaining successful resolution to these issues in the foreseeable future.

MIDWIFERY, A BLEND OF ART AND SCIENCE

Mary Ann Shah, CNM, MS, FACNM

President, American College of Nurse-Midwives (ACNM)

Editor Emeritus, *Journal of Midwifery & Women's Health*

In 2005, the American College of Nurse-Midwives (ACNM) will celebrate its 50th anniversary as the professional organization for certified nurse-midwives (CNMs) and certified midwives (CMs). However, its historic roots date back to 1925 when Mary Breckinridge sent public health nurses to Great Britain for midwifery training, and they returned to the Frontier Nursing Service of Kentucky, serving as the first nurse-midwives in the United States. A few years later, the first formal nurse-midwifery education program within the United States was initiated in New York City, and public health nurses were, once again, targeted for recruitment.

The ACNM has had a long and complex history with nursing. Nurse-midwifery established itself as a profession in the 1920s, separate from but paired with nursing; thus, its hyphenated name. During the mid-1940s, a section for nurse-midwives was created within the National Organization of Public Health Nurses (NOPHN). However, NOPHN was absorbed into the American Nurses Association and the National League for Nursing a few years later, and subsequent efforts to reestablish a niche specific to nurse-midwifery within these nursing organizations were unsuccessful. Thus, nurse-midwives were forced to seek their own professional organization; in 1955, they incorporated in New Mexico as the American College of Nurse-Midwifery (the name was modified to its current one in 1969). Today, midwives are licensed to practice under a variety of midwifery, nursing, medical, and/or other state regulatory agencies. Regardless of how they are credentialed, it seems safe to say that the interrelationship between midwives and nurses will always be a collegial and collaborative one.

The ACNM has also had an evolving relationship with the American College of Obstetricians and Gynecologists (ACOG). Although formal recognition by ACOG in the early 1970s helped bring midwifery care into hospitals, finding language that supported autonomous decision-making has been difficult. This was finally achieved in October 2002, when the current version of the Joint Statement of Practice Relations was approved by both organizations. This document clearly espouses mutual respect and collaboration between physicians and CNMs/CMs while placing professional accountability where it rightfully belongs: on the individual provider of care: "ACOG and ACNM affirm their commitment to promote appropriate standards for education and certification of their respective members, to support appropriate practice guidelines, and to facilitate communication between obstetrician-gynecologists and certified nurse-midwives/certified midwives."[ii]

While the majority of today's midwives have entered the profession through nursing education and have received the CNM credential, a growing number are gaining entry via an approved alternate, but equivalent, education pathway and are qualifying for the CM credential. The ACNM currently represents over 7,100 CNMs and CMs, having certified the 10,000th midwife in 2002. The organization is committed to maintaining the highest standards for the practice of midwifery, the accreditation of education programs, and the certification of practitioners.

It must be underscored that, similar to their nurse peers, non-nurse applicants to ACNM-accredited midwifery education programs must successfully complete university-level prerequisite courses in biology, microbiology, anatomy and physiology, pathophysiology, psychology, sociology, chemistry, human development, epidemiology or statistics, and nutrition. Furthermore, although the ACNM Division of Accreditation did not mandate that all CNMs and CMs possess a minimum of a baccalaureate degree until the 1990s, over 73 percent have earned an additional master's or higher degree. In addition, all must graduate from an accredited midwifery education program that is affiliated with an institution of higher learning and must pass the national certification examination administered by the ACNM Certification Council, Inc.

According to data released by the U.S. National Center for Health Statistics in 2001, CNMs attended 10 percent of all vaginal births in the United States, more than tripling the number reported nationally since 1989. Most notably, 34.5 percent of all vaginal births in New Mexico that same year were attended by CNMs, with Georgia (23.5 percent), New Hampshire (22.1 percent), and Vermont (21 percent) also setting remarkable records. Unfortunately, other aspects of midwifery practice are more difficult to track.

The midwife's scope of practice, as embodied within the ACNM's standards, promotes "individual rights and self-determination within boundaries of safety," comprises "knowledge, skills, and judgments that foster the delivery of safe, satisfying, and culturally competent care," and is supported by the ACNM's Hallmarks of Midwifery,[iii] which espouse, among others, the following high ideals:

- Advocacy of nonintervention in the absence of complications, informed choice, participatory decision-making, and the right to self-determination
- Incorporation of scientific evidence into clinical practice
- Promotion of family-centered/continuity of care, cultural competency, care to vulnerable populations, and a public health perspective
- Recognition of the therapeutic value of human presence
- Empowerment of women as partners in health care
- Skillful communication, guidance, and counseling
- Health promotion, disease prevention, and health education
- Facilitation of healthy family and interpersonal relationships
- Familiarity with common complementary and alternative therapies

The ACNM's Core Competencies for Basic Midwifery Practice[iii] specifically delineate the minimal expectations for CNMs and CMs upon entry into practice and serve as the foundation on which all ACNM-accredited midwifery education programs base their curricula. They stipulate that the CNM/CM must be prepared to independently manage—utilizing consultation, collaboration, and/or referral to appropriate levels of health care services—all of the following:

- Primary health screening and health promotion of women from the perimenarcheal through the postmenopausal periods
- Gynecologic and family planning interventions
- Human sexuality counseling
- Therapies for common health problems/deviations of essentially healthy women
- Care of women during pregnancy, childbirth, and the postpartum period
- Care of the newborn during the first 28 days of life

The ACNM proudly proclaims that midwifery represents the ideal blend of art and science, i.e. "the best of both worlds," offering women "high-touch/low-tech care with high-tech options," and that midwives are "With women, for a lifetime®". As Hattie Hemschemeyer, ACNM's first president, wrote in 1956: "The future looks bright."

CLINICAL NURSE SPECIALISTS: CURRENT CHALLENGES

Brenda L. Lyon DNS, FAAN

Professor, Adult Health Nursing

Indiana University School of Nursing

Past President, National Association of Clinical Nurse Specialists

Over the years, there has been considerable confusion regarding the commonalities and differences among the four different advanced practice nurse (APN) scopes of practice and roles, particularly between those of the clinical nurse specialist (CNS) and nurse practitioner (NP). Although there are some commonalities in competencies and some common concerns across all APNs, each area of advanced practice nursing is responsive to different societal needs for care.

CNSs are registered nurses (RNs) who have graduate (master's or doctoral degree) preparation as a CNS. The CNS is a clinical expert in the application of theory and research-based knowledge in a specialty area of nursing practice. Specialization is at the heart of all CNS practice. Today CNS specialties encompass one or any combination of settings (e.g., critical care, home or community care), general disease or injury categories (e.g., medical-surgical, trauma, neurology, oncology, diabetes, orthopedics, pulmonary, or perioperative), age (e.g., pediatrics or gerontology), life processes (e.g., perinatal or genetic), disease stage (e.g., chronic disease), and health-related phenomena (e.g., pain or stress). Areas of specialization have evolved over time in response to societal needs for CNS services.

The CNS scope of practice encompasses three spheres of influence: patient/client (direct care), nursing personnel (advancing the practice of nursing), and organization/network (interdisciplinary). The second and third spheres are often referred to as the indirect domains of CNS practice. The balance or focus of a CNS practice in these three spheres varies based on client and employer need. Each sphere of influence requires a unique set of core competencies regardless of specialty area. The National Association of Clinical Nurse Specialists (NACNS) Statement on Clinical Nurse Specialists Practice and Education[iv] articulates core CNS competencies in each of these spheres.

Nationally, the RN license authorizes the practitioner independently or autonomously to diagnose (nursing diagnoses) and treat (nursing therapeutics/treatments) health-related problems (symptoms and functional problems). In addition to this autonomous nursing scope of practice, practice acts authorize RNs to implement delegated medical therapeutics via prescriptive delegation or protocol. Since the 1970s, most CNSs have practiced at an advanced level within these scopes of practice. Some CNSs have extended their practice outside the domains authorized by the RN license, e.g., obtaining prescriptive authority. Important regulatory issues need to be addressed regarding CNS prescriptive authority. Specifically, should a second license be required for the CNS who prescribes medications as this practice activity is not authorized in the RN scope of practice?[v]

Today there is a critical shortage of CNSs. The U.S. Department of Health & Human Services (DHHS) estimated that there were approximately 54,000 CNSs in 2000.[vi] This number is lower than estimated in previous years, largely as a result of a reduction in CNS academic programs and positions during the 1990s. Reductions in reimbursements to hospitals in the early and middle 1990s created downward pressures on both RN and CNS staffing. The East and West coasts were particularly hard hit in the reduction of CNS positions. One of the factors contributing to the loss of CNS positions was, unfortunately (despite having a positive impact on outcomes and cost), the fact that most CNSs were documenting time spent in activities rather than outcomes, cost savings, cost avoidance, or revenue generation.[vii] Another factor was the almost exclusive attention placed by policy makers and schools of nursing on the preparation and regulation of NPs.

In 2002, the NACNS received an increasing number of recruiter requests, at least 25 to 50 per month, for open CNS positions. The pressure to increase the number of CNSs is evident in the fact that a 2001 NACNS survey found 183 CNS programs, whereas in 1997 only 147 CNS programs were reported.[vii] The DHHS Division of Nursing, in recent years, has also renewed its priority to include training grants for CNS programs.

Current challenges facing CNSs as APNs arise primarily from the regulatory and educational (academic and continuing professional learning) arenas.

Regulatory Challenges

In the regulatory arena, the challenges are particularly difficult. Specific regulatory challenges include:

- Preventing the creation of credentialing requirements for CNS practice that create unnecessary barriers to the public's access to the full range of CNS services

- Developing a legally defensible alternative to certification for regulatory recognition when no certification examination is available in a CNS specialty

- Achieving a reasonable level of uniformity to the regulation of CNS practice, thereby facilitating reciprocity across state lines

Unnecessary "overregulation" in credentialing CNSs is an immediate concern. Credentialing for regulatory purposes is important to affirm the educational preparation of a CNS, to establish a defined scope of practice, and to ensure patient safety. By 1999, 27 states recognized CNSs in statutes, providing title protection with a defined scope of practice.[viii] The issue is not whether regulation is necessary but what level of regulation is necessary. Some states require a second license; others require registration or certification. When a CNS practices within the domains authorized by the RN license, requiring a second license would create unnecessary practice barriers. However, when a CNS chooses to obtain prescriptive authority or expand the scope of practice, the need to acquire a second license authorizing practice beyond that of the RN license becomes clearer. Currently, state boards of nursing accept certification as a proxy for a second licensure examination. This is not a barrier to practice when there is a CNS certification examination available in a CNS's specialty area of practice. However, when no such examination exists, e.g., in orthopedics, perioperative care, or diabetes, the CNS is denied authorization to practice, and the public is denied access to CNS services. Two possible resolutions have been proposed, including the development of a CNS "core" competencies examination and the use of legally defensible portfolios.[vii] These possible solutions currently are being jointly investigated by the NACNS and the American Nurses Credentialing Center.

Currently, there is wide variation in both statutory recognition of CNSs and regulations governing CNS practice across states. This variation for CNSs and other APNs creates difficult, or even insurmountable, barriers to reciprocity for practice across state lines. This lack of uniformity in regulating APNs must be addressed by the profession as a whole.

Education Challenges

Challenges in the academic and continuing professional learning arena include:

- Implementing educational standards consistent with NACNS standards for CNS academic programs and developing a mechanism to recognize programs that meet these standards or incorporate these standards into accreditation processes.
- Establishing a Web-based continuing education and mentoring network
- Determining whether there is a need for a practice-focused doctoral degree for CNSs to expand knowledge and skill in such areas as action research, e.g., to develop and test models for diffusion of knowledge, testing innovations in practice; and testing the economics and cost-benefits of CNS practice.

The NACNS CNS Educational Standards document was released in early 2004. These standards help assure that CNS academic programs focus on the same learning outcomes while not prescribing a uniform curriculum.

CNSs, like other APNs, are scattered across the country and practice in many different types of settings. Future life-long learning needed for practice and career development will best be met by Web-based continuing education and mentoring.

Currently, there is considerable debate in the discipline about whether there is a need for another doctoral degree; specifically, one focused on nursing practice. The impetus for a practice doctorate is the perceived need to prepare nurses at a higher level for practice as well as to prepare clinical nursing faculty. Currently, many CNSs who seek the doctorate, a research-focused degree, do so because they have been turned on to research and desire to increase their capacity to contribute to knowledge development for the discipline. Questions related to the practice doctorate that must be examined by APNs, educators, and consumers of APN services include what additional competencies are needed and will the market bear the increased cost for a practitioner or APN who has these competencies.

The continuing evolution of CNS practice will be characterized by the sustained development and evaluation of evidence-based innovations in nursing practice and a substantial rise in CNS scholarly publications. There is an increasing need for CNSs to publish scholarly works related to researchable nursing practice problems, best practices, outcomes evaluation, and strategies to enhance diffusion of knowledge into nursing practice. Likewise, there is a tremendous need for systematic evaluation of evidence-based innovations in nursing practice. The systematic demonstration of effectiveness of nursing interventions on patient outcomes and cost-effectiveness will help assure the future inclusion of these activities in CPT coding and therefore reimbursement of CNS autonomous nursing services.

THE NURSE PRACTITIONER: A LOOK AT THE FUTURE

Janet Allan, PhD, RN, NP, FAAN

Dean, University of Maryland School of Nursing

Past President, National Organization of Nurse Practitioner Faculties

A distinguished nursing dean once said, "Nurse practitioners (NPs) are the future of nursing." Time has substantiated this remark. In the nearly 40 years since the NP role was first conceptualized and implemented, the development of the role has in many ways revolutionized nursing education and clinical practice. Although predated by the three other major advanced practice nursing roles, the NP role has served as the major catalyst for changes in education, practice, and policy. NP education is the major component of graduate nursing, with nearly 53 percent of master's level students enrolled in NP programs offered in over 325 institutions.[ix] Curriculum standards, preceptor guidelines, role competencies, and program standards for NP education have been accepted as mainstream in graduate nursing education. NPs have established a well-recognized and respected advanced practice guideline-based direct care role spanning primary care to tertiary care settings. NPs have made a major contribution to improving the health care of vulnerable populations and populations experiencing a disproportionate number of health disparities. By capitalizing on trends in the larger health care system, political activism, and coalition-building, NPs have been able to implement a full primary care scope of practice and receive reimbursement for their services. Despite these successes, many challenges remain for NP education and practice.

I would like to comment briefly on five critical challenges and opportunities facing NP education and practice in the next decade.

Educate the NP for the Future

NP faculty must continue to maintain high educational standards while continuing to evolve curricula to respond to society's needs and health care system changes. There needs to be further elaboration of ways to implement quality improvement methods and national standards. Better data systems need to be developed in order to document and monitor educational outcomes. As the NP role continues to both evolve and diversify from the initial primary care focus, there will be more blended roles, more specialty roles, and further development of the NP scope of practice, particularly within multidisciplinary teams. There needs to be an emphasis on preparing the NP to function in an evolving health care system. Content on cost-effectiveness, work systems, technological supports, quality assessment, leadership, and team-building will need to be incorporated into current educational programs.

Develop Evidence-Based Practices

This has come about given the increasing emphasis on quality of care, guideline-based productivity and evaluation, practice cost outcomes, and the use of evidence-based guidelines to promote equity of care.[x] NPs must fully implement evidence-based practices. NPs, regardless of practice setting, have the opportunity to further develop standardized practice guidelines that integrate nationally accepted interdisciplinary guidelines and practices with nursing's focus on health promotion. Utilization of standardized guidelines provides a basis for evaluation of the contributions of NPs to patient care in multidisciplinary practices. Given a variety of scenarios about future numbers and the role of NPs and physicians in managed care settings, there are opportunities for NPs to develop innovative models of care that expand scope of practice and place the NP in a more dominant primary care management role.

Use Technological Innovations and Practice Support Systems/ Resources to Better Deliver Care

Recent developments in technology and practice systems provide innovative ways to remove barriers and enhance the delivery of care. NPs have the opportunity to incorporate and tailor care support processes and resources to their practice setting and population. Such systems are particularly helpful in primary care settings to maximize the effectiveness of the provider/patient interaction for health behavior change and counseling.[xi] NPs also have opportunities to explore the use of technology to deliver health care to populations at remote sites.

Increase Research on NP Practice

Research on patient outcomes and cost-effectiveness of care is essential to document the value of NP practice and to increase our knowledge base of effective interventions and practice models. We need more knowledge to create effective interventions for populations that differ by ethnicity, gender, and geographic location. Demonstrating improvements in health outcomes and cost-effectiveness will be more and more expected of NPs in the future. We need research on the effectiveness of varying care support systems and technological innovations used to support interventions. NPs in community-based practices need to form more research-based practice networks similar to those of physicians in order to examine clinical problems and practice patterns.[xii] Such networks allow aggregation across many small practices so that NPs can document outcomes of care and study important clinical questions.

Move from Competition to Partnership

The dismal state of our health care system, the lack of consumer satisfaction with health care, the growing elderly population, the growth in community-based care, spiraling costs, and the continuing magnitude of certain populations experiencing major health disparities afford NPs an opportunity to create partnerships, build teams of professional and lay providers, and collaborate with target communities. As a society, we will not be able to provide quality care for the aging population or reduce health disparities effectively without major changes in the way we think about and deliver care. NPs and other disciplines have the opportunity to develop teams and models of care, with the patient at the center. There also is the opportunity to explore interdisciplinary regulation and clinical integration to ensure high standards of care.

SUMMARY

Four nursing leaders have presented their unique perspectives on advanced practice nursing. Similar, yet different, histories, themes, and issues pervade these presentations. APNs are responsible and accountable for practice outcomes. Likewise, we must be accountable for our actions and decisions that influence the policies and events that shape future APN practice. We cannot assume that others, particularly those outside of advanced practice nursing, will assume responsibility for ensuring the future of the profession. The topics addressed in *Advanced Practice Nursing: Emphasizing Common Roles* provide a broad treatment not only of the history of APN roles but also of key issues and events that have impacted the evolution of APN education and practice and continue to present significant challenges to the future of all APN roles.

REFERENCES

[i]American Association of Nurse Anesthetists: Certified Registered Nurse Anesthetists, Nurse Anesthetists at a Glance. http://www.aana.com/crna/ataglance.asp. Accessed 6/26/2003

[ii]American College of Nurse Midwives & American College of Obstetricians and Gynecologists: Joint Statement of Practice Relations, October 2002. http://www.midwife.org/prof/jointstate.cfm. Accessed 11/30/2003.

[iii]American College of Nurse Midwives: Core Competencies for Basic Midwifery Practice, May 2002. http://www.midwife.org/prof/display.cfm?id = 137. Accessed 11/30/2003

[iv]National Association of Clinical Nurse Specialists: Statement on Clinical Nurse Specialist Practice and Education, Harrisburg, PA, National Association of Clinical Nurse Specialists, 2004.

[v]Lyon, BL: The regulation of clinical nurse specialist practice: Issue and current developments. Clin Nurse Specialist 16:239, 2002.

[vi]U.S. Department of Health & Human Services: The Registered Nurse Population. 2000 Fact Sheet. Findings from the National Sample Survey of Registered Nurses. Health Resources & Services Administration. Rockville, MD, Bureau of Health Professions, Division of Nursing, 2001.

[vii]Dayhoff, N, and Lyon, BL: Assessing outcomes of clinical nurse specialist practice. In Kleinpell, R. (ed.): Outcome Assessment in Advanced Nursing, pp. 103–129. New York, Springer Publishing Co., 2001.

[viii]Lyon, BL, and Minarik, P.: Statutory and regulatory issues for clinical nurse specialist practice: Assuring the public's access to CNS services. Clin Nurse Specialist 15:108, 2001.

[ix]Berlin, L, Stennett, J, and Bednash, G. 2002–2003 Enrollment and Graduations in Baccalaureate and

Graduate Programs in Nursing. Washington, DC, American Association of Colleges of Nursing, 2003.

[x]Institute of Medicine: Unequal Treatment: Confronting Racial and Ethnic Disparities in Health Care. Washington, DC, National Academies of Science Press, 2002.

[xi]Solberg, L, et al.: The case for the missing clinical preventive services systems. Effectiveness Clin Pract 1:33, 1998.

[xii]Grey, M, and Walker, PH: Practice-based research networks for nursing. Nursing Outlook. 46:125, 1988.

CHAPTER 1

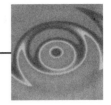

The Evolution of
Advanced Practice
in Nursing

CHAPTER 1

Pauline Komnenich, PhD, RN

Pauline Komnenich, PhD, RN, is currently a Professor in the College of Nursing at Arizona State University. She received her baccalaureate from Stanford University and her master's in nursing from the University of Washington. She also has a master's degree in anthropology and a doctorate in linguistics from the University of Arizona, which she received through the Nurse Scientist Program.

During the past 40 years in nursing, Dr. Komnenich has made contributions to nursing as an educator, researcher in women's health and family caregiving for frail elders in the home, and clinical practitioner in elder care and educational administration. Her major contributions in nursing have been to research, research development, and nursing education. She has provided leadership for care management of the elderly and parish nursing. She has a broad background of experience both nationally and internationally, having participated in nursing education and research in Eastern Europe and primary health care in Argentina. Professor Komnenich participated as a Fulbright Senior Scholar in the School of Health at the University of Sarajevo, Bosnia-Hecegovina, in 1999 to develop a curriculum for nurses and allied health professionals. During that time she also conducted a collaborative study with two Bosnian physiatrists on the cross-cultural factors influencing fall vulnerability in older adults.

Her most current work in the College of Nursing at Arizona State University is expanding the nurse educator track to offer courses that are relevant to teaching and learning in academic and practice settings that are technologically relevant.

Dr. Komnenich has conducted studies on the future of nursing, including perceptions of nurse practitioners and clinical nursing specialists. Her experience in nursing and in both quantitative and qualitative research provides a unique background for a unique chapter on the historical context of advanced practice nursing in four domains.

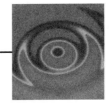

The Evolution of Advanced Practice in Nursing

CHAPTER OBJECTIVES

After completing this chapter, the reader will be able to:

1 Understand the evolution of advanced practice nursing within the historical context of each of the four practice domains—nurse midwives, nurse anesthetists, clinical nurse specialists, and nurse practitioners—by reviewing the written historical accounts and reflections of "the lived experience" of six contemporary nursing leaders.

2 Identify and discuss the sociopolitical forces that stimulated the expanded role for nurses in the four practice domains.

3 Evaluate critical trends in the educational preparation of nurses and the implications of those trends in preparing nurses for advanced practice roles.

4 Distinguish those characteristics that influence the scope of knowledge and skills within the practice domain.

5 Synthesize common or shared role parameters and concerns of advanced practice nurses from a historical perspective.

As Ford,[1] an influential leader in the nurse practitioner movement, pointed out, myths and fallacies surround any movement. Therefore, the opportunity to directly interview those individuals who participated in the specific efforts to change the nursing profession provides a depth of understanding frequently not found in other historical narratives and helps to dispel some of the myths and fallacies. Built around the reflections of six contemporary nurses who have experienced firsthand the evolving role of the certified nurse midwife (CNM), certified registered nurse anesthetist (CRNA), clinical nurse specialist (CNS), and nurse practitioner (NP), this chapter not only provides a written and verbal account of events but also interjects the flavor and energy of the "lived experience" of these advanced practice nurses.

The contributors were selected based on their reputations in their respective practice domains as clinicians, educators, and leaders. Joyce Roberts, PhD, CNM, FAAN, FACNM, and Betty Bear, PhD, CNM, FAAN, FACNM, have worked skillfully through professional organizations to advance nurse midwifery education and professional development. John Garde, MS, CRNA, FAAN, assumed a major role in the American Association of Nurse Anesthetists and continues to provide consultation for the association since stepping down as executive director. Pamela Minarik, MS, RN, FAAN, has practiced as a psychiatric clinical nurse specialist liaison for nearly 20 years. She has contributed to the professional development of the CNS movement through her practice and scholarly publications on the application of theory and research to practice as well as through her publications on political and policy implications for the CNS. Irene Riddle, PhD, MSN, RN, is a professor emeritus in nursing of children; her career as a pediatric nurse, master teacher, scholar, and researcher has included the mentoring of numerous CNS students and professional CNSs. Loretta C. Ford, EdD, MS, FAAN, professor and dean emerita of the University of Rochester, Rochester, New York, is a national leader in the NP movement and one whose contributions and vision of advanced practice for nurses have improved the quality of health care.

Developed through the use of semistructured telephone interviews and documented histories, the chapter describes the evolution of each domain from the perspective of history and sociopolitics, identifies key leaders and events, and discusses common role parameters. It concludes with a discussion of the common themes and distinguishing characteristics of each specific practice domain as well as with some thoughts on the future, drawn from information obtained during the personal interviews.

CERTIFIED NURSE MIDWIVES

According to Dickerson,[59] as of 2003 there were 45 accredited nurse-midwifery education programs in the United States. These programs included 41 master's education programs and 4 certificate programs. In addition to these programs, there are two accredited midwifery programs, which prepare an individual as a certified midwife who is not a nurse. The development of these programs in the United States has a history dating back to the early 1900s. The period from 1900 to 1935 focused on the extension of education of midwives to the growth of nurse midwifery programs, which occurred from 1935 to the present. This development occurred with the placement of nurse midwifery education in post-nursing or post-baccalaureate programs within institutions of higher education.[3] The overall purposes of nurse midwifery education, as stated in the Carnegie Foundation for the Advancement of Teaching report,[4] are the provision of better health care for mothers and babies and the promotion of midwifery as "a quality profession, requiring emphasis on caring, competence and public education" (p. 29).

Historical Context

While the established date for the inception of modern nursing is 1873, there are records of midwifery practice in the North American colonies dating back to 1630 and of attempts to educate midwives dating back to early 1762.[5,6] In these early times, the provision of obstetric care was outside the purview of medical practice and was the exclusive domain of midwives. According to Roberts,[3] efforts to establish formal midwifery schools, such as that of William Shippen, Jr., in Philadelphia in 1762, were unsuccessful, and throughout the 1800s, the native midwife was "self or apprenticeship-taught and was isolated from medicine, nursing or the hospital" (p. 123). Although interest in promoting education for midwifery practice renewed with the immigration of European midwives and physicians to the United States in the latter part of the nineteenth century, it was not sustained.

Many factors are considered by historians as contributing to the demise of midwifery's occupational identity. Of note is the fact that the medical specialty of obstetrics[7,8] arose against the backdrop of the lack of formal midwifery education[5] and the relatively inexact training requirements for midwives. Other social and economic events contributed to the decline of the native midwife.[9] Between 1900 and 1935, midwife deliveries dropped from 50 to 10 percent as the flow of immigration decreased and the emigrant midwife clients became integrated into the dominant society, as home deliveries were replaced with hospital deliveries, and as physicians became increasingly critical of the midwife.

An exception to this pattern of declining midwifery use in the United States existed among the Mormon pioneer midwives. During the late 1800s and early 1900s, the Mormons relied on midwives trained initially in their native lands and then further educated in medical-obstetrics in the United States at that time.[3] In 1874, women who were able to travel to study at the Women's Medical College in Philadelphia returned to Utah and established midwifery courses. Licensure for practice was required in Utah from 1894 to 1932, during which time 208 midwives were licensed in Salt Lake City.

According to Roberts,[3] medical care in the early twentieth century was no better than midwifery care. A 1912 survey, carried out by J. Whitridge Williams, a professor of obstetrics at Johns Hopkins University in Baltimore, found that the lack of preparation of obstetricians rendered their practices as harmful as those of midwives, if not more so, and noted that more deaths occurred from improper operations than from infections at the hands of midwives. Carolyn van Blarcom's 1914 report to the New York Committee for the Prevention of Blindness acknowledged that women may have been better cared for by less educated midwives than by the physicians who were responsible for the eye infections and the puerperal septicemia that were occurring at that time.

Unfortunately, although major reform in medical education began to take place subsequent to the Flexner Report of 1910, no similar efforts to improve the education or preparation of the midwife took place. Roberts[2,3] perceived that the lack of education and opportunity for training further led to diminished opportunities for midwives. Furthermore, because midwives perceived childbirth as a "normal" phenomenon and within the female domain of competence, few of them sought formal education. Moreover, the predominantly male physicians' attitudes toward midwifery were that midwives were unsafe and that no "true" woman would want to learn the knowledge and skills needed for midwifery.[3]

Van Blarcom, instrumental in developing the Bellevue School for Midwives, became known as the first nurse in the United States to be licensed as a midwife.[10] She advocated the training, licensure, and control of midwives, while Williams, ironically, recommended abolishment of midwives and better education for physicians. Even though this controversy led to a decline in midwifery deliveries, Roberts[3] noted that "the negative indicators surrounding childbirth actually rose with the decline of midwives" (p. 128). Lower maternal and infant mortality rates existed only where midwives were retained, notably Newark, New Jersey,[11] and New York.[12] If one considers that midwives were attending to poor, higher-risk women, these findings were even more impressive. Some of the poorer birth outcomes attributed to medicine were thought to be due to physicians' lack of training and experience with childbirth and to the techniques they used to hurry labor.

Fortunately, positive midwifery outcomes in Germany and England were noted by some American nurses who, according to Roberts,[2,3] believed that midwives should play a role in maternity care. This view led to the integration of the roles of the midwife and public health nurse into the preparation of the nurse midwife. American nursing leaders in the early 1900s did not consider midwifery to be a part of nursing preparation or practice. In 1901, Dock,[13] in a report on nursing education, pointed out:

> The nurse never takes up midwifery work and in private practice or district nursing goes only to obstetric cases where a doctor is in attendance. (p. 485)

Because so many births were being carried out in the community, nurses involved in the supervision of midwives worked predominantly in public health and community nursing. During this time, nurses concerned with maternal-child health care who tended to be actively involved in social and health reforms included Lillian Wald, the founder of the New York Henry Street Settlement. One result of these reform efforts was the formation of a federal Children's Bureau. Established between 1909 and 1912, the Children's Bureau, according to Roberts,[3] was a "major force in health reforms and subsequent midwifery practice" (p. 130).

Sociopolitical Context

During World War I, the limited fitness of men for military service resulted in legislative initiatives that were instrumental in leading to social and health care reform and, eventually, to changes in maternity care.[14] The poor physical condition of potential recruits also captured the attention of physicians and public health officials, who noted that if one-half of these men were properly cared for during childhood, they would have qualified for military service. Interestingly, Tom[14] noted that the investment of state and federal funds into public health programs was not stimulated by high maternal and infant mortality rates, but rather by the concern for a fit fighting force to ensure the nation's security. According to Tom:

> For the first time, children were recognized as future members of the military and thus deserving of federal funds. (pp. 4–13)

Childbearing women were considered to be producers of future fighting men; therefore, their health became a national resource.

The need for better maternity services in the context of opposition to midwives by physicians contributed to the controversy in nursing about the role of nurses in the practice of obstetrics. In 1909, the American Society of Superintendents of Training Schools for Nurses (ASSTSN) acknowledged that nurses' training in obstetrics should be included in the program, and in 1911 a resolution was passed to support that position (see Roberts[3] for more detail). However, the association directed that the training be limited to preparing for emergencies, observing symptoms, and reporting problems to a more general practice. In 1911, the ASSTSN passed another resolution to provide training for registration, licensure, and training in the practice of midwifery.

Around the same time, the Bellevue School for Midwives in New York City initiated a program to educate midwives. This occurred largely through the efforts of van Blarcom, who, as noted earlier, was a strong advocate for midwifery. Clara Noyes, Superintendent of Training Schools, Bellevue, and Allied Hospitals, including the School for Midwives, also supported the education of nurses as midwives. The training program for midwives at Bellevue was supported by public monies from 1911 until 1935, when the diminishing need for midwives made it difficult to justify its existence.[3] Basically, the movement of maternity care into the hospitals excluded midwifery. The joint proposal of the Maternity Center Association (MCA) in New York and the Bellevue School of Midwifery to educate nurse midwives was opposed by medical and nursing leaders. Although the need for better maternal-child health services and midwifery practice continued, such opposition inhibited nurses from engaging in the practice of midwifery. Eventually, the continuing need led to the advanced preparation of public health nurses who could supervise midwifery practice and eventually prepare nurse midwives.

In 1921, the controversial Sheppard-Towner Act was enacted to provide money to states to train public health nurses in midwifery.[3] Although there was a major political effort to prohibit passage of the bill, according to Roberts,[3] the joint efforts of women represented "one of the most effective expressions of women's political influence" (p. 131). However, in 1929, major opposition by the American Medical Association (AMA) resulted in the lapse of the bill. Roberts[3] attributed the bill's demise to the desire of the AMA to "establish a 'single standard' of obstetrical care" (p. 131) and also to the AMA's concern that governmental regulation of midwifery would lead to regulation of medical practice.

According to Shoemaker,[15] despite this opposition to midwifery in nursing, the first school for nurse midwifery established in the United States was the Manhattan Midwifery School in 1928. Apparently the school, which was started by Mary Richardson, a public health nursing instructor who had taken a midwifery course in England, was short-lived. Two of the graduates of the school, considered to be the first "unofficial" school[3] (p. 133), were identified as joining the Frontier Nursing Service in 1928.[3] Earlier, in 1925, Mary Breckenridge had brought nurse midwives from England to help establish the Service. The Frontier Nursing Service in Kentucky (service) in 1925 and the MCA (education) in New York City in 1932 were two public health–oriented agencies that characterized the midwifery practice area for public health nurses prepared in nurse midwifery. According to Bear,[16] the Lobenstine Midwifery Clinic was established in 1931 to prepare public health nurses to be midwives. In contrast to the Manhattan School established by Richardson, this clinic was the first recognized nurse midwifery school.

After the opening of the Lobenstine Midwifery Clinic, the School of the Association for the Promotion and Standardization of Midwifery was established in 1932. Priority for attendance in the school was given to nurses from states that had high infant mortality rates and many lay midwives. The intent was for the graduates to return to their home states to establish public health department programs for training and supervising "granny midwives."[3] In 1934, the school merged with the Lobenstine Clinic under the MCA and was known thereafter as The Clinic.

A key figure in the education of nurse midwives was Hattie Hemschemeyer, a public health nurse educator and graduate of the Clinic's first nurse midwifery class. She was later appointed as director of the Clinic, where the emphasis was on the provision of care to women during pregnancy and childbirth in neighborhood settings and staffed by public health nurses and physicians. The MCA, a prototype of this type of service, developed about 30 centers in New York City in 1918.[3] Nurse midwives began to provide services in these centers around 1931 and, hence, the role of the public health nurse as a nurse midwife emerged. At the same time, the role of the nurse in maternity care was evolving but appeared to be quite different from those of midwifery and medical practice.

In 1937, according to Roberts,[3] the National League for Nursing Education (NLNE) description of the role of the midwife in obstetrics was the "overall promotion of the health and comfort of the mother and baby" (p. 135). The obstetric nurse, in contrast, was described as a "bedside assistant" and "teacher of health."[17] Although preparation of the nurse in obstetrics was relatively poor in the early part of the twentieth century, development of programs in nurse midwifery during the 1940s demonstrated progress in the education for the role. According to Diers, as cited by Roberts,[3] nurse midwives have been described as the oldest of the specialized practice roles for nurses [and as providing] an unusually good example of the issues nurses face in addressing public policy considerations of manpower, economics, costs of care, quality and access to care, and interprofessional politics. (p. 136)

World War II had a significant impact on the development of nurse midwives. As a consequence of the war, there was a diminished supply of nurse midwives; thus, another education program, the second in the United States, was initiated as part of the Frontier Nursing Service in Kentucky and was assisted by the MCA in New York. The positive publicity received by the Frontier Nursing Service brought nurse midwifery into public view. Interestingly, this recognition came largely from a Metropolitan Life report describing the first 10,000 Frontier Nursing Service deliveries from its initiation up to World War II. Dublin, as cited by Willeford in 1933,[18] reported that the Frontier Nursing Service protected the life of the mother and baby, saving 10,000 lives a year in the United States, preventing 30,000 stillbirths, and ensuring that there would be 30,000 more children alive at the end of the first month of life. According to Roberts[3]:

> There is an irony in the notion that an insurance company would serve to stimulate the expansion of nurse-midwifery services. (p. 141)

The formalization of nurse midwifery as an extension of public health nursing continued after World War II. With increasing professionalization in nursing and health care services, the progress of nurse midwifery education went hand in hand with the development of public health education, which was considered to be essential for nurse midwifery practice. With the advocacy of clinical nursing specialization within universities, the nurse midwife or advanced maternity nurse became more qualified to work with physicians within a professional framework. Table 1–1 traces significant historical events that helped to shape the midwifery profession.

TABLE 1–1. Significant Historical Events in Midwifery	
Year	Event
1762	Unsuccessful attempt by William Shippen, Jr., was launched to establish formal midwifery schools in Philadelphia.
1874	Mormon midwives who were trained at Women's Medical College in Philadelphia returned to Utah to establish midwifery courses.
1892–1932	License to practice midwifery was required in Utah.
1911	American Society of Superintendents to Training Schools for Nurses passed a resolution to provide for registration, licensure, and training in midwifery.
1921	Sheppard-Towner Act was passed, providing money to states to train public health nurses in midwifery.
1928	Manhattan Midwifery School, the first school for nurse midwifery, was established.
1929	American Medical Association opposition allowed for the lapse of the Sheppard-Towner Act.

Influence of Government Agencies and Professional Associations

In the 1970s and 1980s, efforts of both government and professional associations continued to advance the development of nurse midwifery. The Children's Bureau (later known as the Maternal Child Health Bureau), with leadership from Katherine (Kit) Kendall and Carmella Carvello, and the Division of Nursing, Bureau of Health Professions Education, was instrumental in facilitating the nurse midwifery movement by providing training grants.[2,16] According to Bear,[16] Senator Daniel K. Inouye of Hawaii assisted with lobbying efforts on Capitol Hill and with development of contacts between nursing and other key people. During the same time, Senator Daniel Patrick Moynihan of New York sponsored the Civilian Health and Medical Program for the Uniformed Services (CHAMPUS) in the Omnibus Reconciliation Act of the Defense Appropriations Bill. These activities of both senators had a positive impact on legislation that influenced education and advanced practice initiatives for nurses, nurse practitioners, and nurse midwives

During the mid-1940s, the National Organization of Public Health Nurses (NOPHN) created a section for nurse midwives. This organization was dissolved in 1952; it was absorbed into the American Nurses Association (ANA) and the National League for Nursing (NLN). There was no provision to include nurse midwives as a separate entity within these organizations. Nurse midwives were assigned to the Maternal and Child Health–NLN Interdivisional Council, which included obstetrics, pediatrics, orthopedics, crippled children, and school nursing. The general concern of the membership was that the Council was too broad to represent nurse midwifery, although the nurse midwives assumed much of the leadership of the council. In spring of 1954 at the ANA convention, the Committee on Organization was formed to explore the future organization for nurse midwifery. Through a tedious process and consideration of four options, the Committee voted unanimously to form the American College of Nurse Midwifery (ACNM). The ACNM was officially incorporated in 1955 as an outgrowth of the recommendations of the Committee on Organization.[19] Helen Varney Burst was the first president of the ACNM elected to serve two consecutive terms.[2] This event was particularly significant because her tenure occurred during a time when there were no provisions for nurse midwives in federal programs. Therefore, consistent leadership was needed to maintain intense lobbying efforts for key legislation that influenced programs such as Medicare, Medicaid, and CHAMPUS. These lobbying efforts opened the door for more autonomous nursing practice, the potential for third-party reimbursement, and greater recognition of the CNM as a health care provider.

The medical malpractice crisis was a key sociopolitical event that occurred in 1985 to slow the growth of nurse midwifery. Insurance carriers, fearing financial drains associated with litigation, dropped malpractice coverage for nurse midwives. This created a difficult challenge for the ANA, the ACNM, and the Nurse Association of the American College of Obstetrics and Gynecology, all of which stepped in and worked to assist the ACNM in getting the Risk Retention Act passed. Passage of this law allowed independent carriers to provide malpractice insurance to individuals on a state-by-state basis.

Under Bear's presidency,[16] further movement toward professional development occurred during 1987 to 1989, when the ACNM developed a Division of Research.[16] Joyce Thompson, who succeeded Bear and who was the second person to serve two consecutive terms (1989 to 1993), oversaw marked growth in the number and quality of educational programs. As the deputy director for the International Confederation of Nurse-Midwives (ICNM),[20] Thompson was also involved in the international development of midwifery. During her term, a formal liaison developed between the ICNM and the Royal College of Midwives in London, England.

Among international organizations, the Agency for International Development and the World Health Organization (WHO) were probably most influential in promoting midwifery in developing countries. The ICNM,[20] founded in Europe in 1919, also worked to advance education in midwifery, with the aim of improving the standard of care provided to mothers, babies, and their families throughout the countries of the world. The Confederation is the only international midwifery organization that has official relations with the United Nations and works closely with the WHO and the United Nations International Children's Emergency Fund (UNICEF) to achieve common goals in maternal and child care.

Although its activities were interrupted during World War II, the first World Congress of Midwives began a new era and the start of a series of triennial meetings. These meetings brought together midwives from all over the world to share ideas and experiences and to improve knowledge in the field. The first triennial meeting, hosted by the United States, was held in 1972 in Washington, D.C.[16] during the presidency of Lucille Woodville. Currently, there are nine other organizations that work with the confederation, including the International Council of Nurses and the International Federation of Gynecology and Obstetrics.[20]

Influence of Private Foundations, Colleges, and Universities

The Carnegie Foundation served as a definite stimulus for the nurse midwifery movement. Ernest Boyer, president of the Carnegie Foundation until his recent death and whose wife was a nurse midwife, strongly supported nurse midwifery programs. However, at an exploratory meeting convened by the Carnegie Foundation in July 1989, he posed a critical and continuing question regarding the issue of accreditation of a program designed for individuals who were not first educated as nurses. Basically, the ACNM responded by saying that accreditation of a program for non-nurse midwives would require identification of all the relevant knowledge, skills, and competencies that nurses bring to a nurse midwifery education and would require that those essential competencies be acquired by completion of the midwifery education program.

A key principle underlying the ACNM, Division of Accreditation (DOA) program, was that[3] the ultimate competencies attained in an ACNM-accredited midwifery program for non-nurses would be the same as those required of graduates of DOA-accredited nurse-midwifery programs (p. 151).

However, until recently, the mechanism for taking the ACNM Certification Council (ACC) examinations has not been open to non-nurse midwives, the requirement being that those who took the ACC examination be a registered nurse (RN) licensed in the United States. Now, that avenue is open for both nurses and non-nurses. Although there is some concern by others regarding this issue, the ACNM points out that only those individuals graduating with a minimum of a baccalaureate degree from an ACNM-accredited midwifery program are eligible to take the ACC examination. As of 2003, there are two direct-entry programs, one a certificate and one a master's degree program. Both programs require applicants to hold a baccalaureate degree, but not in nursing, prior to admittance.[59]

Nurse midwifery programs have received notable and growing support from a number of major colleges and universities throughout the United States. Support for doctoral education for nurse midwives who hold positions within university-based programs as well as for the preparation of leaders with the skills of scientific inquiry, knowledge of health policy formulation, educational administration, and research has also become increasingly important.

Forces Influential in Marketing and Effective Utilization

According to Bear,[16] professional associations and legislative support have encouraged consumer use of nurse midwives. Although nurse midwives have been involved in health maintenance organizations (HMOs) since 1980, consumer support was probably the most influential in the marketing and effective utilization of their services. Once the recipients of health care became aware of what nurse midwives could do, earlier misconceptions about midwifery were dispelled. The benefits of midwifery practice, especially among the underserved populations, were appreciated and disseminated.

Key Leaders

There has been a long debate on the content and structure of the curricular content that constitutes adequate education for nurse midwives and an effort by leaders to maintain the quality of education and care of mothers and children. Notable for their contributions to nurse midwifery practice and education were Mary Breckenridge, inducted into the Women's Hall of Fame in 1995,[3,16] and Hattie Hemschemeyer, the first president of the ACNM. These early leaders were dedicated to improving the quality of education for nurse midwives and to establishing institutions for monitoring midwifery care through the ACNM.[2,16] For example, the ACNM has been influential in formulating standards for education and practice that currently reflect the major differences between nurse midwives and traditional midwives.

More contemporary leaders in the discipline include Ruth Lubic, formerly general director of the MCA in New York; Irene Sandvold in the Division of Nursing, Bureau of Health Professions (BHPr), Department of Health and Human Services (DHHS); Dorothea Lang, a former president of ACNM and director of maternal and infant projects in New York City; Joyce Cameron Foster of the University of Utah, who established a nurse midwifery graduate program and certified nurse midwife licensure; Katherine (Kit) Kendall, who was with the Maternal Child Health

Bureau, DHHS; and Elizabeth Sharpe of Emory University and a graduate of Yale University. Joyce Roberts remains an active leader who continues to address nurse midwifery education and practice issues and the challenge to maintain the professional standards of midwifery practice that have been established through the ACNM. Betty Bear is a past leader in nurse midwifery practice and education and continued in this role until her retirement several years ago.[62] Other prominent players featured in the long-standing movement toward the professional status of nurse midwives include Sister Mary Stella, past president of ACNM; Vera Keane, a professor from Yale University who coauthored a book on the perception of patients and their obstetric care providers, *Nurse Patient Relationships in a Hospital Maternity Service;* and Ernestine Weidenbach, author of *Family Centered Maternity Nursing.* Joyce Cameron Foster and Judith Fullerton also were instrumental in developing the National Certification Examination for nurse midwives.[16]

As with every profession, there are many unsung heroes and heroines in the nurse midwifery movement whose commitment, support, and leadership have contributed to its success and are a part of the unwritten history. Among others who worked steadfastly to establish a professional standard for nurse midwifery were Sister Nathalie Elder and Sister Jeanne Meurer, faculty members in the School of Nursing at St. Louis University, St. Louis, Missouri.

Interface with Nurse Anesthetists, Clinical Nurse Specialists, and Nurse Practitioners

According to Roberts,[2] the focus of the nurse midwife is primarily on maternal-infant care within the context of the family and thus differs from the focus of the women's health nurse practitioner (WHNP), who is oriented more toward women's health. Nurse midwives probably identify more closely with nurse anesthetists, who have followed a similar path and positioned themselves within an area of practice that allows them to maintain a degree of autonomy within the medical community. Nurse midwives and nurse anesthetists also have followed a similar avenue by developing specialized accreditation processes for the education programs; both of these APN specialties have traditionally required certification for the practice of the specialty. In contrast, the CNS and NP have only recently begun to examine the need to accredit education programs in addition to the specialized accreditation given to the master's program. Also, NP certification is required by an increasing number of states for practice; however, this requirement is not universal.

Bear[16] has noted that a blending of the roles of advanced practice nurses in maternity care is beginning to occur. Many agree that roles probably overlap, because both the WHNP and the nurse midwife do primary care across the lifespan and prenatal and postnatal care for women. However, the primary focus of the nurse midwife extends from pregnancy through birth, with responsibility for the conduct of the delivery. Nurse midwifery has developed into a professional discipline in the United States and retains its identity as a specialty practice in nursing. In addition, the nurse midwife retains an identity with midwifery internationally,[2] in contrast with the other specialties that constitute advanced practice nursing. In other words, APNs are identified only with a specialty with the general rubric of advanced practice nursing, whereas the certified nurse midwife identifies with advanced practice nursing through nurse midwifery as a specialty and identifies with non-nurse midwifery through the focus of care of pregnant women and newborns.

NURSE ANESTHETISTS

Although midwifery as a vocation dates back to the 1600s, nurse anesthesia predates nurse midwifery as a specialty area of nursing in the United States. From the perspective of world history, the history of women attending other women in labor can be documented in pre-Christian times. Nurses attending patients in surgery to administer anesthesia is more recent.

Historical Context

Anesthesia in the United States reportedly dates back to the mid-nineteenth century, with rival claimants to its discovery. Allegedly, William T. G. Morton successfully demonstrated anesthesia in surgery on October 16, 1846, at a centennial event held at Massachusetts General Hospital. This demonstration was followed by a number of reported studies, all of which failed to mention any involvement of nurse anesthetists. In response to this apparent oversight, Thatcher[21] emphasized the role of the nurse specialist in her book *History of Anesthesia*. In the preface to the book, she stated:

> If the place of the nurse as an anesthetist receives special emphasis in this history, it is because she has been derogated or ignored. (p. 15)

Bankert[23] also described the difficulty associated with identifying the first nurse anesthetist and the limited recognition of the prominence of nurses in anesthesia.

According to Thatcher,[21] church records of 1877 identify Sister Mary Bernard as being called on to function as an anesthetist within a year of enrolling in St. Vincent's Hospital, in Erie, Pennsylvania. As a result of this record, Sister Bernard has been recognized as the first nurse anesthetist to practice in the United States. The further contributions of members of the religious orders to the development of the field of anesthesia include those of Sister Aldonza Eltrich (1860–1920) and certain religious nursing orders.

According to Bankert,[23] the Hospital Sisters of the Third Order of St. Francis managed five hospitals that served employees of the Missouri Pacific Railroad between 1884 and 1888. During this period, nuns from the order served as anesthetists for the five hospitals. In 1912, Mother Superior Magdalene Wiedlocher, an anesthetist, developed a course in anesthesia for sisters who were graduate nurses. In 1924, this course was made available to secular nurses. Based on Thatcher's research, Bankert[23] has detailed the contributions of Catholic and Protestant nursing orders whose members served as nurse anesthetists since the 1850s, providing poignant narratives of these committed women. Included in this group are Alice Magaw, known as the "Mother of Anesthesia," and Sister Secundina Mindrup (1868–1951), both of whom were described as most "touching figures."

The emergence of nurse anesthesia in the United States cannot be considered outside the context of the development of nursing itself. In 1873, three nurse training schools were established in New York, New Haven, and Boston. These American schools were referred to as "Nightingale Schools" and were credited with bringing the art of nursing into a more reputable view. At that time, there was some controversy over the philanthropic desire to make nurses' training attractive to the middle-class American woman. Some physicians supported the idea, while many did not. According to Starr, as quoted by Bankert,[23] physicians were concerned that

> educated nurses would not do as they were told—a remarkable comment on the status anxieties of nineteenth-century physicians. (p. 20)

Fortunately, women reformers paid little attention to these remarks and, like Florence Nightingale, moved forward. The schools were established to attract respectable women and were modeled after the Saint Thomas Hospital Training School for Nurses founded in 1860 by Nightingale.

Eventually, physicians were forced to accept nurses who were trained to carry out the more complex work that hospitals were assuming. Shyrock, as quoted by Bankert,[23] described this change in attitude toward nurses rather vividly:

> All of this related to the public opinion of medical service in general, since the nurses came into more continuous contact with the patient than did any other figure in the whole range of medical personnel. Good nursing was invaluable from a technical point of view. It might make all the difference in the outcome of the individual case, and patients sometimes realized this. Better nursing was an essential feature in the gradual improvement of hospitals, and this in turn modified the earlier popular attitude toward these institutions. ... The whole spirit of hospitals changed. (p. 21)

Baer, as quoted by Bankert,[23] made yet a stronger statement when she asserted that "nursing made medicine look good" (p. 21). She goes on to further illustrate this point:

> Medicine's ultimate success, technological advances, and subsequent impressive social power were achieved through hospitals, and nurses made those hospitals work. Nurses made them reasonable choices for sick-care, providing the environment in which patients felt safe enough to permit medical instrumentation to occur. The development of medical practice, education, therapeutics, etc. proceeded from that point. Happily, one prominent physician understood that and reminded his contemporaries in 1910: "Now one must have some understanding of the value of the profession of nursing in modern medicine. ... It has changed the face of modern medicine: it is revolutionary in its influence upon the progress of modern medicine." (p. 21)

Sociopolitical Context

The advent of anesthetics occurred simultaneously with the acceptance and promotion of asepsis and the emergence of nursing in hospital care[23]; thus, the elements "were in place for a removal of the remaining obstacle in the path of the advancement of surgery" (p. 22). Discussion concerning problems associated with anesthesia delivery began at the time of Morton's first successful induction and continued without resolution for some 40 years. Most anesthesia was given by novice interns who were more interested in the surgery than in the safe administration of anesthesia. In 1898, Saling, as quoted by Bankert,[23] illustrated the rather nonchalant attitude toward anesthesia characteristic of the times:

> Unfortunately, in most hospitals one of the younger interns is, as a rule, selected to administer the anaesthetic. The operator accustomed to having a novice give chloroform or ether for him is kept on the qui vive while performing the operation and watching the administration of the anaesthetic. Such a condition of affairs is not conducive to the best work of the surgeon. (p. 23)

One of the hospitals established by the Sisters of St. Francis played a particularly noteworthy role in the development of anesthesia care. Established in 1889 as St. Mary's Hospital, it later became known as the Mayo Clinic. During the early years at the Mayo Clinic, no interns were available to assist in surgery. Therefore, the clinic relied on nurse anesthetists, initially as a matter of necessity and later as a matter of choice.

The Mayo Clinic's first nurse anesthetists were Dinah and Edith Graham, sisters who had graduated from the school of nursing at the Women's Hospital in Chicago. To train the Graham sisters while continuing to support the work of the clinic, five staff nurses took over the patient care nursing and housekeeping duties while the Grahams administered anesthesia and did general office and secretarial work. According to Bankert,[23] Dinah's career as a nurse anesthetist at the clinic was brief, but her sister Edith continued there until she married William W. Mayo in 1893. Edith was succeeded by Magaw (1860–1928), reported to be brilliant not only as an anesthetist but also as a scholar and researcher.

Bankert[23] noted that although Magaw "won more widespread notice than that of any other member of the Rochester group apart from the [Mayo] brothers" (p. 30), because she was a nurse she was not given membership in the medical society. According to Garde,[24] Magaw administered anesthesia, kept data, and wrote articles. She was a meticulous data collector, and although her papers are not listed in the Physicians of the Mayo Clinic Bibliography, one of her studies was included in the Collected Papers by the Staff of St. Mary's Hospital, Mayo Clinic, Rochester, Minnesota, 1905–1909.[22] A 1941 catalogue by Clapesattle of Magaw's papers revealed that her first comprehensive paper, reporting more than 3000 cases, was titled "Observations in Anesthesia" and was published in Northwestern Lancet in 1899.[22] In 1900, the St. Paul Medical Journal published Magaw's update of the year's work, which included observations of 1,092 cases reported. In 1906, Magaw published another review of more than 14,000 successful anesthesia cases. According to Bankert,[23] Magaw made numerous recommendations that shaped contemporary anesthesia practice. She stressed individual attention for all patients and identified the experience of the anesthetist as a critical element in quickly responding to the patient. Magaw's success was also attributed to her attention to the psychological dimension of the anesthetic experience. In her words, she believed that "suggestion" was a great help "in producing a comfortable narcosis" (p. 32).

The model of nurse anesthesia at the Mayo Clinic drew the attention of medical people from all over the United States and the world. The Mayo Clinic's reputation gave credibility to the movement, and Magaw's efforts provided a particular advantage to careful documentation and publication. As Garde[24] noted:

> We lose so many opportunities in clinical areas because people do not take the time to write articles that could be major contributions to the literature. [By her writing], ... Alice Magaw really made a name for the nurse anesthetists.

In 1936, Crile,[25] hailed as one of America's greatest surgeons, praised the nurse anesthetist movement. In these nursing professionals, he found a special quality of "finesse" for administration of anesthesia not present in medical interns. His choice for the prototype nurse anesthetist was Agatha Cobourg Hodgins, a native of Canada. According to Bankert,[23] she "proved herself to be not only a brilliant anesthetist, but a woman of vision" (p. 39) in her dedication to the development of professional nursing and the establishment of a national nurse anesthesiology association.

A graduate of the Boston City Hospital Training School for Nurses, at age 21, Hodgins went to Cleveland to work as a head nurse at Lakeside Hospital. There she was selected by Crile to administer anesthesia. She avidly read all she could about anesthesia, and she "walked the wards" at night listening to sleeping patients' breathing to detect subtle differences. According to Crile, as quoted by Bankert[23]:

> Miss Hodgins made an outstanding anesthetist for she had to a marked degree, both the intelligence and the gift. (p. 41)

Crile and Hodgins inaugurated the Lakeside School of Anesthesia, which at once was recognized as an organized center for teaching anesthesiology, contributing to the education of nurse anesthetists and furthering the work of the graduates.[23]

Not surprisingly, World Wars I and II, the Korean conflict, and the Vietnam War all had a significant impact on the development of anesthesia. Crile and Hodgins were part of the Lakeside Unit at the American Ambulance at Neuilly in 1914.[23] After 2 months, Crile returned to the United States to present a plan to the U.S. Surgeon General for the creation of hospital units composed of doctors, nurses, and anesthetists for service internationally. Hodgins stayed on in Neuilly to teach nurses, dentists, and physicians how to administer anesthesia. She returned to Cleveland to resume her work at the Lakeside School of Anesthesia. The first graduating class consisted of 6 physicians, 2 dentists, and 11 nurses. After the formal declaration of war by the United States on April 6, 1917, the Lakeside Hospital Unit, Base Hospital No. 4, was mobilized. Hodgins did not accompany the unit at the time, instead remaining as director of the school and engaging in training nurse anesthetists for military service.

In addition to training at the Mayo Clinic, preparation of nurse anesthetists was also occurring in other parts of the country.[23] For example, Sophie Gran Winton (1887–1989), a graduate of Swedish Hospital in Minneapolis, had trained as an anesthetist. After garnering 5 years of anesthesia experience and having established a record of more than 10,000 cases without a fatality, she joined the Army Nurse Corps. Winton and other nurses from the Minneapolis Hospital Unit No. 26

were assigned to Mobile Hospital No. 1 in the Chateau-Thierry area of France. Working with the physician anesthetist James T. Gwathmey, the unit succeeded in pioneering anesthesia in mobile hospital units.

As suggested, a repeated theme in the nurse anesthetist movement has been that of an acknowledgment of the intelligence and dedication of women while pointing out, with some bias, that the gender differences made anesthesia a natural place for women to display their intelligence and feminine attributes. Bankert[23] described the following expectations as characteristic of persons administering anesthesia in 1896. She notes that these qualities were found in women who were recruited into a field shunned by physicians. According to Bankert, women of that period, as perceived by physicians such as Dr. Frederic Hewitt, should:

(a) have been satisfied with the subordinate role that the work required

(b) not have made anesthesia their one absorbing interest

(c) not have looked on the situation of anesthetist as one that put them in a position to watch and learn from the surgeon's technic

(d) have accepted comparatively low pay

(e) have had the natural aptitude and intelligence to develop a high level of skill in providing the smooth anesthesia and relaxation that the surgeon demanded. (p. 50)

As Bankert[23] suggested, this "glorified handmaiden" image was part of the expectation of the surgeon and was one that came to be associated with nursing. The first battle between nurse anesthetists and medicine was waged in the 1920s. At that time, Francis Hoeffer McMechan, a third-generation Cincinnati physician, began to promote the organization of physician anesthesia. But before nurse anesthetists could assume McMechan's challenge to "cease and desist" practice, they first had to win a battle of acceptance within the profession of nursing. Again, it was Hodgins who led the movement to integrate nurse anesthetists into mainstream nursing through the ANA.

For years, the nurse anesthetist movement had met resistance from organized nursing. In 1909, nurse anesthetists were stunned when Florence Henderson, a successor of Magaw, was invited to present a paper at the ANA, with the unmet expectation of an invitation to join the association. In 1931, Hodgins initiated a formal effort for nurse anesthesia to become a section within the ANA (see Bankert,[23] p. 65, for a comprehensive account of this effort). According to notes in Bankert,[23] Hodgins mobilized the Lakeside alumnae as well as other nurse anesthetists around the country to "attend a meeting for the purpose of considering the organization of [a] nurse anesthetist group" (p. 67). She was committed to separating nurse anesthetists from hospital service but retaining nurse anesthesia within the ANA framework. The ANA eventually rejected this proposal, accepting nurse anesthetists only into the Medical-Surgical Nursing section. According to Bankert,[23] when the ANA rejected the affiliation of nurse anesthetists, Hodgins made a profound statement that led to an alliance with the American Hospital Association (AHA). The following words, excerpted from Bankert, are part of the speech Hodgins made to nurse anesthetists:

It seems to us that anesthesia, being in no sense nursing, could not be absorbed into a strictly nursing group such as the ANA, as we hope to include in our sustaining membership surgeons, hospital superintendents, and others interested in advancing the cause. (p. 73)

The nonacceptance by organized nursing stimulated nurse anesthetists to form the International Association of Nurse Anesthetists (later changed to the National Association of Nurse Anesthetists [NANA] in an effort to merge with the ANA). By 1938, the NANA had changed its name to the American Association of Nurse Anesthetists (AANA) and had moved to its new one-room office at the AHA's offices in Chicago. The affiliation with the AHA proved to provide a home that fostered the profession of nurse anesthesia.

The recognition by the AHA and the subsequent onset of World War II, with its need for an increased number of military nurses trained in anesthesia, stimulated further development of the nurse anesthetist movement and later prompted other efforts to standardize nurse anesthetist education and to establish a national certification examination.[23] According to Bankert,[23] Gertrude Fife addressed the first national convention of the NANA in 1933, calling for a committee to

investigate nurse anesthesia schools for the purpose of accreditation and for a national board examination for nurse anesthetists. (p. 96)

Fife's stand on the direction for nurse anesthetist education was different from that of Hodgins and ultimately was opposed by Hodgins. Although Fife had the support of prominent physicians and the help of Dr. Howard Karsner, professor of pathology at Western Reserve University, in the development of national accreditation and procedures, opposition by Hodgins was based on the perception that, under Fife's plan, the nurse anesthetist would not have a separate legal status.

Despite being ill and semiretired, Hodgins continued to influence the progress of the professional movement of nurse anesthetists. However, it was Fife who carried the ball, later giving credit to John Mannix, assistant director of University Hospitals at Western Reserve. At the urging of Mannix, Helen Lamb and Walter Powell joined Fife to produce a nurse anesthesia program and move forward to achieve the following objectives[23]:

(a) advance the science and art of anesthesiology

(b) develop educational standards and techniques in the administration of anesthetic drugs

(c) facilitate efficient cooperation between nurse anesthetists and the medical profession, hospitals, and other agencies interested in anesthesiology

(d) Promulgate an educational program to help the public understand the importance of the proper administration of anesthetics. (pp. 76–77)

Although Hodgins died before the first qualifying examination for membership in the AANA was held on June 4, 1945, and before the first Institute for Instructors of Anesthesiology was convened in Chicago later that same year, her efforts, along with those of other leaders, came to fruition in peacetime after World War II. Education became the primary goal of the association, and an increased effort was made to form standards and to develop a standardized curriculum to teach nurses to be nurse anesthetists.

The move toward accreditation of schools of anesthesia was approved in September 1950 with the encouragement of the AHA's Council on Professional Practice and under Lamb's leadership as chair of the Advisory Committee of the AANA.[23] The AANA accreditation program for schools of nurse anesthesia became effective on January 19, 1952. Although the program allowed for an interim period during which schools in existence could meet the accreditation criteria, new schools were required to meet accreditation requirements from the outset.

Unfortunately, the rift between organized nursing and nurse anesthesia continued as deans of nursing schools and colleges resisted inclusion of nurse anesthetist academic programs into their curricula. According to Garde,[24] this dilemma of nonacceptance led to the development of many anesthetist programs in colleges of allied health and education. Although allied health was most receptive to nurse anesthesia, the profession wanted and needed more than a certificate program.

The 1970s witnessed pivotal and profound changes in society: the nation's economic recession, the energy crisis, inflation, involvement in Vietnam, and President Nixon's articulation of a "health care crisis," to name a few. The general direction of nursing education preparation was changing as well. As the educational requirement in nursing moved from diploma to a baccalaureate degree, the requirement for nurse anesthesia moved from certification to a baccalaureate and master's framework. A major breakthrough in nurse anesthesia preparation occurred when Rush University decided to offer a master's of science in nursing for anesthesia through its Graduate School. Another major move to higher education for nurse anesthetists was the establishment of the first master's program in nurse anesthesia through the Department of Nursing at California State University,[24] an effort promoted by the leadership of Joyce Kelly, a nurse anesthetist affiliated with Kaiser Permanente. Currently, nurse anesthesia is considered to be an advanced clinical nursing specialty. Requirements for admission to a nurse anesthesia program are a bachelor's of science in nursing or another appropriate baccalaureate degree, a license as a registered nurse, and a minimum of 1 year of acute care nursing experience (determined by the individual program). Following completion of and graduation from an accredited nurse anesthesia education program, the nurse must pass a national certification examination to become a Certified Registered Nurse Anesthetist (CRNA). All nurse anesthesia education programs now offer a master's degree, which can be in nursing, allied health, or the biological and clinical sciences.[26]

In the 1970s, the AANA experienced a change in leadership and a continued controversy with organized medicine. Although Florence A. McQuillen ("Mac") had single-handedly held the organization together since 1948, the time had come for a new approach, marking the end of an era for the Association. The conflict between the American Society of Anesthesiologists (ASA) and the AANA centering on issues of control and autonomy has not yet been fully resolved.

Influence of Government Agencies

The various state boards of nursing, which worked closely on licensing issues with the National Council of State Boards of Nursing and the U.S. Department of

Health, were most influential in supporting nurse anesthesia. Controversy over the authority and licensing of nurse anesthetists continues to the present day. The consensus was that state boards of nursing should regulate nursing, including advanced practice nursing. According to Garde,[24] the AANA monitored the recommendations of the Pew Commission very closely as they pertained to advanced practice. The AANA viewed the report as a way of collapsing barriers and opening doors to allow nurse anesthetists to practice unencumbered. Currently, CRNAs are qualified and permitted by state law or regulations to practice in every state of the nation."[26] CRNAs can practice solo, in groups, and collaboratively. In addition, CRNAs have the legal authority to practice anesthesia without anesthesiologist supervision in all 50 states, typically in every setting where anesthesis is administered. Some states have placed restrictions and supervisory requirements in some settings.[60] CRNAs may have independent contracts with physicians or hospitals. They are the sole anesthesia providers in more than two-thirds of rural hospitals in the United States.

In 2001, at the very end of the Clinton Administration, a Medicare regulation was signed that would have removed the federal physician supervision requirement for nurse anesthetists. Both the American Hospital Association (AHA) and the National Rural Health Association (NRHA) supported Medicare's ruling. However, when the Bush Administration took over later that month, a freeze was placed on the enactment of all regulations signed at the end of the Clinton Administration. Subsequently, in November 2001, a Medicare Rule was enacted that allowed state governors to opt out of the supervision requirement by sending a written lettter to the Centers for Medicare and Medicaid Services (CMS). Prior to sending the letter, the governor must consult with the state boards of medicine and nursing, determine that removal of the supervision requirement is in the best interests of the citizens of that state, and determine that opting out of the requirement is consistent with state law.[22] As of January 2004, 12 states opted out of the Medicare supervision requirement.[22]

Key Leaders

The succession of key national leaders began with Alice Magaw, who was recognized for her techniques in the administration of anesthesia as well as for her brilliant documentation of anesthesia. Her papers, though not identified as research, probably merit being identified, along with Nightingale's, as an early effort to systematically document patient outcomes and report those outcomes in scholarly publications.

Agatha Hodgins, the second most prominent nurse anesthetist, was noted for contributions stemming from her work with and support of Crile and for their combined efforts to improve the education and professional status of nurse anesthetists. She was the impetus behind the movement for professional development of nurse anesthetists and was elected the first president of the AANA (1931–1933). Other leaders who appeared repeatedly in the literature included not only Fife (Hodgins' successor) but also the following past presidents of the AANA: Hilda Solomon, Helen Lamb, Hazel Blanchard, Lucy Richards, and Verna Rice.

In addition, the following were recipients of the association's Award of

Appreciation for their contributions to the profession: Barnes Hospital, part of Washington University in St. Louis, Missouri, a site where much of the educational progress for nurse anesthetists took place (1948); and individuals such as George W. Crile, MD (posthumously, 1948); Gertrude L. Fife (1956); Mae B. Cameron (1951); Agnes McGee (1953); Hospital Sisters of the Third Order of St. Francis, Springfield, Illinois (1954); Helen Lamb and Lucy Richards (1956); Hilda Solomon (1958); and Verna Rice (1959). Honorary memberships (nonanesthetist) were extended to Cameron W. Meredith and Betty A. Colitti for their contributions, and a special recognition award was given to John R. Mannix for his assistance in establishing licensing examinations.[63]

Interface with Certified Nurse Midwives, Clinical Nurse Specialists, and Nurse Practitioners

Although the role of nurse anesthetists has been more akin to that of nurse midwives, who struggled to maintain an identity with nursing while preserving their own practice in an autonomous role outside medicine, there are shared goals with other advanced practice nurses. Garde[24] in 1998 envisioned commonly shared roles, with advanced practice nurses practicing to their fullest potential without artificial barriers, with direct and fair reimbursement, and with services marketed to managed-care organizations.[26] As health care is becoming more business-oriented, nursing in general and advanced nurse practice in particular will be facing major challenges to identify the breadth and depth of advanced practice nursing. Garde's[24] vision of a united effort to keep medicine and hospital administration on the same path with advanced practice nursing that will have a positive impact on health has come to fruition. As sole anesthesia providers to some 70 million rural Americans, it is evident that CRNAs provide a significant amount of anesthesia in rural as well as inner city areas.[26]

CLINICAL NURSE SPECIALISTS

According to Hamric and Spross,[27] the concept of nurse specialties is not new in the profession of nursing. Minarik[28] referred to DeWitt's article in the American Journal of Nursing (see Bibliography), in which DeWitt attributed the development of nursing specialties to present civilization and modern science (p. 14).

According to Sparacino, Cooper, and Minarik,[29] DeWitt's view of specialty nursing follows the medical model, basically responding within a limited domain to nursing patients with certain types of conditions or "working for a specialty physician" (p. 4).

Historical Context

During the first half of the twentieth century, the term "specialist" implied[29]

> a nurse with extensive experience in a particular area of nursing, a nurse who completed a hospital-based "postgraduate" course, or a nurse who performed with technical expertise. (p. 3)

Although, at that time, such nurses were recognized for their expert knowledge regarding nursing practice in a specific area, most postgraduate nursing courses before World War II were limited to functional courses that prepared a nurse administrator and/or nurse educator. There is some controversy about when the title "clinical nurse specialist" was first used; there is clear agreement that in 1943 Frances Reiter promoted the idea of the nurse clinician.[27,28,30] According to Hamric and Spross,[27] her perception of the nurse clinician was that of

a nurse with advanced knowledge and clinical competence committed to providing the highest quality of nursing care. (p. 3)

She did not believe that a master's degree was the distinctive qualification to be a nurse clinician, but she did recognize that graduate education was the most efficient means of preparing such practitioners.

Norris[31] dated the inception of the CNS to 1944 and the NLNE's Committee to Study Postgraduate Clinical Nursing Courses. Smoyak[32] credited a national conference of directors of graduate programs, sponsored by the University of Minnesota in 1949, for the genesis of the clinical-nurse specialty. Even though the NLNE had recommended a plan to develop nurse specialists, urging qualified universities to undertake the experiment, one major difficulty with advancing the concept of the CNS was that the predominant level of education for nurses at the time was the diploma. Another was that many nurses in baccalaureate- and master's-level courses shared the same classroom in the 1950s. Eventually, psychiatric nursing was credited with being the first specialty to develop graduate-level clinical experiences.

Sociopolitical Context

Several factors inhibited the growth of specialization in nursing. After World War II, there was both an increased demand for nurse generalists and an increased demand for the advanced education of such nurses because of the numbers of veteran nurses who were eligible for educational benefits under the GI Bill. Factors such as these, as well as the focus of preparation of the early graduate leaders in nursing at Teachers' College, Columbia University, and the post–World War II increase in hospital care, resulted in nursing shifting from a private duty model to a supervisory model within a hospital bureaucracy. In response, the National Mental Health Act was passed, which provided research and training funds for advanced study in core mental health disciplines. Because psychiatric nursing was identified as a core discipline, both undergraduate and graduate education in this specialty were eligible for funding. Hildegarde Peplau,[33] a psychiatric nurse leader, educator, and clinician, developed the first master's program focused on advanced practice in psychiatric nursing.

Oncologic nursing was another area that early on developed graduate education for specialization. These efforts were spearheaded by the American Cancer Society and the National Cancer Institute. According to Hamric and Spross,[27] the American Cancer Society has continued its interest in the development of CNSs in oncology into the 1990s. The Oncology Nursing Society is credited with establishing cancer nursing as a specialty and with contributing to the development of the oncology CNS role and refining of the advanced practice role in oncology.

The Professional Nurse Traineeship Program of 1963 was a major force that stimulated the inclusion of education in the development of the CNS movement. This expansion, along with the increasing numbers of baccalaureate-prepared nurses and with the profession's interest in graduate education, led to the establishment of education for clinical specialization within graduate programs.[29] The shortage of physicians in the 1960s helped to create a milieu for expanding clinical specialization in nursing; in addition, opportunities were opening up within the health care environment for more competent professionals prepared for advanced practice. By the 1970s, there were master's-level programs to prepare CNSs for a variety of practice settings and specialty areas. However, without a clear mandate for entry-level preparation, confusion remained over the use of multiple-role titles such as nurse clinician, nursing specialist, expert clinician, clinical nurse scientist, and CNS. Also during this time, questions were raised regarding the purpose, preparation, function, responsibility, and practice setting for the CNS.

According to Minarik,[28] the role confusion began to resolve somewhat with the publication of the ANA Social Policy Statement, which defined specialization in nursing. Clarification of the various issues provided a public declaration of criteria for the title of CNS. Other groups embraced the definition and supported the characteristics; but without a doubt, the strongest support came from the ANA in 1980.[34] Specialty organizations and state nurses' associations then reinforced this definition by formally describing the requisites and competencies of nurses assuming the CNS role (e.g., American Association of Critical Care Nurses' [AACN] position statements [1987],[35] ANA [1986],[36] and California Nurses' Association [1984][37]). According to Sparacino, Cooper, and Minarik,[29] further validation of acceptance of the CNS role within the ANA became a reality with the publication of a study undertaken by the Council of Clinical Nurse Specialists reporting that 19,000 RNs functioned as CNSs. A clear definition of the CNS role appeared in the ANA publication *The Clinical Nurse Specialist,* published in 1986 when Sparacino was chair of the CNS Council.[38]

Funding for advanced-nursing education occurred through federal government agencies, such as the National Institute of Mental Health and the BHPr, Division of Nursing. Private foundations, such as The Robert Wood Johnson Foundation (RWJF), also provided funding.

Minarik's[28] perception of the evolution of the CNS role was that it grew out of needs recognized by nurse educators and clinicians, in contrast to the NP role, which grew out of recognition of a need to provide services for well children in primary care. Before the development of the CNS role, there were no rewards or opportunities for advanced study and practice in clinical nursing; a graduate student had two role selections: educator or administrator.

The social forces noted by Minarik[28] that had a significant impact on the CNS movement included growing specialization, growing use of technology, growing acuity of care and, in a phrase coined by Cooper,[39] a growing need for "attendance" in nursing. The CNS was similar to the attending nurse who, by virtue of confidence and skills gained through years of direct clinical contact with patients, was a refined expert in providing care and guidance to others. Unlike the generalist nurse, the CNS had to be more than just a safe practitioner. As the ANA Social Policy Statement[34] emphasized, the CNS was expected to have attained competence in a clinical specialty over time. In addition, the role reflected the additional components of educator, consultant, and researcher. In early conversations with Minarik[28] and Riddle,[30] one gains a view of the CNS as a special kind of nurse who is able to view the patient from a well-developed knowledge base in a specialized area of nursing. According to Riddle,[30] who is not a CNS but a master teacher and clinician in nursing of children, the CNS could be viewed as a pioneer. These clinicians learned how to present themselves in a professional manner and how to work with nursing services in innovative and creative ways. The CNS programs helped nursing students learn to upgrade the quality of the care they delivered. The CNS has a broader set of responsibilities than the non-CNS in the service setting and, thus, needs a broader educational experience.

According to Minarik's[28] personal experience, inherent and invaluable in the CNS educational experiences are collegial relationships that can be sustained over time. Minarik described her experience as follows:

> The beautiful thing that happened to me was being at the University of California at San Francisco because of the colleague relationship. … There were strong clinicians, strong thinkers. This resulted in my colleagues being editors for each other's work. We struggled through the thinking involved, it was a wonderful exciting process of co-mentorship, editing and learning together.

These comments by Minarik[28] reflect the collegiality, collaboration, and creativity that developed as these clinicians worked together to provide expert patient care in teams of nurses and physicians. Emerging from these collegial, creative, and collaborative relationships was a need to communicate through writing what occurred with patients. The shared experience resulted in innovative nursing care in which individuals learned from one another and shared that knowledge with others.

Boyle[40] attributes CNS continuity to a history rich in problem-solving and other skills responsive to change in the practice settings. Basically, she perceives the persistent involvement of the CNS with patients across the continuum of care as providing a special view of assessment of needs, concerns, and omissions that will aid in providing for continuity of care. Shifting of care from the acute hospital setting to outpatient and home care provides an ideal milieu in which the CNS can translate the need for nursing care in a more contemporary context.

In 1998, the National Association of Clinical Nurse Specialists (NACNS) Legislative and Regulatory Committee completed a critical analysis of state statutes and developed a model of statutory and regulatory language governing CNS practice. The model was driven by the expansion of nurse practitioners and the need to define qualifications for practice and scope of practice for CNSs. The model recognizes the CNS scope of practice as encompassing three spheres of influence identified in the NACNS statement on CNS Practice and Education (1998). These spheres include direct patient care, advancing the practice of nursing through nursing personnel; and system interventions to improve patient care cost-effectively.[41]

Influence of Government Agencies, A Private Foundation, and Professional Associations

In the 1970s and 1980s, the RWJF was a major funding agency, as was the Division of Nursing of the BHPr for CNS education. A particular influence in the marketing of the role has been the students themselves.[28, 30] CNSs have generated a vast number of publications in which they have described patient care within their specialties and have attempted to clarify areas of responsibility, specialization, and the multiplicity of the roles. However, according to Minarik,[28] because they did not write about their roles as CNSs, they remained invisible as CNSs. The ANA remained a strong marketing force, working hard to increase the visibility of the CNS. The Oncology Nursing Society and the AACN also focused on clinical practice problems and efforts.

The more recent history of the CNS role depicts a shift in the role of the CNS from its traditional focus to a broader scope of practice as the local and national health institutions changed. The environment of the late 1980s and early 1990s created new challenges and a need for definition and conformity with the Advanced Practice Registered Nurse (APRN) Model. Downsizing of hospitals and budget constraints coupled with increasing role ambiguity as the nurse practitioner gained increasing visibility led to a need for a clearer definition of the the CNS.[58] The following definition of the CNS emerged in January 2001: A clinical nurse specialist (CNS) is a registered professional nurse who has a graduate degree (master's or doctorate) or post-master's certificate from an accredited nursing program that prepares students for the CNS role; is nationally certified in a designated or relevant specialty to the preparation or meets waiver requirements if no certification examination is available for that specialty. In addition, the CNS must meet all Board of Nursing requirements to practice as a clinical nurse specialist.[41]

Key Leaders

A list of the key leaders in the CNS movement begins with Frances Reiter,[27,28,30] who introduced the title "nurse clinician." Hildegarde Peplau is known for opening the door to clinical specialization in psychiatric nursing. Riddle[30] also includes on this list the many students who should be credited for opening doors by marketing their skills and collaborating with other health care providers. The students were risk-takers and innovators.

Minarik,[28] after 20 years of experiencing the role, has identified other influential contributors to the CNS movement. For example, Pauline Beacraft was recognized for the creation of the CNS journal and for providing a forum for discussion of CNS issues. Beverly Malone implemented the role and a consultation service of CNSs at the University of Cincinnati. Linda Cronenwett was a key player in introducing the use of research in practice. Pat Sparacino provided leadership through her practice and publications as well as through her activities as chair of the ANA Council of Clinical Nurse Specialists. Helen Ripple, director of nursing at the University of California Hospitals in San Francisco and former president of the

American Organization of Nurse Executives, strongly supported the CNS role and, as an administrator, implemented mechanisms within the service setting to fully use the expertise of CNSs. She also actively supported 14 years of annual CNS conferences, sponsored by the University of California at San Francisco, that brought together leaders in the field to grapple with key issues and promote the CNS role.

Other notable contributors to the role include Joyce Clifford at Beth Israel Medical Center in Boston and, more recently, Brenda Lyon and others in the NACNS. Barbara Safriet, a lawyer, has focused on the professional question and scope of practice for APNs, and Dorothy Brooten has focused on research outcomes.

Interface with Certified Nurse Midwives, Nurse Anesthetists, and Nurse Practitioners

Minarik[28] believes that the four roles of nurse midwife, nurse anesthetist, CNS, and NP have more similarities than differences. The expertise of the CNS is in the identification and intervention of clinical problems and in the management of those problems within the larger health care system. The challenge of the future will be the ability of the APN to be prepared to serve in a variety of roles. Leadership, flexibility, responsiveness to change, and depth and breadth in theoretical knowledge, all combined with fully developed expertise and advanced clinical judgment, are critical in all four areas of practice. According to Minarik,[28] defining the expertise and how students are educated will be the greatest challenge. She believes strongly that it cannot be done without graduate preparation and that it is important to understand that preparation of the expert is not only in learning facts and content but in developing critical thinking and judgment.

NURSE PRACTITIONERS

The NP movement—the most modern of the four advanced practice roles—arose against the backdrop of the 1960s and in response to needed changes in the health care environment and in the education of graduate nurses.

Historical and Sociopolitical Context

The time of transition from the post–World War II generation to the baby boomers' developmental years was one of social activism and scientific advancement. The assassination of President John F. Kennedy created a sense of deep national commitment to public service among young people, and according to Ford,[42] a national leader in the NP movement, there was a true concern for both the "haves and have nots." While the war in Vietnam was accelerating, President Lyndon Johnson declared the war on poverty. As the increase in technology was driving the need for knowledge, information systems began to emerge, and the pace of life began to accelerate.

During this time, society exhibited a sincere concern about the maldistribution of health resources, especially of physicians. The increasing concerns relating to health care and the emerging emphasis on health promotion made it a good time for change in the profession of nursing. Ford[42] described the time as one in which nurses were able to try new things. Although there was some uncertainty and resistance to change, the window of opportunity was clearly open.

In a candid interview reported in the *Journal of the New York State Nurses Association,* Ford[1] described the NP movement as an

> outgrowth (a) of the Western Interstate Commission on Higher Education for Nursing (WICHEN) Clinical Content study on Master's preparation in Community Health Nursing in which I was involved from 1963 to 1967 and (b) an experience that pediatrician Henry K. Silver had at a Child Health Nursing Conference which was organized in the mid-1960s by the public health nurses and the Colorado State Health Department. (p. 12)

The WICHEN project provided the stimulus for the change needed in the health care environment and the education of graduate nurses, and Dr. Silver's involvement provided the mechanism for that change.

Ford[1] has identified seven myths that have hampered the NP movement and that continue to the present day. The first myth is that the development of the NP role was solely in response to a proclaimed physician shortage existing at the time. The reality is that the rationale for the development of the NP role came from nursing leaders who were committed to preparing graduate nurses for clinical specialization. Four groups of faculty, representing 13 western states, had worked together to identify the clinical content for a master's degree in nursing. Stimulated by both social and professional developments and aided by the maldistribution of medical personnel, an "opportunistic" environment for changes in well-child care in ambulatory settings was created.[1,41] The aim of the clinical-content model was not only to prepare graduate students for clinical specialization but also, according to Ford,[1] to "reclaim a role that public health nurses had historically held" (p. 12).

To reclaim that role, nurses needed to be able to work in an autonomous and collegial way with physicians. The experience with Silver provided an opportunity for Ford and Silver to promote an experiment that would allow nurses to reclaim the role. Dr. Silver, who had been introduced to Ford by Henry Kemp, a pediatrician known for his identification of the battered-child syndrome, had not been enthusiastic about the idea of NPs. However, he returned from his attendance at the Child Health Nursing Conference with a new and enthusiastic view of nurses. Thus, the liaison began.[1,42]

This association between Ford and Silver led to a collegial relationship in which the role of nursing in well-child care was tested to determine if nurses could competently care for well children in community-based settings. The NP model was far from the "medical model" that is frequently attributed to the practitioner program; it was fashioned after the nursing profession's criteria for clinical practice, as set forth by the ANA. The emphasis was on professional, direct client care, health and wellness, collegiality with physicians, and prevention-oriented care, including consumer education.

The initial NP program at the University of Colorado began as part of a demonstration project in which a post-master's student worked in an expanded role for nursing. Ford[42] dated the inception of the practitioner program to the admission of the first student to the University of Colorado's program in the fall of 1965. The demonstration project tested the scope of practice by building on what had existed as part of community health nursing and doing it more thoroughly. A survey of health needs identified major problems commonly encountered by nurses in the community.

More than just collecting data, the survey also focused on data interpretation and management of the well child. Results of the demonstration project helped to extend the focus of practice toward[43]

> testing a nursing role in well-child care to determine whether nurses could competently deliver care to well children in community-based settings.

Included in the project were efforts to increase the sensory input of nurses and to increase the nurse's ability to share that input with parents, thus assisting the parents in making decisions for themselves that were based on an informed consideration of both options and consequences.[43] As a result, the observations of the nurse and her decision-making abilities were sharpened.

The intent of the project was not only to teach nurses how to provide care competently and confidently but also to establish an advanced nursing practice grounded in, and held to, a post-baccalaureate academic standard. The program was successful and led to the establishment of nine accredited programs, with the standard for entry being a baccalaureate in nursing. Initially, the first programs awarded certificates given jointly by the American Academy of Pediatrics and the ANA. However, by 1973, the number of master's degree programs began to increase and soon outnumbered the certificate programs.[44] The early NP programs attracted nurses with international experience, including mission work and broader community experience.

Although the myths about the program may have been negative, the outcomes were very positive. It was not, as suggested by the second myth identified by Ford, a medical model with nurses performing as junior physicians. According to Ford,[1,42] the model was anything but medical: it was based on well-child care, health promotion, and disease prevention, and it afforded the nurse an opportunity to assess autonomously, innovate, and work collaboratively with physicians and families in providing care. Ford also considered the National League of Nursing's statement[45] that the early programs

> have been considered a means of controlling costs by introducing lower-paid health care providers ... as an answer to distribution problems in geographic areas short of physicians. (p. 2)

Ford[1] believed that the distribution problems provided an opportunity to test the expanded role of nurses.

The third myth focuses on the educational pattern followed to prepare NPs, suggesting that[1] short-term continuing education courses were the educational pattern used to prepare nurse practitioners from any nursing background. (p. 12)

Ford[1] clarified that the first pediatric NP program at the University of Colorado, which had been funded through the Medical Research Fund at the University of Colorado and began admitting students in 1965, required a baccalaureate in nursing and qualifications to meet graduate school admission requirements. Findings from this experimental program were to be incorporated into collegiate nursing programs at the appropriate degree level.[45] It is not clear in the literature when and why a change occurred. From Ford's comments and her debunking of myths surrounding the NP programs, the intent all along was to expand the role of the public health nurse and to build the NP role on a nursing model.[1] The development of the NP role according to Fenton and Brykczynski[47] paralleled development of the CNS role and was viewed as a "clinical option to the more traditional educator or administrative role in graduate nursing programs." Probably, increase of federal support in the 1970s accelerated the development of both CNS (educator-oriented role) and NP (practice-oriented role) programs. The fourth myth, according to Ford,[1] is that the "innovations in expanded roles came from professionals other than nurses" (p. 12). The fifth myth addresses the issue of laws governing practice. Ford emphasized that the model was within the practice of nurses and did not necessitate changing nurse-practice acts. The sixth myth, according to Ford,[1] is that "physician supervision was necessary for nurse practitioners" (p. 12). Ford pointed out that the University of Colorado program was collegial; it was only when academic standards were compromised that the NP role became confused with the physician assistant role and control by the medical profession became an issue.

The seventh myth surrounds the acceptance or lack of acceptance of the NP by physicians and patients. Again, according to Ford,[42] once collegiality was experienced, problems between or among groups apparently diminished, resulting in the mutual acceptance of roles.

Influence of Government Agencies

Federal support came a little late to the movement, mainly for political reasons. Without the strong support of the professional organizations, it was difficult to promote the developing programs. The first attempt to gain federal support for the demonstration project at the University of Colorado was through the Children's Bureau. However, this approach was unsuccessful because the perception was that the project did not fit the mold or mission of the Children's Bureau. According to Ford,[41] the bureau's rejection turned out to be fortunate because it motivated a search for other funding sources that proved to be very productive. The other source of federal funding was through the Division of Nursing of the BHPr. Following the initiation of the Colorado program in 1965, the 1970s opened up to a significant increase in master's programs for NPs. By 1977 there were 84 programs, 75% of which required a thesis and 20% had support of what was then the Department of Health, Education and Welfare (HEW). There were 131 certificate programs at that time. Length of time for completion of the programs ranged from

9 to 18 months and required 270 to 1,440 hours of experience under the supervision of a preceptor.[48]

Influence of Private Foundations, Colleges, and Universities

Despite the lack of support and the resistance of the professional associations, the practitioner movement made continued progress through the support of private foundations and specialty organizations. The RWJF and The Commonwealth Fund were very supportive of the NP role. Through their efforts, including both moral and financial support, the program, according to Ford, was "put on the map."[42] Unfortunately, university nursing faculty were slow to do more than challenge the ideas; it appeared that faculty were more interested in preparing the CNS. In addition, the few faculty who were in practice feared medical control.

Curriculum was the most important aspect of this movement, according to Ford[42]; however, in many schools, that preparation did not include physiology, had a behavioral focus, and did not include research. Ford[42] thought that the practitioner movement was doing what it should be doing: testing the "boundaries of knowledge." The ANA stated that clinical studies should be undertaken, but it was using the model of the CNS, including the nursing process with a focus on clinical judgment and nursing management.

Given that the ANA and the schools did not support the early NP effort, the NP movement went to the American Academy of Pediatrics for sponsorship and certification. From 1970 and into the 1980s, NPs persisted in their attempts to be recognized by nursing organizations and academies, making repeated demands of the traditional organizations. In the 1990s, according to Ford[1]:

> The goals of the first nurse practitioner educational programs—to be integrated and institutionalized in collegiate nursing programs—are coming to fruition. (p. 13)

The NP is clinically competent, well accepted by patients and health care professionals, cost-effective, and professionally credentialed.[42,43] The NP has continued to expand into new settings and new specialty areas as needs, demands, and opportunities have increased. The NP has also been influential in academic settings, introducing the concept of faculty practice and influencing graduate and undergraduate curricula.[46] The breadth of the role has expanded from a 3-month formal preparation beyond the basic nursing education program to master' level NP preparation in family health, pediatrics, gerontology, adult health, women's health, neonatal care, acute care, and psychiatric/mental health.[49] In an article addressing blending of the CNS and NP roles, Lynch describes the NP role as not only providing direct, holistic, and comprehensive care but as one that includes assessment and treatment within the scope of practice.[50]

Forces Influential in Marketing and Effective Utilization

From Ford's perspective,[42] the use of pilot projects, spurred by the academic credentials and success of Ford and Silver, helped to keep programs afloat. The Colorado

Health Department and private pediatricians helped to study the process and to identify outcomes by following students into the practice areas. Ford served on the State Board of Nursing in Colorado and, as president, helped to keep the health community informed. She made visits to the medical and nursing boards and described what NPs were doing, reassuring the boards that nurses were not changing the nature of practice but remaining within its scope.

The students themselves were probably most influential in marketing and communicating the effective use of NPs.[42] Articles, published books, personal testimonies, and invitations to visitors for direct observation at practice sites contributed to highlighting the progress and distributing the message of the NP. As health care issues assumed a larger part of the public agenda, newspapers began to pick up on the trend.

An obstacle to the marketing and effective use of NPs has been the lack of uniform credentialing. Ford[1] prefers that the ANCC or other nursing organizations confer NP certification and that the states' nurse-practice acts not be altered. Ford[1] believes that every professional nurse should be required to read Safriet's scholarly analysis (see Bibliography) of the legal "mishmash created by nurse practitioner legislation" (p. 13).

Key Leaders

The movement toward expanding the NP role included leadership from nurses and physicians alike. In addition to Ford and Silver, the following is a brief list of some of the prominent figures who were engaged in the expanding scope of practice through collaboration with physician colleagues: Priscilla Andrews, RN, John Connelly, MD, and others in Massachusetts[51]; Barbara Resnick, RN, and Charles Lewis, MD, in Missouri[52]; and Harriet Kitzman, RN, and Evan Charney, MD, in Rochester, New York.[53] According to Ford[1]: "These maverick nurses were pioneering innovators; but most of all, they were nurses." (p. 12)

Ingeborg Mauksch, PhD, FAAN,[54] who became an NP in 1972, published a paper with a physician colleague on joint practice and later became an ANA representative to the National Joint Practice Commission, where she served for 4 years. She also served as director of the Robert Wood Johnson Faculty Fellowships in Primary Care program, helping to prepare 100 fellows in primary care leadership, teaching, and practice. In addition, many nursing leaders in key positions throughout the country supported the movement. These leaders include Margaret Arnstein, Fay Abdellah, Mary Kelley Mullane, Florence Blake, and Esther Lucille Brown, whose favorite quote regarding NPs was "I have seen nursing in its finest."[42] The Center for Human and Child Development also strongly supported the development and positioning of the NP movement.

Leaders such as these served to explode the last four myths about the NP, which implied that practice laws would need to be expanded, that increased supervision of NPs would be necessary, that patients and physicians would have a difficult time accepting the NP, and that NPs would become extinct once the physician shortage was over. Again, according to Ford,[1,42] due in part to the leadership of such nurses, none of these notions was true. In addition to the positive pilot projects, publicity, and the rapidly changing health environment that were a continuous stimulus to the movement's development, these nurses committed the NP to a high quality of education during a time when government and professional support was lacking. For a more comprehensive list of exceptional NPs and "Who's Who" among NPs, refer to the special anniversary issue of *Nurse Practitioner,* September 1990.[55]

Interface with Nurse Midwives, Nurse Anesthetists, and Clinical Nurse Specialists

According to Ford,[42] the nature of nursing is "timeless and enduring." The role of the NP is similar to that of the other three advanced practice roles in its emphasis on practice autonomy and interdisciplinary collaboration and its continuing efforts toward a barrier-free practice. At the same time, there are distinguishing characteristics among the three role components. In general, the NP is focused on health and wellness in a community-based primary care setting, autonomy in clinical decision-making, systematic and orderly collection of data through history-taking and provision of feedback to the client, and advocacy on the client's behalf. The collaborative element of the NP role affords not only an opportunity for consumer choice but also for effective resource allocation and follow-up.

JOINING FORCES: ROLE PARAMETERS AND CONCERNS

Within the historical and sociopolitical contexts of the evolution of the four advanced domains of CNM, CRNA, CNS, and NP, certain similarities and differences are evident. From the educational perspective, the most common theme is the fact that all four domains were influenced by the early development of nursing, which, through the Nightingale schools, stimulated better education and professional development for nurses. As each practice area has evolved, education has been a significant force in enabling greater autonomy in practice.

Trends in educational preparation gradually have moved toward postbaccalaureate preparation, with the CNS, NP, and CRNA almost universally requiring master's-level preparation and a strong move in the CNM-APN domain, although not supported by the ACNM,[61] toward a similar level of preparation. Nonetheless, controversy surrounding entry-level education for nursing continues to persist. Moreover, because there were no clear paradigms for advanced practice, each role has evolved within its own framework. For instance, faculty in the western United States have not yet agreed on a definition of advanced practice nursing and its scope in health care. However, in the past 5 years the professional organizations have made great strides in identifying competencies for advanced practice nursing, particularly for the NP and CNS. There have been conflicting discussions in the literature about blending the NP and CNS roles. Each role, however, retains a distinctive definition with some blurring of functions. Lynch[50] proposes that it is time to merge the CNS and NP roles under one APN model, taking into account that NPs need additional educational preparation in systems management, consultation, and research in additional to a minimum of master's-level preparation. CNSs on the other hand need additional preparation in assessment skills and primary care management techniques. There is increasing clarity by the specialty organizations in defining CNS and NP role and scope of practice.[50]

As has been illustrated, progress in advanced practice nursing has been hampered by the profession's history, medicine's concern for competition, the lack of acceptance of nursing both externally and internally as a discipline with its own body of knowledge, and by the tendency toward a lack of mutual support and collaboration as each movement has moved forward. As Minarik[28] pointed out, nurses tend to be territorial, holding on to their areas of practice. Even nursing faculty have been separated by their own agendas in these advanced practice areas, with each having a strong orientation or bias. In more recent years, however, collaboration and mutual support among the APN organizations have been evidenced.

Table 1–2 compares historical information and the views of the nursing leaders interviewed for this chapter. The historical developments of nurse midwifery and nurse anesthesia are clearly more alike in their association with the medical community and their competition with medicine. The CNS movement and the NP movement are more recent and have been focused on comprehensive health care in acute and primary care settings.

In each of the four practice areas, interviewees noted the recognition of the move toward autonomy in decision-making and professionalism by the medical community as consistently important in operationalizing each role. For nurse midwives, nurse anesthetists, and NPs, acceptance of the autonomous nature of their roles by the medical community helped connect responsibility and accountability to authority in independent decision-making in areas of assessment and care normally requiring medical management under the purview of the physician. The CNS, in contrast, needed similar autonomy but was not so closely aligned to medical management as were the other three. Responsibilities of the CNS were broader within the specialty and focused more on nursing management of illness in acute care, consultation, education, and research.

In all four domains, support from medicine, from state and federal legislatures, and, most important, from the consumer, was of significant consequence. The nurse midwives' primary source of consumer support came from the underserved populations who benefited from their attendance at home deliveries. Nurse anesthetists gained recognition through physicians and patients, especially because of their impeccable records with survival rates through surgery. Similarly, but in different practice arenas, CNSs and NPs have been their own best advocates. Consumer satisfaction and physician advocacy have proved to be powerful stimuli for both of these movements. Unlike the NP and CRNA movement, the CNS movement had the benefit of unyielding support from the ANA. All four groups were actively involved in scholarly and lay publications as their specialties developed, keeping both professionals and the public informed.

With the exception of the NP role, a state of war acted as a catalyst to the expanded use, and consequential favorable opinion, of the advanced practice

TABLE 1–2. **Comparison of Four Specialty Domains**				
Characteristics	**Certified Nurse Midwife**	**Certified Registered Nurse Anesthetist**	**Clinical Nurse Specialist**	**Nurse Practitioner**
Mechanisms that helped operationalize the role	Autonomy Professional development War Medical support Access to consultation Legislative support Consumer support (dealing with underserved populations) Publications	Autonomy Professional development War Medical support Access to consultation Publications	Autonomy Professional development War Medical support Access to consultation Legislative support (primarily ANA lobby) Publications Managing illness in acute care Growing specialization Increased use of technology in acute care created need for an attending nurse	Autonomy Professional development Medical support Access to consultation Legislative support Consumer support Publications Academic support of Ford and Silver Communication with state board (Colorado) Pilot projects
Forces that influenced marketing and effective utilization	Wars Focus on improving education Federal initiatives (Frontier Nursing Service) Development of the American College of Nurse-Midwives Malpractice crisis 1985 Consumer support	Wars Focus on improving education Certification Department of Health National Council of State Boards Private Foundations Pew HCFA	Federal initiatives Private foundations (Robert Wood Johnson) Students Consumer support Support of nursing service administration	Federal initiatives (not initially but later) Private foundations (The Commonwealth Fund and The Robert Wood Johnson Foundation) Students Consumer support

(Table continued on following page)

TABLE 1–2. Comparison of Four Specialty Domains (Continued)

Characteristics	Certified Nurse Midwife	Certified Registered Nurse Anesthetist	Clinical Nurse Specialist	Nurse Practitioner
Distinguishing characteristics	Health and comfort of mothers and babies Distinctive medical support Development of core competencies in 1978 Well grounded in childbirth Community-based and hospital-based	Medical focus nature of Distinctive medical support Systematic and orderly data collection Hospital-based	Direct care broad within the specialty Filled the gap for the need for attending nurse to coordinate care within the specialty in the acute care setting Depth and breadth of clinical knowledge in one specialty Fully developed specialty	Good public relations Health and wellness focus within a community-based primary care context Systematic and orderly data collection with feedback Consumer advocacy within the independent role
Interaction with other specialties	National Organization for Specialty Nurses Frontier Nursing Service	National Organization for Specialty Nurses	National Organization for Specialty Nurses	National Organization for Specialty Nurses
Common shared roles	Autonomy in practice Interdisciplinary emphasis and sharing of each other's skills Joint effort to practice without artificial barriers Recognition of each other's areas of expertise Practice in acute-care and community-based settings Movement to graduate preparation	Autonomy in practice Interdisciplinary emphasis and sharing of each other's skills Joint effort to practice without artificial barriers Recognition of each other's areas of expertise Shared role in selling services in managed care Movement to graduate preparation	Autonomy in practice Interdisciplinary emphasis and sharing of each other's skills Joint effort to practice without artificial barriers Recognition of each other's areas of practice Movement to community-based care, potential for merging of role with NP Graduate preparation	Autonomy in practice Interdisciplinary emphasis and sharing of each other's skills Joint effort to practice without artificial barriers Recognition of each other's areas of practice Movement to acute care, potential for merging of roles with CNS Movement to graduate preparation

HCFA = Health Care Financing Administration

nursing role. Other significant outside influences included both public and private initiatives. The Children's Bureau was significant in the nurse midwifery movement. The National Council of State Boards was important for maintaining standards for the CRNA, and Robert Wood Johnson, Pew, and the Division of Nursing, BPHr, helped to support educational programs that moved the CNS and NP movements forward. While the ANA focused its support on the CNS movement, The Commonwealth Fund was a particularly helpful source of support for the NP movement. In addition, advancing technology and growing acuity in care gave further impetus to the need for clinical specialization, thus assisting the CNS movement. In contrast, the current emphasis on primary care and community-based illness prevention and health promotion have created greater opportunities for the NP.

Each of the domains has experienced its own struggle in establishing credibility and acceptance by the profession and public. Educational preparation, certification, licensure, and credentialing are overriding concerns for all four domains. Increasing competition in the health care market in the 1970s and 1980s was a concern to those practicing in each of the areas, but especially to the emerging NP, who is particularly susceptible to the issues of equitable economic reimbursement for services, hospital privileges, and prescriptive authority. Collaboration, interdisciplinary emphasis, and mutual support are emerging as key common elements in a changing health care environment. Garde[24] pointed out that it will be necessary for artificial barriers to communication within the profession to be removed and for each practice area to join forces in identifying the best ways to provide services in a managed care environment in a way that recognizes each other's area of practice.

The distinguishing characteristics of the four domains are presented from a multitude of perspectives in the literature. Roberts[3] does an excellent job of summarizing the various events influencing CNMs and their move to professionalism. Bankert[23] and Thatcher[21] are two authors who have done an outstanding job in capturing the history of the CRNA from its inception. Sparacino, Cooper, and Minarik,[29] Hamric and Spross,[27] and Menard[56] have provided historical and clinical descriptions of the role of the CNS. Ford[1] has contributed to dispelling myths that have been perpetuated in the literature regarding the NP, as well as clearly articulating the NP's role.

The distinctive feature of the nurse midwifery practitioner is the focus on the health and comfort of mothers and babies during the birthing experience, both in the home and in the hospital. CRNAs and nurse midwives have engaged in systematic data collection through key leaders to demonstrate competency. Direct care is probably the most distinctive feature of the CNS role, followed by coordination, evaluation, and planning for the individual within the broader context of acute and, to some extent, community-based health care. According to Sparacino, Cooper, and Minarik,[29] the CNS role incorporates theory, clinical practice content, and research in a particular specialty area, thus promoting the "integration of education, consultation, and leadership with the clinical practice component" (p. 7). The early hallmarks of the NP role were an emphasis on primary care and health promotion that occur in an independent or collegial setting and the fact that the NP role provides an excellent opportunity for independence and innovation in practice.

Trends indicate that the future of advanced practice nursing will contine to expand, including the emphasis on community-based primary care in a managed care environment. For the NP and the nurse midwife, this trend will probably increase the scope of practice and the potential for new growth. The nurse anesthetist has been, and will continue to be, affected by the health care changes, with more emphasis on one-day outpatient surgery. The implications of this type of surgical experience in a changing environment will create a need for continuity and better communication between providers. The future of the CNS is less clear.

Twenty-five NPs were interviewed about the movement's evolution and the future challenges for the role. The question of the appropriate curriculum for NPs has resulted in mixed opinions. While the need for "advanced practice" preparation has always been recognized, the question of integration of the CNS and NP roles continues to result in differing opinions. Mauksch[54] envisioned a retitling of NP to CNS in primary care for consistency with ANA nomenclature for the appropriate master's-level preparation in the specific field. Ford,[57] along with others,[38] saw the need to merge these two roles, with a general effort made to increase the assessment skills of all nurses and to provide for additional clinical learning at the undergraduate level. Ford[57] also promoted postmaster's-level continuing education for CNSs and a "retooling and retraining [of] faculty" (p. 28).

Within the last 3 years, there has been increasing discussion about the APRN role and the symbiotic relationship between the NP and CNS. There is also a remergence of the CNS in acute care settings, with a new emphasis on the value of patient education and consultation, key characteristics of the CNS role. The nursing shortage has led to a reconsideration of the role of the CNS and the signifcant contributions that can be made to improving the quality of care. As the health care system responds to the nursing shortage, the clarification of definitions and competencies may help the NP and CNS gain new ground in the health care delivery system.[58]

Minarik[28] and Riddle[30] held a different view of the future of the NP and CNS roles. Although many NPs originally foresaw the CNS role eventually being absorbed into the NP role, Minarik and Riddle questioned who "will provide direct care in the acute care setting" and expressed concern that the "broad responsibility and creative nursing care of the CNS" may be lost in the transition. Whether there will be a true blending of CNS and NP roles or an emergence of a coordinator of health care based on the scholarly, sensitive, patient-centered approach that has been so much a part of the CNS role has yet to be determined, although the second alternative is becoming more prevalent.

The nursing shortage and changes in the state of the nation and the world have created a new focus for health providers. In recent years, nursing and the nation have faced some major crises. With the occurrence of the terrorist attack on America, September 11, 2001, and the subsequent concerns regarding bioterrorism, war and the potential for future attacks on the nation, the readiness of first responders prepared to maintain the health integrity of the populace is critical. APNs have a major role to play in providing the resources to meet the demands of a nation in crisis. As APN roles continue evolving, the public's expectations for nurses to join forces within the health field and provide leadership for maintaining the welfare of communities will provide new opportunities and challenges.

The current state of uncertainty surrounding the American health care delivery system may present the greatest window of opportunity for advanced practice nurses to unite and be heard as a vital force in care during health and illness. A response to the rapid changes in medical technologies worthy of nursing's history, the concerns over health care resources, and the ethical considerations inherent in the pressure to deliver high-quality, cost-effective health care will require collective strength that demands a joining of forces of these four autonomous domains of practice. Although, in the past, disputes over nursing's "identity" created internal conflicts and diverse opinions on what is best for nursing, these histories reflect a collective commitment by the profession to remain true to its essence while continuing to develop. With our predecessors as prototypes, the secure and successful future of nursing in the emerging model of health care can best be accomplished by collaboration and cooperation and by drawing on the intellect, integrity, and vigor that has marked the best of nursing's past.

SUGGESTED EXERCISES

1. Briefly trace the historical development of the four domains of advanced practice nursing discussed in this chapter. From an historical perspective, identify the forces that have influenced progress in each of these areas of practice. From your perspective, which of these forces do you view as having the most significant impact, and why?

2. Identify three key players in each of the domains, and discuss their major contributions to the advanced practice movement.

3. Describe the role of the federal government and private foundations in the advanced practice movement. Compare and contrast the similarities and differences of these organizations in moving advanced practice forward in each of the four domains.

4. After reading this chapter and thinking about the four domains of practice and your personal experience, where do you perceive the need for joining forces, and what mechanisms would you identify as critical in enabling these four areas of practice to move forward in a unified way?

5. Create a scenario in which representatives from each of these domains have been called forward to testify at a congressional hearing to convince members of Congress to continue to support advanced practice nursing. What points should each representative make unique to each domain and relevant to all four domains that would support continued funding?

6. Consider yourself a consumer advocate for each of the four domains. Describe what you consider the strengths of each of these specialties and how they contribute to improving health care of the U.S. population.

7. How would you respond to a layperson who asked you why one might select an APN as a provider?

8. On the basis of this chapter, what roles, if any, do you see merging, and which do you view as remaining separate? In your thinking, take into account the historical context in which these roles emerged.

9. This chapter incorporated interviews from the "lived experience" of key players in each of the four domains of practice. What role does the lived experience play in historical

documentation of nursing movements, and what did you learn that you might not have learned if the chapter included only written documentation versus personal communication?

10 In what ways can our lived experiences be preserved to document the historical progress of nursing?

REFERENCES

1. Ford, LC: Nurse practitioners: Myths and misconceptions. J New York State Nurses Assoc 26:12, 1995.
2. Roberts, J: Personal communication, March, 1996.
3. Roberts, J: The role of graduate education in midwifery in the USA. In Murphy-Black, T (ed): Issues in Midwifery: 119. Churchill Livingstone, Tokyo, 1995.
4. American College of Nurse-Midwives: Background on the ACNM/MANA Interorganization workgroup on midwifery education (IWG). Quickening 24:29, 1993.
5. Hiestad, WC: The development of nurse-midwifery education in the United States. In Fitzpatrick, ML (ed): Historical Studies in Nursing. Teachers' College Press, Columbia University, New York, 1978.
6. Chaney, JA: Birthing in early America. J Nurse Midwifery 25:5, 1980.
7. Litoff, JB: American Midwives: 1860 to the Present. Greenwood Press, Westport, CT, 1978.
8. Litoff, JB: The midwife throughout history. J Nurse Midwifery 27:3, 1982.
9. Stern, CA: Midwives, male-midwives, and nurse-midwives. Obstet Gynecol 39:308, 1972.
10. Hawkins, JW: Annual Report of the ANA Council on Maternal-Child Nursing. American Nurses Association, Kansas City, June 1987.
11. Levy, J: The maternal and infant mortality in midwifery practice in Newark, NJ. Am J Obstet Gynecol 77:42, 1918.
12. Baker, J: The function of the midwife. Woman's Med J 23:196, 1913.
13. Dock, LL: In Robb, IA, Dock, LL, and Banfield M (eds): The Transactions of the Third International Congress of Nurses with the Reports of the International Council of Nurses. JB Savage, Cleveland, Ohio, 1901.
14. Tom, SA: The evolution of nurse-midwifery 1900–1960. J Nurse Midwifery 27:4, 1982.
15. Shoemaker, MT: History of Nurse-Midwifery in the United States. The Catholic University of America Press, Washington, DC, 1947. Dissertation.
16. Bear, B: Personal communication, February, 1996.
17. Hall, CM: Training the obstetrical nurse. Am J Nursing 27:373, 1927.
18. Willeford, MB: The frontier nursing service. Public Health Nurs 25:9, 1933.
19. The History of the American College of Nurse-Midwives. Adapted from Varney's Midwifery, 3rd ed, from http://www.midwife.org/about/history.cfm
20. International Confederation of Midwives. Fact sheet. nd.
21. Thatcher, VS: History of Anesthesia with Emphasis on the Nurse Specialist. Lippincott, Philadelphia, 1953
22. American Association of Nurse Anesthetists. Capitol corner. http://www.aana.com/capcorner/factsheet_111301.asp. Accessed April 2004.
23. Bankert, M: Watchful Care: A History of America's Nurse Anesthetists. Continuum, New York, 1989.
24. Garde, J: Personal communication, February, 1996.
25. Crile, GW (ed): George Crile: An Autobiography. Lippincott, Philadelphia, 1947.
26. Questions and Answers: A Career in Nurse Anesthesia, from http://aana.com/crna/careerqna.asp. Accessed May 2003.
27. Hamric, AB, and Spross, JA: The Clinical Nurse Specialist in Theory and Practice, ed 2. WB Saunders, Philadelphia, 1989.
28. Minarik, PA: Personal communication, March, 1996.
29. Sparacino, PA, Cooper, DM, and Minarik, PA: The Clinical Specialists: Implementation and Impact. Appleton & Lange, Stamford, CT, 1990.
30. Riddle, I: Personal communication, February, 1996.
31. Norris, CM: One perspective on the nurse practitioner movement. In Jacox, A, and Norris, C (eds): Organizing for Independent Nursing Practice. Appleton-Century-Crofts, New York, 1977.
32. Smoyak, SA: Specialization in nursing: From then to now. Nurs Outlook 24:676, 1976.
33. Peplau, HE: Specialization in professional nursing. Nurs Sci 3:268, 1965.

34. American Nurses Association: Nursing: A Social Policy Statement. American Nurses Association, Kansas City, 1980.
35. American Association of Critical Care Nurses: AACN Position Statement: The Critical Care Clinical Nurse Specialist: Role Definition. American Association of Critical Care Nurses, Newport Beach, CA, 1986.
36. American Nurses Association: Clinical Nurse Specialists: Distribution and Utilization. American Nurses Association, Kansas City, 1986.
37. California Nurses' Association: Position Statement on Specialization in Nursing Practice. California Nurses' Association, San Francisco, 1984.
38. Sparacino, P: The clinical nurse specialist. Nurs Pract 1:215, 1986.
39. Cooper, DM: A refined expert: The clinical nurse specialist after five years. Momentum 1:1, 1983.
40. Boyle C. Lesson learned from clinical nurse specialist longevity. J Adv Nurs 26:168, 1997.
41. Lyons, B.L (2003). NACNS Model Statutory and Regulatory Language Governing CNS Practice, from http//www.nacns.org/legis. Accessed May 2003.
42. Ford, LC: Personal communication, February, 1996.
43. Ford, LC, Cobb, M, and Taylor, M: Defining Clinical Contact Graduate Nursing Programs: Community Health Nursing. Western Interstate Commission for Higher Education, Boulder, CO, 1967.
44. Bullough, B: Professionalization of nurse practitioners. Ann Rev Nurs Res 13:239, 1995.
45. National League of Nursing: Position Statement on the Education of Nurse Practitioners. National League of Nursing, publication 11–1808, New York, 1979.
46. Ford, LC: The contribution of nurse practitioners to American health care. In Aiken, LH (ed): Nursing in the 1980s: Crises, Opportunities, Challenges. Lippincott, Philadelphia, 1982.
47. Fenton, MV, and Brykczynski, K. Qualitative distinctions and similarities in the practice of clinical nurse specialists and nurse practitioners. J Prof Nurs 9:313, 1993.
48. Malasanos, L.: Health assessment skills in nursing: From conception to practice in a single decade. In McCloskey, JC, and Grace, HK: Current issues in nursing. Pennsylvania: Blackwell Scientific Solutions, 1981.
49. Snyder, M, and Yen, M: Characteristics of the advanced practice nurse. In Snyder, M, and Mirr, M.(eds). Advanced Practice Nursing: A Guide to Professional Development. New York: Springer Publishing Company, 1995
50. Lynch, A. M. (August 1, 1996). At the Crossroads: We must Blend the CNS + NP Roles. [Electronic Version] from http://www.nursingworld.org/ojin/tpc1/tpc1_5.htm. Accessed May 2003.
51. Ford, LC, and Silver, HK: The expanded role of the nurse in child care. Nurs Outlook 15:43, 1967.
52. Lewis, CE, and Resnik, BA: Nurse clinics and progressive ambulatory patient care. N Engl J Med 277:1236, 1967.
53. Charney, E, and Kitzman, H: Child-health nurse (pediatric nurse practitioner) in private practice: A controlled trial. N Engl J Med 285:1353, 1971.
54. Mauksch, I: Special anniversary issue: 25 years later 25 exceptional NPs look at the movement's evolution and consider future challenges for the role. Nurse Pract 15:28, 1990.
55. Special anniversary issue: 25 years later 25 exceptional NPs look at the movement's evolution and consider future challenges for the role. Nurse Pract 15:28, 1990.
56. Menard, SW: The Clinical Nurse Specialist: Perspectives on Practice. John Wiley & Sons, 1987.
57. Ford, LC: Special anniversary issue: 25 years later 25 exceptional NPs look at the movement's evolution and consider future challenges for the role. Nurse Pract 15:28, 1990.
58. Quaal, SJ: Clinical nurse specialist: Role restructuring to advanced practice registered nurse. Crit Care Nurs Q 21:37, 1999.
59. Dickerson, N: Personal communication, June, 2003.
60. Tobin, Mitch: Personal communication, June, 2003.
61. American College of Nurse-Midwives: Position Statement on Mandatory Degree Requirements for Midwives, latest revision November 1998. http://www.midwife.org/prof/display.cfm?id=102. Accessed June 2003.
62. Williams, Deanne: Personal communication, June, 2003.
63. American Association of Nurse Anesthetists. Archives Library, Historical Resources. http://www.aana.com/archives/awards/honorary_member.asp. Accessed April 2004.

ADDITIONAL REFERENCES

Aiken, LH: Health Policy and Nursing Practice. McGraw-Hill Book Co, New York, 1981.
American Association of Colleges of Nursing: Nursing Education's Agenda for the 21st Century. American Association of Colleges of Nursing, Washington, DC, March 22, 1993.

American Association of Colleges of Nursing. The Essentials of Master's Education for Advanced Practice Nursing. American Association of Colleges of Nursing, Washington, DC, 1996.

American Association of Nurse Anesthetists: Guidelines and Standards for Nurse Anesthesia Practice, Park Ridge, IL, 1992.

American College of Nurse-Midwives: Background on the ACNM/MANA Interorganization Workgroup on Midwifery Education (IWG). Quickening 24:29, 1993.

Baker, J: The function of the midwife. Womans Med J 23:196, 1913.

Bankert, M: Watchful Care: A History of America's Nurse Anesthetists. Continuum, New York, 1989.

Barry, PD: Psychosocial Nursing Care of Physically Ill Patients and Their Families, ed 3. Lippincott, Philadelphia, 1996.

Bear, B: Personal communication, February 1996.

Breckenridge, M: Wide Neighborhoods, p. 117. Ross Laboratories, Columbus, OH, 1967.

Burnside, I: A scarce professional: The geropsychiatric clinical nurse specialist. Clin Nurse Specialist 4:122, 1990.

California Alliance of Advanced Practice Nurses: October 1, 1995.

California Nurses' Association: Position Statement on Specialization in Nursing Practice. California Nurses' Association, San Francisco, 1984.

Campbell, ML, et al: An advanced practice model: Inpatient collaborative practices. Clin Nurse Specialist 9:175, 1995.

Chaney, JA: Birthing in early America. J Nurse Midwifery 25:5, 1980.

Charney, E, and Kitzman, H: Child-health nurse (pediatric nurse practitioner) in private practice: A controlled trial. N Engl J Med 285:1353, 1971.

Clapesattle, H: The Doctors Mayo, p. 427. University of Minnesota Press, Minneapolis, 1941.

Clinical Nurse Specialist Survey: State of California, Board of Registered Nursing, Sacramento, December, 1994.

Cooper, DM: A refined expert: The clinical nurse specialist after five years. Momentum 1:1, 1983.

Corbin, H: A nurse looks ahead. Am J Obstet Gynecol 59:899, 1946.

Crile, GW (ed): George Crile, An Autobiography, p. 168. Lippincott, Philadelphia, 1947.

DeWitt, K: Specialties in nursing. Am J Nurs 1:14, 1900.

Diers, D: Future of nurse-midwives in American healthcare. In Aiken, L (ed): Nursing in the 1980s: Crises, Opportunities, Challenges. JB Lippincott, Philadelphia, 1982.

Dock, LL: In Robb, IA, Dock, LL, and Banfield, M (eds): The Transactions of the Third International Congress of Nurses with the Reports of the International Council of Nurses. p. 485. JB Savage, Cleveland, OH, 1901.

Education and Practice Collaboration: Mandate for Quality Education: Practice and Research for Health Care Reform. American Association of Colleges of Nursing, Washington, DC, October 25, 1993.

Faut-Callahan, M, and Kremer, M: Nurse anesthesia: An established advanced practice nursing specialty. Unpublished manuscript, 1996.

Fenton, MV, and Brykczynski, KA: Qualitative distinctions and similarities in the practice of clinical nurse specialists and nurse practitioners. Professional Nurse 9:313, 1993.

The first nurse anesthetist. BNANA 7:63, 1939.

Fitzpatrick, ML (ed): Historical Studies in Nursing, p. 68. Columbia University, New York, 1978.

Forbes, KE, et al: Clinical nurse specialist and nurse practitioner core curricula survey results. Nurse Pract 15:43, 1990.

Ford, LC: The contribution of nurse practitioners to American health care. In Aiken, LH (ed): Nursing in the 1980's: Crises, Opportunities, Challenges, p. 231. JB Lippincott, Philadelphia, 1982.

Ford, LC: Nurse practitioners: Myths and misconceptions. J New York State Nurses Assoc 26:12, 1995.

Ford, LC: Personal communication, February, 1996.

Ford, LC: Special anniversary issue: 25 years later 25 exceptional NPs look at the movement's evolution and consider future challenges for the role. Nurse Pract 15:28, 1990.

Ford, LC, Cobb, M, and Taylor, M: Defining Clinical Contact Graduate Nursing Programs: Community Health Nursing. Western Interstate Commission for Higher Education, Boulder, CO, 1967.

Ford, LC, and Silver, HK: The expanded role of the nurse in child care. Nurs Outlook 15:43, 1967.

Freeland, T: Letters to the editor. Clin Nurse Specialist 8:289, 1994.

Galloway, DH: The anesthetizer as a specialist. The Philadelphia Medical Journal, p 1175, May 27, 1899.

Garde, J: Personal communication, February, 1996.

Gleeson, RM, et al: Advanced practice nursing: A model of collaborative care. MCN 15:9, 1990.

Guyette, MI: Letter to the editor. Clin Nurse Specialist 9:424, 1995.

Hall, CM: Training the obstetrical nurse. Am J Nursing 27:373, 1927.

Hamric, AB, and Spross, JA: The Clinical Nurse Specialist in Theory and Practice, ed 2. WB Saunders, Philadelphia, 1989.

Hawkins, JW: Annual Report of the ANA Council on Maternal-Child Nursing. American Nurses Association, Kansas City, June, 1987.

Hemschemeyer, H: A training school for nurse-midwives established. Am J Nurs 32:374, 1939.

Hiestad, WC: The development of nurse-midwifery education in the United States. In Fitzpatrick, ML (ed): Historical Studies in Nursing. Teachers' College Press, Columbia University, NY, 1978, p 86.

Hoyer, A: Sexual harassment: Four women describe their experiences: Background and implications for the clinical nurse specialist. Arch Psychiatr Nurs 8:177, 1994.

Is primary care the answer? Nurses respond. The American Nurse, 1994.

Jackson, PL: Advanced practice nursing: II. Opportunities and challenges for PNPs. Pediatr Nurs 21:43, 1995.

Keane, A, and Richmond, T: Tertiary nurse practitioners. Image J Nurs Sch 25:281, 1993.

Kobrin, FE: The American midwife controversy: A crisis of professionalization. Bull Hist Med 40:350, 1966.

Kupina, PS: Community health CNSs and health care in the year 2000. Clin Nurse Specialist 9:188, 1995.

Lerner, G: The Majority Finds Its Past: Placing Women in History. Oxford University Press, New York, 1979.

Levy, J: The maternal and infant mortality in midwifery practice in Newark, NJ. Am J Obstet Gynecol 77:42, 1918.

Lewis, CE, and Resnik, BA: Nurse clinics and progressive ambulatory patient care. N Engl J Med 277:1236, 1967.

Litoff, JB: American Midwives: 1860 to the Present. Greenwood Press, Westport, CT, 1986.

Litoff, JB: The midwife throughout history. J Nurse Midwifery 27:3, 1978.

Long, KA: Master's degree nursing education and health care reform: Preparing for the future. Prof Nurs 10:71, 1994.

Magaw, A: A review of over fourteen thousand surgical anesthesias. BNANA 7:63, 1939.

Magaw, A: Observations in anesthesia. Northwestern Lancet 19:207.

Mauksch, I: Special anniversary issue: 25 years later 25 exceptional NPs look at the movement's evolution and consider future challenges for the role. Nurse Pract 15:28, 1990.

Mason, G, and Jinks, A: Examining the role of the practitioner-teacher in nursing. Br J Nurs 3:1063, 1994.

Medicaid Waiver Programs: Lessons for the Future or Time-limited Experiments. State Initiatives in Health Care Reforms, May/June, 1994.

Menard, SW: The Clinical Nurse Specialist: Perspectives on Practice. John Wiley & Sons, New York, 1987.

Minarik, PA: Alternatives to physical restraints in acute care. Clin Nurse Specialist 8:136, 1994.

Minarik, PA: Cognitive assessment of the cardiovascular patient in the acute care setting. Cardiovasc Nurs 9:36, 1995.

Minarik, PA: Collaboration between service and education: Perils or pleasures for the clinical nurse specialist? Clin Nurse Specialist 4:109, 1990.

Minarik, PA: Editor's response. Clin Nurse Specialist 8:289, 1994.

Minarik, PA: Federal action on prescriptive authority. Clin Nurse Specialist 7:46, 1993.

Minarik, PA: Graduate education and health care. Clin Nurse Specialist 246:10, 1996.

Minarik, PA: Health Care Financing Administration (HCFA) instructions clarify Medicare reimbursement eligibility. Clin Nurse Specialist 8:16, 1994.

Minarik, PA: Incorporating imagery in clinical practice. Clin Nurse Specialist 7:234, 1993.

Minarik, PA: Legislative and regulatory update: DEA registration for midlevel practitioners. Clin Nurse Specialist 7:319, 1993.

Minarik, PA: Legislative and regulatory update: Federal reimbursement revisited. Clin Nurse Specialist 7:102, 1993.

Minarik, PA: Legislative and regulatory update: Health care reform and managed competition: Implications for CNSs. Clin Nurse Specialist 7:105, 1993.

Minarik, PA: Legislative and regulatory update: Priorities for clinical nurse specialists. Clin Nurse Specialist 6:168, 1992.

Minarik, PA: Legislative and regulatory update: Reimbursement and health care reform legislation introduced. Clin Nurse Specialist 7:245, 1993.

Minarik, PA: Legislative and regulatory update: Second license for advanced practice? Clin Nurse Specialist 6:1, 1992.

Minarik, PA: Medwatch: Medical products reporting program. Clin Nurse Specialist 8:74, 1994.

Minarik, PA: Mind-body connection: Enhancing healing through imagery. Clin Nurse Specialist 7:169, 1993.

Minarik, PA: Personal communication, March, 1996.

Minarik, P, and Learith, M: The angry demanding hostile response. In Riggel, B, and Ehrenreich, D (eds): Psychological Aspects of Critical Care Nursing. Aspen Publishers, Rockville, MD, 1989.

Montemurd, MA: The evolution of the clinical nurse specialist: Response to the challenge of professional nursing practice. Clin Nurse Specialist 1:106, 1987.

National League for Nursing: Position statement on the education of nurse practitioners, publication 11–1808. National League for Nursing, New York, 1979.

New York Adopts Pure Community Rating: Other States Take Incremental Approach. State Initiatives in Health Care Reform, July/August, 1994.

Norris, CM: One perspective on the nurse practitioner movement. In Jacox, A, and Norris, C (eds): Organizing for Independent Nursing Practice, p. 21. New York, Appleton-Century-Crofts, 1977.

Nursing's Agenda for Health Care Reform: Final Draft. Lf:021. American Nurses Association, Kansas City, Mo, April 24, 1991.

Owen, H, and Wangensteen, SD: The Rise of Surgery, p 353. University of Minnesota Press, Minneapolis, 1978.

Peplau, HE: Specialization in professional nursing. Nursing Science 3:268, 1965.

Pew Health Professions Commission: Health Professions Education for the Future: Pew Professions Committee, UCSF Center for the Health Professions, San Francisco, February, 1993.

Pew Health Professions Commission: Policy Papers. UCSF Center for Health Professions, San Francisco, April 1994.

The professional anesthetizer (editorial). Medical Record, p 522, April 10, 1897.

Public Education Crucial to Health Care Reform: Citizens Bombarded with Special Interest Messages. State Initiatives in Health Care Reform, September/October 1994.

Qualifications and Capabilities of the Certified Registered Nurse Anesthetist. American Association of Nurse Anesthetists, Park Ridge, IL, 1992.

Reid, ML, and Morris, JB: Perinatal care and cost effectiveness: Changes in health expenditure and birth outcome following the establishment of a nurse midwife program. Med Care 17:491, 1979.

Riddle, I: Personal communication, February, 1996.

Robb, IAH: Nursing: Its Principles and Practice for Hospital and Private Use. WB Saunders, Philadelphia, 1893.

Roberts, J: The role of graduate education in midwifery in the USA. In Murphy-Black, T (ed): Issues in Midwifery: 119. Churchill Livingstone, Tokyo, 1995.

Roberts, J: Personal communication, March, 1996.

The Role of the Clinical Nurse Specialist. American Nurses' Association, Kansas City, 1968.

Roush, RE: The development of midwifery: Male and female, yesterday and today. J Nurse Midwifery 24:27, 1979.

Safriet, BJ: Healthcare dollars and regulatory sense: The role of advanced practice nursing. Yale J Regul 9:417, 1992.

Shoemaker, MT: History of nurse-midwifery in the United States. The Catholic University of America Press, Washington, DC, 1947. Dissertation.

Shoultz, J, Hatcher, PA, and Hurrell, M: Growing edges of a new paradigm: The future of nursing in the health of the nation. Nurs Outlook 40:58, 1992.

Shyrock, R: The Development of Modern Medicine, pp. 346–347. Knopf, New York, 1947.

Sloan, PE: Commitment to equality: A view of early black nursing schools. In Fitzpatrick, ML (ed): Historical Studies in Nursing. Columbia University, New York, 1978.

Smoyak, SA: Specialization in nursing: From then to now. Nurs Outlook 24:676, 1976.

Sparacino, P: The clinical nurse specialist. Nurs Pract 1:215, 1986.

Sparacino, PA, Cooper, DM, and Minarik, PA: The Clinical Specialists: Implementation and Impact. Appleton & Lange, Stamford, CT, 1990.

The Specialist Role of the ICN. Nursing Times 90:63, 1994.

Spenceley, SM: The CNS in multidisciplinary pulmonary rehabilitation: A nursing science perspective. Clin Nurse Specialist 9:192, 1995.

Starr, P: The Social Transformation of American Medicine, p. 155. Basic Books, New York, 1982.

Stern, CA: Midwives, male-midwives, and nurse-midwives. Obstet Gynecol 39:308, 1972.

Strunk, BL: The clinical nurse specialists as change agent. Clin Nurse Specialist 9:128, 1995.

Thatcher, VS: History of Anesthesia with Emphasis on the Nurse Specialist, pp. 27–28. Lippincott, Philadelphia, 1953.

Tierney, MJ, Minarik, PA, and Tierney, LM: Ethics in Japanese health care: A perspective for clinical nurse specialists. Clin Nurse Specialist 8:235, 1994.

Tom, SA: The evolution of nurse-midwifery 1900–1960. J Nurse Midwifery 27:4, 1982.

Van Blarcom, CC: Midwives in America. Am J Public Health 4–6:197, 1914.

Webster's New Collegiate Dictionary. G and C Merriam, Springfield, MA, 1979.

Willeford, MB: The frontier nursing service. Public Health Nurs 25:9, 1933.

Williams, JW: Medical education and the midwife problem in the United States. J Am Med Assoc 58:1, 1912.

CHAPTER 2

Advanced Practice Nursing in the Current Sociopolitical Environment

Lucille A. Joel, EdD, RN, FAAN

Lucille Joel is a Professor at Rutgers—The State University of New Jersey College of Nursing and was Director of the Rutgers Teaching Nursing Home from 1982 to 1998. Dr. Joel has served as president of the American Nurses Association (ANA) and First Vice-President of the International Council of Nurses (ICN), headquartered in Geneva. She holds official status as ICN's representative to UNICEF and the UN and serves on the International Advisory Board of the *American Journal of Nursing*. Dr. Joel has served as a professional-technical advisor to the Joint Commission on the Accreditation of Healthcare Organizations (JCAHO) and chaired the Federal Drug Administration's (FDA) steering committee on nursing and medical devices. She continues as ANA's liaison to Centers for Medicare and Medicaid Services (CMS), formerly the Health Care Financing Administration (HCFA) in work on quality and case mix reimbursement for long-term care. She is currently Vice-President of the Board of Trustees of the Commission on Graduates of Foreign Nursing Schools (CGFNS). Dr. Joel is a certified clinical specialist in psychiatric–mental health nursing and maintains a private practice. She has been involved in the education of advanced practice nurses since 1976.

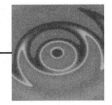

Advanced Practice Nursing in the Current Sociopolitical Environment

CHAPTER OBJECTIVES

After completing this chapter, the reader will be able to:

1 Estimate those qualities of the advanced practice nurse (APN) most valued by the public.

2 Articulate current barriers to advanced practice that may become more formidable obstacles as the health care delivery system evolves.

3 Formulate a strategy for facilitating the practice of APNs.

4 Critique the sociopolitical tactics used by organized nursing to promote the advanced practice nursing agenda.

What advanced practice nursing is and what it will become depend largely on the choices that the American people make about their health care. Ideally, public opinion is a major force in determining governmental policy and, consequently, the form and function of the health care delivery system. However, with the dramatic shift in public opinion from the urgent call for government-initiated health care reform in 1993 to the clarion call for balancing the budget, it is clear that the public vision for its health care system remains in a formative stage.

With the election of President Clinton in 1992, dramatic and immediate reforms in the American health care system were predicted. Commissions were formed, congressional committees were convened, and the electronic and paper media reported constantly on the public's demand for health care reform. Then in 1994, the American people handed control of the Congress to the Republicans and, indirectly, endorsed that party's "Contract with America." Waste in government was condemned, balancing the budget became a priority, and social welfare programs were scrutinized with an eye to cost containment. Health care ceased to be a concern, except to the extent that public entitlement programs represented a large target for budget cuts.

The sequence of events by which the sociopolitical environment forges public policies is familiar. These policies or their absence will shape the health care industry, including the role of APNs as participants in the industry. That being the case, we must move cautiously to assure a future for advanced practice nursing. An understanding of the preferences of American consumers, their attitudes toward health services, and an appreciation of the economic and political forces that continue to influence the form and function of our emerging health care delivery system can enable the nursing profession to decide how and if it fits into the emerging delivery system. The focus of this chapter is advanced practice, but the implications go well beyond this one segment of nursing.

THE AMERICAN PEOPLE AND THEIR HEALTH

A health care system is the product of political, sociological, economic, cultural, and demographic trends. Change in every aspect of our lives is the norm, but change has never been as quick and penetrating as in recent years. Given this reality, it is amazing that the health care industry has not undergone an even more radical transformation. It is impossible to identify all the factors that have conspired to maintain the status quo and equally challenging to define all the reasons for those that have compelled the recent changes. Political, sociological, and economic perspectives provide the backdrop for this chapter.

Demographics are presented here, albeit briefly, to illustrate current population trends, because any discussion of health care services must begin with an appreciation of the people they serve.

Our Aging and Changing Society

The U.S. population is aging rapidly, with the greatest future population growth predicted to be among the old-old, those over 85 years, who numbered 3 million in

1994 and are expected to increase to 19 million by 2050.[1] More than 22 percent of Americans over 85 years live in nursing and convalescent homes. On a given day, such facilities are caring for 1 out of every 20 Americans over 65 years.[2] Americans have become more urbanized over time, but there is some indication that this trend has slowed. More generous public assistance and agricultural subsidies, the decline of industry and manufacturing, and the negative image of many cities are said to have caused a disenchantment with migration to the cities.[3]

Our Economic Issues and Problems

The new millennium has represented a period of restabilization for the American family, which has shrunk to its smallest size ever, 2.62 people in 1992 and rebounded to 3.14 people in the 2000 census. Of 70.8 million children under 18 years, 69 percent live in households with two parents, and 27 percent live with one parent. Where children live with one parent, 38 percent of those parents are divorced, 35 percent were never married. In two-parent families, it continues to be common for both parents to work outside the home, and the single-parent family is usually headed by a working woman. The number of families headed by single mothers has increased 25 percent since 1990 to more than 7.5 million households. For most of the past decade, about a third of all babies were born to unmarried women, compared with 3.8 percent in 1940.[4]

The last 50 years have been an economic roller coaster in the United States, with more highs than lows. There have been several periods of unparalleled prosperity interspersed with periodic recession. Since 1995, there have been fewer poor people, and median family income has been higher. About one half of the nation's poor are either under 18 or over 65 years. There were about 12 million children (16.1 percent) living in poverty in the year 2000. By race and ethnicity, 30.6 percent were black children, 28 percent were Hispanic, 14.4 percent were Asian and Pacific Islanders, and 12.9 percent were white children. Poor children are twice as likely as non-poor children to suffer stunted growth or lead poisoning and to be kept back in school. Two of five, or 39.8 percent, of children in families headed by a single woman were poor in 2000, whereas only 8.2 percent of children in married families were poor.[5]

About 3.4 million elderly persons (10.2 percent) were below the poverty level in 2000. Another 2.2 million, or 6.7 percent, of the elderly were classified as "near-poor" (income between the poverty level and 125 percent of this level). One of every 12 (8.9 percent) elderly whites was poor in 2000, compared with 22.3 percent of elderly African Americans and 18.8 percent of elderly Hispanics. Older women had a higher poverty rate (12.2 percent) than older men (7.5 percent) in 2000.

Poverty is also associated with homelessness. At any one point in time, 600,000 people are homeless in this country, and 7 million people will be homeless at some point during their lifetime, with the fastest growing group being single mothers and children.[6] Where middle-class Americans once had a great deal of sympathy for these needy people, sympathy has turned into backlash, with financial pressures, crime, unemployment, and international hostilities all testing their patience.

Our Ethnic Makeup

The United States is also experiencing a dramatic shift in ethnic and racial diversity. Immigration is at an all-time high, rivaling the numbers of people who entered this country around the turn of the century. One notable difference is that, unlike the great European migrations of earlier times, the new immigrants are primarily of Hispanic and Asian origins. Between 1990 and 2000, about 33 million people were added to the U.S. population. Hispanics were the fastest-growing racial/ethnic group, adding almost 13 million people to the population (Table 2–1). Hispanic Americans tend to be relatively young, with one-third being younger than 18 years and one-half being younger than 26 years. For the first time in history, most immigrants speak one language—Spanish. Many of the newest immigrant groups tend to live in ethnic enclaves or neighborhoods, where they sometimes are immune to assimilation. This creates a population that is more a "mosaic" than a "melting

TABLE 2–1. Countries of Birth of the US Foreign–Born Population, 1970–2000 (resident population)				
10 leading countries by rank[1]	1970	1980	1990	2000
1.	Italy 1,009,000	Mexico 2,199,000	Mexico 4,298,000	Mexico 7,841,000
2.	Germany 833,000	Germany 849,000	China 921,000	China 1,391,000
3.	Canada 812,000	Canada 843,000	Philippines 913,000	Philippines 1,222,000
4.	Mexico 760,000	Italy 832,000	Canada 745,000	India 1,007,000
5.	United Kingdom 686,000	United Kingdom 669,000	Cuba 737,000	Cuba 952,000
6.	Poland 548,000	Cuba 608,000	Germany 712,000	Vietnam 863,000
7.	Soviet Union 463,000	Philippines 501,000	United Kingdom 640,000	El Salvador 765,000
8.	Cuba 439,000	Poland 418,000	Italy 581,000	Korea 701,000
9.	Ireland 251,000	Soviet Union 406,000	Korea 568,000	Dominican Republic 692,000
10.	Austria 214,000	Korea 290,000	Vietnam 543,000	Canada 678,000

In general, countries as reported at each census. Data are not totally comparable over time due to changes in boundaries for some countries. Great Britain excludes Ireland. United Kingdom includes Northern Ireland. China in 1990 includes Hong Kong and Taiwan. Source: Profile of the Foreign-Born Population in the United States: 2000, U.S. Census Bureau, 2001.

pot." These observations provide insights essential for the design and location of health care services and for the education and recruitment of providers.

Our Future Selves

To anticipate the future of our health care delivery system from socioeconomic and sociopolitical perspectives, it is important to remember that each generation is a product of its times. Today's "twenty-something" adults are the subject of much commentary. Many were raised by surrogates while their "baby-boomer" parents were caught up in the perceived need for dual incomes and the all-too-common eventuality of divorce and the "supermom" phenomenon. At least half of these Generation X'ers are college-educated and have expressed resentment at having to pay the price for the uncontrolled spending and environmental indiscretions of their parents. Also labeled "13ers" because they are the 13th generation in American history, most analysts predict that the 13ers have fought to regain what they claim they have lost. They have strengthened the family, looked suspiciously on public assistance, supported conservative public policy, and favored the needs of the young over the old, who, ironically, will be their boomer parents. They have supported volunteerism, long-term commitment as opposed to "adhocracy," and have a no-nonsense attitude about social welfare programs.[7]

The rising millennial generation, called Generation Y, is another factor in the intergenerational equation, bringing with it values and attitudes that are more aligned with the baby boomers than with Generation X. Where the Generation X'ers were disillusioned and pessimistic, Generation Y seems to embody the optimism and idealism that baby boomers themselves hold dear. Generation Y is of particular interest because, by 2020, this group will comprise 32 percent of the population. Generation Y is ethnically diverse, with minorities constituting 34 percent of its total. It is intensely computer-driven, skeptical of government and the media, although well aware of societal issues and problems.[8] Although it is still too early to characterize it properly, Generation Y seems to look to their parents and admire their accomplishments. Each generation has characteristics that will affect their employer/employee and client/provider relationships.

Our Health and Lifestyle

In the midst of all this turbulence, some things remain constant. Heart disease, cancer, stroke, chronic obstructive pulmonary disease, diabetes mellitus, pneumonia, and accidents continue to claim the most lives. Minority distinctions in morbidity and mortality rates continue to be notable in all areas and become an ethical issue. Although the statistics are confusing, some general statements can be made. All Americans have shared in life expectancy gains, although life expectancy for the black male population is 68.3 years, in contrast to 74.8 years for white males. In 2000, deaths from heart disease, stroke, and diabetes were 20 to 60 percent more prevalent in minority populations.[9] The largest discrepancies in health outcomes for minorities came in the areas of cardiovascular disease,

HIV/AIDS, cancer, and diabetes. Minorities were less likely to receive sophisticated treatments such as angioplasty, bypass surgery, kidney transplantation, or combination drug therapy for HIV disease.[10] Similar ethnicity-based differences are evident in maternal-child health statistics, such as the high incidence of low-birth-weight babies.

Factors contributing most significantly to death and disability in this country are associated with lifestyle: smoking, diet, lack of exercise and activity, substance use, stress, firearms, risky sexual behavior, vehicular accidents, and environmental pollution. Appreciating the wisdom of investing in health, the U.S. Department of Health and Human Services in 1991 initiated the Healthy People 2000 project.[11] The aim of the project was to increase the years of health and to decrease the disparities in health among the American people. The project involved periodic monitoring of quality-of-life indicators. By the middle of the decade, decreases were noted in cigarette smoking and alcohol-related vehicular accidents and deaths. Americans were noted to be consuming less fat and salt and were using more supplementary vitamins and minerals. At the same time, industrial accidents, homicides, and teenage pregnancies had increased, and Americans were more overweight than ever before. Deaths were down slightly from heart disease, cancer, and stroke, but deaths from chronic obstructive pulmonary disease and AIDS, which had become the leading cause of death for women between ages 25 and 45 years, had increased. By 1993, almost 11 percent of the population was disabled by chronic disease,[12] a direct result of the sophisticated medicine we practice and the lives we lead.

The new phase of Healthy People began in January 2000. With Healthy People 2010, the emphasis is health status and the nature of life—quality years, not just longevity.[37] A broadened perspective has come from the development of the science of prevention, improved data systems and surveillance activities, consumer demand for promotion of health, and a renewed appreciation of public health. Healthy People 2000 put a participatory and decentralized process into operation; Healthy People 2010 capitalizes on those dynamics. The agenda continues to be a variation on the theme: to increase quality and years of healthy life and to eliminate health disparities between America's people. Our unique American health care system, with its blend of private- and public-sector resources, its taste for specialization, and its state-of-the-art technology, is envied here and abroad. At the same time, consumers' expectations of freedom of choice in health care and our allegiance to states' rights have created serious problems with regard to access, cost, and quality. Roughly 41.2 million people, or 14.6 percent of U.S. residents, lacked health coverage for all of 2001, compared with 14.2 percent the previous year.[13] These observations have not escaped the notice of the public. Americans are highly critical of this country's health care system, and that criticism is creating an awakening of conscience.

The American public's attitude about health care and the health care industry is well documented. There is agreement that the health care system is flawed and needs to be fixed. Many consumers believe that the major problems are greed and waste. There is general suspicion of all traditional leaders, including doctors, lawyers, clergy, and politicians. More Americans feel powerless once they enter the health care delivery system. Because of the prevalence of employer-based health insurance, many Americans feel trapped in their jobs, often afraid to seek more challenging and satisfying work because of preexisting conditions that jeopardize insurance coverage if there is a gap in coverage and because of fear that an illness will threaten their financial security. The Medicare "final directives" requirement and the Congress's request that the U.S. Agency for Health Care Research and Quality (AHRQ) develop clinical guidelines are no coincidence. The result of both is pressure on the federal government to return to consumers some control over decisions influencing their life and death in the health care delivery system.

Despite apparent discontent with the system, most Americans seem to prefer inaction. For the most part, the voting public has access to health care, even if it is limited and of questionable value. President Clinton's Health Security Act of 1993 provided the vehicle for broad, sweeping change. After much debate, this legislation failed in September 1994. However, there are lessons to be learned from the experience. To begin, Americans are not willing to jeopardize one-sixth of the domestic economy. According to Joel[14]: "Incremental reform—proceeding with caution, building on successes, allowing one change to be assimilated before requiring that another be accommodated—may be the only option, however distasteful to some" (p. 7).

Furthermore, Americans also tend to guard tenaciously their freedom of choice in health care, even though most do not realize that their health care choices have already been limited. States Joel[15]:

"They want options, but they also want the safe haven associated with relinquishing some of those options" (p. 7).

Managed care plans have responded to this sensibility by offering the opportunity to "buy out at the point of service"—the assured access to health care services with the right to choose providers outside the plan's network for an additional out-of-pocket cost. The American passion for freedom of choice in health care is closely associated with a distaste for the heavy hand of government. The Clinton plan seemed to guarantee a bloated bureaucracy and federal mandates that would have preempted states' rights. The plan seemed to call for a mushrooming social-welfare state, funded by heavier taxation on the middle-class majority. The government's response was to propose reduced funding for entitlement programs, notably Medicare and Medicaid. An intuitive public recognized that the private sector would ultimately be required to subsidize the funding deficit created in these programs.

The 107th Congress, which ended January 2003, although responding to public sentiment, had cause for concern and displayed confusion. There were attempts to reinstate some of the deep financial cuts made to both Medicare and Medicaid, and block grants were created to fund health care insurance for near-poverty children. Both Democrats and Republicans voiced sympathy regarding the need to introduce some type of a drug program for the elderly, based on a sliding scale. Further talk of health care or cost containment was at least temporarily upstaged by international affairs and the threat to American security.

THE HEALTH CARE DELIVERY SYSTEM: ORIGINS OF CHANGE

Enactment of Titles 18 and 19 of the Social Security Act created Medicare and Medicaid almost 40 years ago. After a very few years of experience operating the programs, the federal government began to anticipate a serious financial crisis. Hoping to find some solution that would contain the rapidly accelerating cost of health care, the government supported a variety of demonstration projects. By 1982, this period of experimentation had produced the Medicare prospective payment system incorporating diagnostic-related groups (DRGs) as the "case-mix" model for payment to hospitals. Targeted at hospitals, the most costly offenders in the system, this model's use began an era of technical game-playing to reduce cost, while the issue of quality care became secondary.

Although the financial pressure on hospitals was first applied by Medicare, other public and private sector insurers quickly adopted the same or similar reimbursement strategies. The health care industry responded with a rapid migration to community-based services. The variety of clinical situations managed in physicians' offices and the supportive technology in those settings grew rapidly and probably was the first stage in restructuring. Many office-based practices began to resemble mini-hospitals, although largely unregulated. Concentrating their practices in these settings allowed physicians to circumvent the utilization constraints and oversight of hospitals.

The all-inclusive DRG rate for one hospitalization made internal monitoring of the prescriptive practices of physicians a necessity. Physicians who remained insensitive to the length-of-stay limitations and who ordered expensive diagnostic tests and therapeutic regimens, when less expensive options were available and appropriate, were considered a liability and pressured to rethink their practice patterns. Yet, physicians continued to be essential to hospital survival, given their virtually exclusive ability to admit patients.

Observing the escalating cost of Part B of Medicare, the Health Care Financing Administration began the search for algorithms (similar to DRGs) that would place reimbursement limits on the activities of providers. Common procedural technology codes and the resource-based relative value scale (RVS) were developed for this purpose. So far, these algorithms have been unsuccessful; they do not appear to control volume but only seem to fuel discontent in the medical community.

Still lagging in its ability to control cost, government looked to private-sector models, notably managed care. While fee-for-service (payment for each activity or service) and episode-of-illness (DRG) models continued, further economies were deemed unachievable. The long-standing success of managed care in the private sector piqued the interest of government and politicians. Although managed care comes in many structural forms and financial arrangements, the goal is to encourage (more often require) the least costly (and sometimes the least aggressive) diagnostic and treatment approaches. A transition to managed care was a major ingredient in the Clinton administration's Health Security Act.

DOMINANT TRENDS IN AMERICAN HEALTH CARE

The nature of health care delivery continues to change in response to economic and social forces at work in the community. The prescriptive practices of providers are being reshaped to ration limited resources. This comes as a harsh blow to an American public that reveres specialization and technology and that has come to expect aggressive clinical management. Attempts to introduce reason into clinical decision-making have been branded as rationing. Unwilling to accept any scrutiny of their practice, many physicians with a robust following, in turn, have rejected managed care arrangements. In contrast, physicians with fewer patients often see managed care as an opportunity, resulting in a stereotype of managed care as a second-class option.

Ignoring an initial (and often persistent) negativism, managed care plans continue to flourish as the only option that promises a more cost-efficient future. Medicare and Medicaid have contributed to a growing managed care market by offering incentives to relinquish most of traditional fee-for-service insurance in favor of managed care. Although not all managed care plans are capitated, this form appears to promise the best value. Whether quality will be sacrificed remains an unanswered question. By the end of 2001, 87.6 percent of Americans with private-sector health plans, 56.8 percent of Medicaid recipients, and 14.5 percent of those with Medicare were using managed care.[16]

Primary care is the backbone of most managed care programs regardless of their form. The literature contrasts older models of primary care with a hybrid that incorporates a broader view of health, patient, and community. Contemporary practice should include the intense use of information systems, active patient participation, appreciation of limited resources vis-à-vis the concept of value (the relationship of quality to cost), and an interdependence among a variety of providers. Providers will be as concerned with populations as with individuals, promising a renewed commitment to public health.[17]

The primary care provider (PCP) is the linchpin in many managed care systems, filling the subroles of direct care provider, first contact at point of entry into the system, and coordinator of continuing care. Referral to a specialist is the exception rather than the rule. The PCP is expected to shape the health behavior of patients. Often gaining access to patients through the management of minor acute illness and chronic conditions, the PCP seizes the opportunity to prevent disease and develops consumers' attitudes and skills for healthy living. Although this philosophy may be inconsistent with the medical model, it is totally consistent with the orientation of nursing.

In the managed care environment, multiple levels of care come together in a vertically integrated system. Primary and specialty, acute, subacute, long-term, ambulatory, home care, and rehabilitation services are combined into a seamless continuum of services. Patients may enter at any point and move with fluidity in and out of any component in the system. This essential characteristic creates the need for alliances and has prompted an industry merger-and-acquisition frenzy to build a full range of services.

THE ADVANCED PRACTICE NURSE
AND THE EMERGENT DELIVERY SYSTEM

The form of tomorrow's health care system is certain but not firmly set. All the actors have not yet been cast, and statements of philosophy and beliefs are often contradictory. The system is still maturing, and part of that process requires public education about, and socialization into, managed care. The value of health promotion, disease prevention, and self-sufficiency is gaining momentum. Consumers are demanding more control over their health care decisions, even if the freedom of choice in providers is limited to those with the financial ability to seek and purchase care outside of a provider's plan.

For many, access to the system will be through the PCP, who will continue to coordinate services and manage those problems that can be resolved at the PCP's level of competence. In the ideal situation, the PCP is not only a skilled clinical generalist but also a developer of people. Counseling and teaching must be the forte, and consumer satisfaction is a requisite outcome. Managed care plans strive to guarantee the consumer a sound relationship with a PCP, but these relationships can often be strained by the emphasis on appropriate, but not unlimited, care. Adequate enrollment in the plan is always a concern: a testy encounter with a PCP could result in the loss of a plan subscriber. The inability to retain subscribers and to develop self-reliance ultimately increases costs. APNs are well suited to the PCP role, given their clinical competence, their philosophy of health promotion, and their commitment to the goal of increasing the independence of their clients.

Although a window of opportunity still exists for APNs in managed care arrangements, it may close soon. Historically, physicians have been more interested in specialization and subspecialization than in generalist practice and health. This is not a criticism, but a simple observation based on the past. APNs, more specifically nurse practitioners (NPs), clinical nurse specialists (CNSs), and certified nurse midwives (CNMs), are the natural competitors with physicians for the PCP role. While only a handful of physicians select primary care practice, the government has been offering incentives for them to select this option. These incentives and the current physician surplus must be considered in any strategy to increase the presence and prominence of APNs in managed care. The policies of these plans should also be monitored carefully. For example, it is becoming common to allow female subscribers to have a relationship with two PCPs, one for women's health and a second for general health concerns. This trend has strategic implications and should cause the APN to reflect on the CNM role and the nature of our specialty preparations. Women's health becomes an attractive clinical choice, and CNMs are logical as PCPs.

The future of APNs is closely associated with the concept of value: the value of caring in its own right, the economic value of APNs as physician substitutes, and the inherent value of primary care and APNs' exceptional suitability for the PCP role. Given the urgency implicit in today's health care debate, APNs must be open to a broad range of interpretations of value. The efficacy of nurses in advanced practice has been proved many times over. APNs are safe and therapeutically effective.[18] Although nursing should continue to support research that verifies APNs' credibility and value, efforts should not end there. The research focus should shift to the value of caring in its own right and, more specifically, the value of nursing's performance in the PCP role.

Advance Practice Nursing: Beyond Primary Care

The acceptance of primary care as a valued component of an evolving health care system is significant but should not cause nursing to ignore traditional markets for nursing services. The increased complexity of patients at every level of care creates the need for APNs in a variety of direct care roles, including case management, patient advocacy, triage, and development of the practice of staff nurses. Neither is the APN role restricted to community practice; it has become established in acute and critical care, rehabilitation, and long-term care settings. Satisfaction and success in these roles require certain requisite skills. A "mental set" that integrates clinical and financial information is necessary. Information systems that justify the APN's salary must be established. If patient outcomes cannot be attributed directly to their practice, APNs must become masters of inference. Much of the frustration facing those who practice in the CNS role derives from the fact that it is a highly mediated role. Positive patient outcomes are frequently accomplished by other nurses but only because the CNS has developed the nurses' capacity for more sophisticated practice.

The advanced practice role often removes the "critical mass" advantage that staff nurses have found so useful in their campaign for a higher quality workplace. The educational and experiential background of the APN should result in peer status in a multidisciplinary environment. This background also assumes that the practitioner is above parochialism and ready to join in interdisciplinary practice. Seeing some role activities as equally fit for a number of providers is a relatively novel attitude for many nurses. Case management is a good example of a situation in which the physician, nurse, or social worker (among others) may be equally suited to the role.

BARRIERS TO ADVANCED PRACTICE NURSING

Internal Disputes

Advanced practice nurses include the CRNA, CNM, CNS, and NP. Today's APN requires the knowledge, skills, and supervised practice that comes only through graduate study in nursing (the master's or doctorate). In the past, these educational requirements were often satisfied through certificate programs, with no specific entry requirements other than licensure. Nurses from these certificate programs continue to practice today and should be commended for their leadership contributions to the advanced practice movement. All CNS and most NP educational programs award the master's degree. For the NP, preferential federal funding and certification requirements have hastened the movement toward graduate education.

Although the trend is toward the master's degree, four post-licensure certificate programs that require a baccalaureate degree but not in nursing still exist for the study of nurse midwifery.[19] Of the 89 accredited nurse anesthesia educational programs nationwide, all offer a master's degree, and some offer clinical nursing doctorate options for CRNAs.[20]

The CNS and NP roles are in a state of transition. These roles evolved almost simultaneously. The CNS established the credibility of clinical-nursing practice at the graduate level, and the NP legitimized the concept of practice autonomy in those border areas of practice shared with medicine. NPs were most commonly found in primary care, and CNSs in secondary and tertiary settings. Over time, these roles have started to overlap in response to consumer need.

An apparent merger of these roles was responsible for the consolidation of the American Nurses Association's (ANA) councils of NPs and CNSs into the Council of Nurses in Advanced Practice. This merger was significantly influenced by a 1990 curriculum study that found the education for these roles to be more alike than different.[21] Many APNs also saw the roles as interchangeable and claimed that maintaining the distinction was an impediment to career mobility. Whether those who clamored for change were a representative sample of APNs is subject to challenge. Further, the rigor with which the survey's validity and conclusions were scrutinized is subject to debate. I am not implying that nursing has taken the wrong route, but I am suggesting that milestone events often go unrecognized.

The merger of the CNS and NP roles originated with the legislative and regulatory strategy of the ANA. In the 1980s, the ANA began to link the NP and CNS in public policy language. Legislators already understood the NP role and its benefit to the public. This appreciation was based largely on the NP's ability to substitute for the physician, offering the same services at a lower cost. Linking the less commonly understood CNS with the NP in public policy hastened progress toward recognition of both groups. In the early 1990s, the term "advanced practice nurse" was chosen to additionally include the CRNA and CNM. The purpose of this language was political and directed largely toward the reimbursement agenda.

While there is agreement that both the CNS and NP are advanced practitioners, there is less support for the use of the single title of APN. Debate continues over the body of knowledge and skills common to both. Many of the most prestigious university schools of nursing have ignored these internal debates and have begun to blur the distinctions between these two roles. Meanwhile, APNs in one category or another continue to question whether role crossover is possible without additional education. The disparity in the views of educators and practicing APNs surfaces, one basing action on logic (as they see it) and the other on experience (as they live it). Meanwhile, the good job market for NPs has created a demand for post-master's and second-master's-degree programs for the CNS preparing for NP practice. Some of these changes can be traced to state laws that require graduate education to specify NP preparation. In this case, role crossover is no longer left to the discretion of the profession or the professional. These observations tend to highlight the critical need for advisory relationships between education and practice and a combined effort to control the sometimes illogical behavior of government agencies.

Such internal disputes are a part of the politics of nursing. NPs question the ability of CNSs to diagnose and treat the common illnesses that are a major part of generalist practice. CNSs suspect that NPs are socialized into the medical model and therefore are less able to negotiate and manipulate systems of care on behalf of their patients or to develop the clinical sophistication of the nursing staff. No such disputes have arisen around CRNA or CNM practice; each of these groups seems to be in control of its clinical area.

Such differences of opinion have seriously hampered the ability of APNs to move into the vanguard of health care. Foresight is often rare. While nursing debates the details, it ignores the fact that the merger of NP and CNS roles is becoming more useful as society is confronting growing numbers of the chronically ill who need primary care. The best PCP for these situations may be the CNS because the patient also needs the sophistication of a specialist. NPs are valuable in acute, critical, long-term, ambulatory, and home care for their abilities in health assessment and clinical management. The market for NPs in acute care has increased as graduate medical education funding has decreased. Rather than responding with arrogance or infighting regarding the assumption of some medical responsibilities, nursing should seize the opportunity to bring advanced practice nursing to new populations and to establish further autonomy in border areas of practice.

External Obstacles

Most external obstacles to advanced practice have, in one way or another, been associated with public policy. Although doors open slowly, nurses have achieved good legislative and regulatory gains. The goal has been for the APN to secure direct access to the public. In our fragmented, litigious, and medicalized system, this requires direct reimbursement and presence on managed care panels of providers, prescriptive authority, clinical privileges, adequate professional liability insurance, and nursing practice acts and credentialing systems that attest to our competency. Anticipating the future, providers who bring these indicators of autonomy with them will assume roles of clinical prominence in managed care. Many of our efforts have been frustrated by the resistance of other health professionals, particularly organized medicine, to expanding the scope of practice of the APN.

Reimbursement

Achieving reimbursement for advanced practice nursing services has been a torturous and costly agenda. Progress has been slow but steady. All categories of APNs are reimbursable in the Federal Employee's Health Benefits Program (FEHB). Similar provisions are included in TRICARE/CHAMPUS. TRICARE is the government's "managed care" program for active and retired members of the military. CHAMPUS is the acronym for the Civilian Health and Medical Program for the Uniformed Services. It shares the costs of inpatient and outpatient medical care from civilian hospitals and doctors when care is not available through a military hospital or clinic. NPs, psychiatric CNSs, CNMs, and CRNAs are authorized to provide TRICARE/CHAMPUS services and are directly reimbursed.[22]

There is a federal mandate for the reimbursement of pediatric and family NPs and CNMs through Medicaid (at 70 to 100 percent of the physician rate), but state discretion prevails for other NPs, CRNAs, and CNSs. Mandatory in terms of federal legislation means that a provider must be reimbursed through Medicaid (or other federal programs as specified) for services within the provider's scope of practice as recognized within that state. None of the federal reimbursement laws supersede the states' responsibility for health and safety.

Medicare has been the most resistant program but was opened to direct reimbursement of APNs with the provisions of the Balanced Budget Act of 1997, although at only 85 percent of the fee received by physicians. Before the Balanced Budget Act, NPs and CNSs were limited to serving Medicare recipients in rural and medically underserved areas. This restriction has been removed. Nursing homes had been able to receive Medicare reimbursement for NPs who provided periodic medical monitoring and recertification services, but the NP could not receive any fee directly. CNMs and CRNAs were already recognized in Medicare. A noteworthy gain has been the federal Department of Transportation's recognition that NPs and CNSs may perform and be reimbursed for the physical examination needed to qualify for a commercial driver's license.

On March 9, 2000, HCFA announced that removal of the federal requirement that CRNAs must be supervised by physicians when administering anesthesia to Medicare patients was forthcoming. Delays continued until July 5, 2001, when Centers for Medicare and Medicaid Services (CMS), formerly HCFA, published a proposed rule that would maintain the existing supervision requirement but allow a state's governor the right to petition CMS requesting exemption from this requirement once (s)he had: consulted with the state's boards of medicine and nursing, determined that opting out of the requirement was consistent with state law, and decided that it was in the best interests of the state's citizens. By January 2004, 12 states had opted out of the federal physician supervision requirement.[23] In the rule comments, the CMS directed the Agency for Healthcare Research and Quality (AHRQ) to conduct a study addressing anesthesia outcomes in those states that selected to "opt out" of the CRNA supervision requirement compared with those states that did not.[24]

In many states you will find the NP preferentially recognized but not the CNS. Of course, this circumstance should not be treated lightly, but it can be best understood if analyzed in its sociopolitical context. Primary care is assured prominence in the emergent delivery system, and NPs have established themselves in that area. CNSs have had less visibility and are seen by many as an add-on cost as opposed to a more cost-efficient option. The laws or statutes of 40 states include CNSs within the APN category, but 7 of those only recognize the CNS in psychiatric–mental health nursing.[25]

Indemnity and commercial insurance is governed by state laws, and these laws recognize advanced practice nursing in varying amounts. The picture is confusing, however, and changes from day to day. APNs report reimbursement in 37 states,[26] and many APNs report reimbursement "incident to" the practice of a physician by both federal and state programs, as well as private-sector plans. In this situation, the nurse is paid a fee equal to what a physician would have received for the same services. If the APN bills independently, the fee is anywhere from 65 to 85 percent of the physician's reimbursement amount. This continues to be a controversial issue.

Reimbursement is honeycombed with social bias and self-serving behavior. A particularly blatant example can be seen in the work of the Physician's Payment Review Commission (PPRC). Charged with proposing a rate structure for Part B of Medicare, the PPRC based its fee-setting techniques on the service to the patient, as opposed to the identity of the provider. The commission justified this move by alleging the need to increase the attractiveness of primary care for physicians by reducing the financial differential between generalists and specialists. However, when it came time to apply the same standard to nonphysician providers, the PPRC recanted and proposed that the extent of the provider's education should be built into the reimbursement formula for this group.

There has been a recent surge in the NP job market associated with growth in community-based services and primary care. The fact that NPs are very comfortable in the employee role and excel in their ability to work within systems has not been lost on employers. Furthermore, NPs are seen as lower-cost physician substitutes. In contrast, the CNS is often undervalued, even by nurses themselves, and is considered expendable when money gets tight in health care institutions. The fact that CNSs are not a luxury but a necessity is theirs to prove. It is painful but true that the activities sanctioned by nursing licenses traditionally have not been reimbursable, but priorities are changing as the medical model becomes less dominant. Managed care could be the catalyst for this metamorphosis. Disease prevention, health promotion, and self-care promise more value than earlier paradigms. Reimbursement may soon become a nonissue, with the rapid domination by managed care. APNs must be included within managed care networks and as members of approved provider panels. State prohibitions that limit the ownership of medical offices to physicians and other select providers must be challenged.

Prescriptive Authority

Almost every American entering the health care system receives a prescription for drug therapy. Historically, the right to prescribe medications has been the exclusive domain of the physician. Even as NPs become more established, many continue to manage illness, including the prescription of medication, in a joint practice or a collaborative relationship (sometimes a euphemism for supervision) with a physician. The reasoning is warped. NPs are proposed as a physician substitute because they represent a better value at lower cost but with equal or better outcomes. This rationale loses its credibility when medical management cannot proceed without physicians' approval. Physicians who accept the responsibility for an APN's practice are sometimes confronted with an increase in their liability-insurance premiums. Naturally, the cost is passed on to the consumer. If APNs are to be PCPs, they must have full prescriptive authority and the right to prescribe medications (including controlled substances) on their own signature.

The authority to prescribe independent of any physician involvement exists for one or more categories of APNs in 13 states (the District of Columbia is treated as a state for this analysis); 38 others maintain the caveat of physician oversight of some type. No state totally rejects prescriptive authority.[27] Prescriptive authority for nurses may be controlled in a variety of ways. The range of drugs permitted to be prescribed by nurses is sometimes limited to a formulary developed jointly by state boards of nursing, medicine, and/or pharmacy. Prescriptive authority may be limited to drugs common to a specialty area. The variety of constraints is creative and often obviously self-serving. It appears that the medical community is bound and determined to maintain as much control as possible over access to drug therapy.

There are almost 150,000 nurses who are likely candidates to move into the PCP role and, consequently, pursue prescriptive authority. While physicians direct their energy and money toward foiling the attempts of APNs to expand their practice into the once-exclusive domain of medicine, other non-nursing professional groups are making inroads that could ultimately establish precedent. Psychologists and pharmacists argue that they are qualified to prescribe. Many states now allow pharmacists some variety of prescriptive ability. PAs are authorized to prescribe in 47 states.[28] As each occupational group evolves, it will expand its scope of practice and seek more rights and responsibilities.

With characteristic patience and tenacity, nursing has made progress related to prescriptive authority by accepting physician oversight. Strategically, this can be a first step toward autonomy. In 1990, New Hampshire nurses were successful in "carving out" the requirement for physician supervision from their prescriptive authority statute. This scenario, which could be repeated often in the future, is contingent on electing legislative representatives sympathetic to nursing, thus creating a public demand for nurses to offer these services. The best source of detail on state-to-state variations in prescriptive authority can be found each year in the January issue of *The Nurse Practitioner*.

In the interim, prescriptive authority contingent on oversight can be workable. Joint practice arrangements between nurses and physicians could be the expected norm in primary care centers. The inherent value of this arrangement may be appealing, particularly where these centers are owned, operated by, or contracted with managed care plans. Community nursing centers usually employ a medical director, who could be relied on to fill the oversight requirement until the time when such oversight is unnecessary.

Professional Staff Privileges

Criteria for the approval and accreditation of health care programs and facilities have been fairly consistent in adopting an expanded definition of the term "professional staff." This expanded definition awards professional staff privileges to a variety of providers. However, health care systems often impose more specific restrictions for the expressed purpose of denying privileges to emerging or nontraditional providers, such as APNs, podiatrists, chiropractors, and dentists. According to Kelly and Joel[29]: "It remains to be tested whether the withholding of privileges is an act of discrimination or restraint of trade" (p. 326).

Because the survival of any health care organization will depend on its ability to negotiate managed care contracts, nursing must now be willing and able to educate managed care plan administrators to the value of APNs as full-fledged professionals.

Professional staff privileges often recognize the right to admit, discharge, treat, visit, or consult on the clinical management of patients. In effect, withholding privileges denies patient access to excluded providers once they are admitted to a particular system. The nursing staff organization has been proposed by some as the counterpart of the medical staff organization (currently renamed the professional staff organization). However, such arrangements could be confused with the organized nursing staff who come together for purposes of negotiating conditions of employment (with or without a formal collective bargaining agreement). This is an unacceptable solution for many reasons. One reason is parity and a need for appropriate recognition within a multidisciplinary environment. A second concern is a technicality of labor law. An organized effort such as this could be misconstrued and later create a challenge to the right of nurses to choose a collective bargaining agent and/or unionize.

Several beginning prototypes can provide the APN some guidance. APN hospital privileges are becoming more common. Access to these privileges does not include all APNs but is usually limited to a specific category (NP, CNS, CRNA, or CNM). In some situations, privileges are associated with joint or collaborative practice with a physician. Specialty-dependent limitations remain (e.g., psychiatric–mental health CNS, gerontological nurse practitioner, and so forth). Other dynamics and dilemmas will be contingent on whether the APN with privileges is an employee or an independent contractor. Physicians are empowered by their ability to admit patients to a system, thereby contributing to its financial stability. To the extent that an APN is viewed by an institution as a "mere employee," the power of the admitting privileges could be minimized. This issue is more important as APNs become prominent in rural and medically underserved areas.

CNMs are a contrasting story of success. Just 25 years ago, few states permitted nurse midwives to practice. Between 1975 and 1991, the number of hospital births attended by CNMs increased sevenfold. CNMs' mandatory access to Medicaid recipients ensures practice viability in every state and territory. The preferred practice setting for CNMs has become the hospital, perhaps due to the legal requirement to maintain a collaborative arrangement with an obstetrician.

CRNAs have the legal authority to practice anesthesia without anesthesiologist supervision in all 50 states, typically in every setting where anesthesia is administered. The most restrictive proposals concerning CRNA practice in recent years have tended to occur in the context of laws, rules, or guidelines or position statements regarding physician office practice, but many of the proposed restrictions have been rejected.[30] These observations also support the prevalence of hospital practice privileges among both CNMs and CRNAs.

Assuring Competency

The issue of assuring competency has surfaced with a vengeance as APNs and, more specifically, NPs and CNSs have become more aggressive in the pursuit of reimbursement and prescriptive authority. Leaders in medicine and nursing caution that specialty practice should be regulated internally by the profession as opposed to externally by the government. This opinion is based on the clinical complexity of specialization and the fact that the science advances through research conducted in specialty areas. For the discipline to advance, the specialty edge must remain unencumbered by public policy and the inevitable bureaucracy that it attracts.

For nursing, it is already too late to hold firm to this standard of autonomy for the practice. Forty-nine states currently address advanced practice in public policy. For the most part, state boards of nursing hold the authority, and 31 of them currently require a nationally recognized certification in the specialty.[31] Sometimes additional education in pharmacology is expected where the prescription of medications is a sanctioned activity. By this arrangement, many state boards of nursing have deferred to the profession's right to recognize its specialists through certification and to develop and promulgate the standards of practice on which certification is based. This position had been actively questioned. Critics saw the standards as vague and called for precise competency statements on which to build certification. They demanded examinations that were rigorous and procedures that were reliable. At its annual meeting in summer 1995, the National Council of State Boards of Nursing (NCSBN), an association of state and territorial boards of nursing, postponed action on a motion to move forward on a certification program for NPs and CNSs under the aegis of the state boards themselves.

The regulatory process for CNMs and CRNAs seems to have attracted less scrutiny. This could be in part due to the fact that the CNM is commonly recognized in the law through amendment to the Medical Practice Act, which legally requires CNMs and CRNAs to practice collaboratively with a physician. The CRNA has a long history of credibility but is currently defending against medicine's attempts to require anesthesiologist supervision of their practice. Some attempts at regulatory change have proposed a one-on-one supervisory relationship between the CRNA and the anesthesiologist. Rather than inserting this oversight requirement in the CRNA licensing law, an alternate tactic has been to insert language in the regulations for facility licensing. Obviously, this degree of dependency would make the use of CRNAs inefficient and, at the very least, would result in increased cost to the consumer and, more ominously, loss of anesthesia practice to nurses.

Motivated primarily by a sense of public stewardship and to some extent by the aggressive position of the NCSBN, both the American Association of Colleges of Nursing (AACN)[32] and the National Organization of Nurse Practitioner Faculties (NONPF)[33] have developed program standards for NP and advanced practice nursing education that give direction for competency statements. Building on this work, in October 2002 the AACN and NONPF completed work on nurse practitioner primary care competencies in the specialty areas of adult, family, gerontological, pediatric, and women's health. These competencies were identified by a national panel including organizations that represent the five NP specialties as well as by credentialing and certifying agencies. A validation panel composed of leaders from nursing practice, education, and accreditation organizations confirmed the relevance of the national panel's work.[34] In this same year, Core Competencies for Basic Nurse Midwifery Practice were authored by the ACNM, and revised standards of practice were completed by the AANA. Additionally, in 2001, NONPF and AACN moved forward vigorously with the reconvening of the National Task Force on Quality Nurse Practitioner Education (NTFC) and the revision of the Criteria for Evaluation of

Nurse Practitioner Education.[35] This landmark work was accomplished collaboratively with certification, accreditation, and education organizations.

The logic follows that nursing educational accreditation boards should incorporate these competencies in their program evaluation, and/or certification boards should design their examinations based on these competencies. This is not merely an option but a necessary step for the profession to maintain any control over advanced practice. Application of the same standard by both the accrediting and the certifying agencies would provide the best assurances for the consumer. The fact that these competency statements originated with practitioners would show a united front and enhance credibility.

Based on input from a broad constituency, the Board of Commissioners of the Commission on Collegiate Nursing Education (CCNE)—a nationally recognized accrediting body for baccalaureate and higher degree nursing education—acted in October 2003 to amend its accreditation standards. In doing so, effective January 1, 2005, all NP programs that are affiliated with CCNE will be required to meet the NTFC.

Medicine has assured the credibility of its specialists (advanced practitioners) by the creation of an oversight board, the American Board of Medical Specialties (ABMS). The ABMS recognizes specialty boards that conform to specific standards defined by their specialties, the process and testing instruments used to ensure the competency of their diplomates, and the quality of their residencies, among other program aspects. In 1992, nursing established the American Board of Nursing Specialties (ABNS) for the purpose of assuming a similar leadership role in certification. However, the ABNS has not become prominent. Given the threat of increased government oversight, the ABNS could be a vital link between internal and external regulation of the specialties.

Professional Liability Insurance

A liability insurance crisis occurred in 1985 when CNMs sustained an increase in their premiums so great that it could not be absorbed by their incomes. CNMs were assumed to represent a liability risk equal to obstetricians, who have the highest claims experience in the medical field. Nurse midwives, with their long-standing mandatory relationship with physicians to ensure backup in the event of intrapartum complications, have been tainted by physicians' malpractice experience. The ANA, negotiating on behalf of CNMs, secured temporary and affordable coverage through the ANA carrier until a more permanent solution was possible. That solution was a self-insured arrangement involving the ACNM and a consortium of insurance companies. CRNAs, NPs, and CNSs have not had similar experiences. Their claims experience is low, and coverage is available at reasonable rates, although they are beginning to experience similar increases in premium rates.

The National Practitioners Data Bank (NPDB) provides some hard evidence about the claims experience of APNs. Almost two-thirds of the malpractice payments against nurses were made on behalf of RNs, not APNs. Of the 1,127 payments reported for APNs for the period September 1990 to December 2000, CRNAs were the most frequently sued, accounting for 65 percent of the reported payments. CNM and NP payments were 22 percent and 13 percent of the total, respectively.

For calendar year 2000 only, the number of payments for all nurses was 364, with a mean value per claim of $269,090. The median payment reported for all nurses in 2000 was $82,700. Even adjusted for inflation, the mean and median payments for claims for nurse malpractice have not risen markedly.[36]

Many skeptics choose to ignore the safe, effective, and satisfying service provided by APNs. Instead of interpreting their low claims experience as an indication of quality, critics prefer to agree that a litigant will target providers with assets ("deep pockets") in hope of greater financial recovery. Regardless of the past, we are entering an era of tort reform in which financial recovery may be based on a new standard. The personal danger that litigation holds for the provider will also be different in a managed care environment where many providers are employees.

SUMMARY

To date, NPs have achieved the greatest autonomy working with underserved populations. CRNAs are the sole anesthesia providers in the majority of rural hospitals but have been less dominant in areas where physicians' presence is high. CNSs are the unsung heroes, best known for their work with the seriously ill. Today, it is the middle-class majority (many, from urban areas, are relatively healthy and financially secure) whose acceptance and demand for APNs could establish their credibility. The difficulty is that these potential clients do not know about APNs and advanced practice nursing. The exception may be the CNM, whose popularity has grown with Americans of moderate and substantial means. Because midwifery services are not always reimbursable, those who can pay out of pocket represent a large share of midwifery clients. In resisting challenges to midwifery practice and the operation of birthing centers, CNMs have succeeded in mobilizing the support of the influential middle and upper classes on their behalf.

Many APNs who wish to serve the middle-class market have joined physicians in their practices as employees. These opportunities are readily available but must be initiated and developed. Often, positions appear to be cast in the medical model, and therefore, many APNs may be reluctant to secure them. The decision for the APN remains whether to walk away from a challenge or to work for change from within.

In presenting themselves to the middle class, the clinical competency of APNs must be beyond question. Resentment over the need to be better, brighter, and more giving holds little weight. There is no one so condemning as the advocate for advanced practice nursing who provides APNs with access to patients and then receives reports of inept clinical management. The most painful incidents occur when APNs are displaced in favor of physicians, unfortunately a frequent occurrence with today's physician surplus. APNs often do not document the value they represent, nor do they routinely mobilize patients or the community in communicating their value.

Nurse-managed centers are an ideal setting in which to prove and promote APN excellence. These centers are managed and staffed by nurses. Nurse-managed centers may be free-standing, entrepreneurial enterprises or affiliated with a college of nursing or a health care institution. They are strong candidates for partnerships with managed-care networks. A fuller discussion of nurse-managed centers can be found in *Dimensions of Professional Nursing.*[38]

Educated risk-taking, a commitment to excellence, and the courage of one's convictions must become watchwords as APNs shape a future that is good for nursing and good for the American public.

SUGGESTED EXERCISES

1 Propose a strategic plan to ensure the competency of APNs to the public. Include the roles of the profession and the government.

2 Develop a career plan for an APN in a geographic area that has never experienced an advanced nursing practice.

3 Identify the reimbursement and prescriptive authority rights of APNs in your state. What should be the next stage in policy development to increase APNs' access to the public?

4 Anticipate the opportunities for advanced practice nursing in the emerging health care delivery system and the areas of resistance that APNs will encounter.

5 Propose a plan to create an American middle-class following for APNs.

REFERENCES

1. Census 2000. Retrieved June 14, 2002, from http://www.usatoday.com/graphics/census2000/United States/state.htm
2. Marshall RT: Nursing Home Issues. Retrieved June 1, 2002, from http://www.elderweb.com
3. Joel, LA: Kelly's Dimensions of Professional Nursing. McGraw-Hill, New York, 2003.
4. Census 2000, ibid.
5. Children's Defense Fund. Retrieved June 17, 2002, from http://www.childrensdefense.org
6. Homelessness: Programs and the People They Serve. Retrieved June 17, 2002, from http://www.huduser.org/publications/homeless/homelessness/content.html
7. Quinn, JB: The Luck of the Xers. Newsweek, p. 66, June 1994.
8. Northwestern University. Faces of the New Millennium. Retrieved May 28, 2002, from http://pub-web.acns.nwu.edu/
9. National Center for Health Statistics. Retrieved August 15, 2000, from http://www.cdc.gov/nchs/about/otheract/hp2000/2000indicators.htm
10. Connolly C: US minorities get lower quality health care: Moral implications of widespread pattern noted. Washington Post, March 21, 2002.
11. Institute of Medicine, National Academy of Science. Healthy People 2000: Citizens Chart the Course. National Academy Press, Washington, DC, 1990.
12. McGinnis, JM, and Lee, PR: Healthy People 2000 at mid-decade. JAMA 273:1123, 1995.
13. After decline, the number of uninsured rose in 2001. The New York Times. September 30, 2002, A21.
14. Joel, LA: Health care reform: Getting it right this time. Am J Nurs 95:7, 1995.
15. Ibid.
16. Department of Health and Human Services. Retrieved July 30, 2002, from http://www.medicarehmo.com
17. Geoppinger J: Renaissance of primary care: An opportunity for nursing. In Hickey, JV, et al (eds): Advanced Practice Nursing. Lippincott, Philadelphia, 1996, p 70.
18. Brown, S, and Grimes, D: Meta-Analysis of Process of Care: Clinical Outcomes and Cost-Effectiveness of Nurses in Primary Care Roles: Nurse Practitioners and Nurse Midwives. American Nurses Association, Kansas City, 1992.
19. Personal communication, Nancy Dickerson, ACNM, June 11, 2003.
20. Personal communication, Rita Rupp, AANA, July 20, 2002.

21. Forbes, KE, et al: Clinical nurse specialist and nurse practitioner core curricula survey results. Nurse Pract 15:43, 1990.
22. Mittelstadt, P: Federal reimbursement of advanced practice nurses' services empowers the profession. Nurse Pract 18:43, 1993
23. American Association of Nurse Anesthetists. Retrieved April 7, 2004, from http://www.aana.com/capcorner
24. Bruton-Maree, N, and Rupp, R: Federal healthcare policy: How AANA advocates for the profession. In Foster, SD, and Faut-Callahan, M (eds): A Professional Study and Resource Guide for the CRNA. AANA Publishing, Park Ridge, IL, 2001, pp 357–379.
25. Pearson, LJ: Annual update of how each state stands on legislative issues affecting advanced nursing practice. Nurs Pract 27:1, 2002.
26. Ibid.
27. Pearson, LJ: Sixteenth annual legislative update: How each state stands on legislative issues affecting advanced nursing practice. Nurs Pract 29:1, 2004.
28. Personal communiction, Liz Roe, AAPA, June 13, 2003.
29. Kelly, L, and Joel, L: Dimensions of Professional Nursing, 8th ed. McGraw-Hill, New York,1999.
30. Personal communication, Mitch Tobin, AANA, June 9, 2003.
31. American Nurses Association. Retrieved October 1, 2002, from http://nursingworld.org/gova/charts
32. American Association of Colleges of Nursing: The Essentials of Master's Education for Advanced Practice Nursing. American Association of Colleges of Nursing, Washington, DC, October 1996.
33. National Organization of Nurse Practitioner Faculty. Advanced Nursing Practice: Curriculum Guidelines and Program Standards for Nurse Practitioner Education. National Organization of Nurse Practitioner Faculty, Washington, DC, 1995.
34. National Organization of Nurse Practitioner Faculties & American Association of Colleges of Nursing. Nurse Practitioner Primary Care Competencies in Specialty Areas: Adult, Family, Gerontological, Pediatric, and Women's Health. U.S Department of Health and Human Services, Health Resources and Services Administration, Bureau of Health Professions, Division of Nursing, Rockville, MD. April 2002.
35. National Task Force on Quality Nurse Practitioner Education. (2002). Criteria for Evaluation of Nurse Practitioner Programs, 2nd ed. Washington, DC: Author.
36. National Practitioner Data Bank. (2001). Fact Sheets. Washington, DC Retrieved August 3, 2002, from http://www.npdb-hipdb.com
37. Office of Disease Prevention and Health Promotion, U. S. Department of Health and Human Services: Healthy People. Retrieved April 2004, from www.healthypeople.gov
38. Joel, L. Kelly's Dimension's of Professional Nursing, 9th ed. NewYork: McGraw-Hill, 2003, pp 146–148

ANNOTATED BIBLIOGRAPHY

American Nurses Association. Nursing's Agenda for Health Care Reform. American Nurses Association, Washington, DC, 1991.

This agenda has been endorsed by over 80 nursing and allied health associations and remains the public policy agenda of the profession.

Dochterman, J, and Grace, HK (eds). Current Issues in Nursing, 6th ed. Mosby, St Louis, 2001.

A variety of papers on current issues organized in sections that are introduced by a debate relevant to the particular topic area.

Harrington, C, and Estes, CL (eds). Health Policy and Nursing. Jones and Bartlett, Boston, 1997.

Good chapters on finance, the delivery system, outcomes of care, the nurse labor market, and implications for nursing in every issue area.

Howe, N, and Strauss, B. The 13th Generation: Abort, Retry, Ignore, Fail? Vintage Books, New York, 1993.

Presentation of the unique characteristics, history, and predicted future of today's 20-something adults.

Joel, L. Kelly's Dimension's of Professional Nursing, 9th ed. NewYork: McGraw-Hill, 2003.

A compendium of the nonclinical aspects of nursing. It includes a history of the APN and a discussion of contemporary issues.

Kovner, A, and Jonas, S. (eds). Health Care Delivery in the United States. New York: Springer, 1999.

An overview of the U.S. delivery system, its providers, and settings for care, funding, historical development, and emergent trends.

Lee, P, and Estes, CL (eds). The Nation's Health, 6th ed. Boston: Jones and Bartlett, 2001.

Recent statistics and chapters that allow basic understanding of the delivery system and its issues.

Mason, DJ, et al (eds). Policy and Politics for Nurses, 4th ed. WB Saunders, Philadelphia, 2002.

Chapters on policy and politics in a broad range of situations, including the politics of nongovernmental organizations and workplace policies.

Shea,C, et al. Advanced Practice Nursing in Psychiatric and Mental Health Care. St. Louis: CV Mosby, 1999.

A state-of-the-art analysis of the transforming mental health care environment, issues in advanced clinical practice, and developments in professional scholarship within psychiatric nursing. These trends and issues are easily bridged to other specialty areas.

Shi, L, and Singh, D. Delivering Health Care in America: A Systems Approach. Aspen, Gaithersburg, MD, 2001.

The authors present the conceptual basis for the U.S. health care delivery system, its historical origins, the health care structures, and a translation of these structures into health services, being mindful of their impact on cost and quality.

Stanfield, P, and Hui, Y. Introduction to the Health Professions, 4th ed. Boston: Jones and Bartlett, 2002.

A review of contemporary health professions, their history, issues, and futures.

Sultz, H, and Young, K. Health Care USA. Aspen, Gaithersburg, MD, 2001.

An overview of significant changes that have occurred in health care over recent years.

CHAPTER 3

The American Health Care System: Implications for Advanced Practice Nursing

Mary Knudtson, MSN, NP

Mary Knudtson, MSN, NP, is Professor of Family Medicine at the University of California, Irvine. Ms Knudtson is prepared as both a family and a pediatric nurse practitioner. Ms Knudtson has completed a Robert Wood Johnson Exectutive Nurse Fellowship and a Department of Health and Human Services Primary Health Care Policy Fellowship. Ms Knudtson has practiced in a variety of settings as an advanced practice nurse for over 14 years. Currently, she is involved in clinical practice in primary care and is the Director of the Family Nurse Practitioner program at the University of California, Irvine. She is a past president of the American College of Nurse Practitioners and is currently serving as a practice consultant, answering member questions on practice issues.

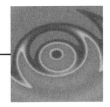

The American Health Care System: Implications for Advanced Practice Nursing

CHAPTER OBJECTIVES

After completing this chapter, the reader will be able to:

1 Analyze the influence of economics on the restructuring of the health care delivery system in the United States.

2 Compare and contrast various challenges facing health care, both publicly and privately financed.

3 Synthesize information regarding cost-containment efforts as they affect advanced practice nursing.

4 Compare and contrast various models proposed for the delivery and financing of health care.

5 Debate the advantages and disadvantages of different reimbursement strategies as they might apply to the advanced practice nurse (APN) in a managed care environment.

6 Delineate strategies that can be used by APNs to gain entry into health care markets.

In Dr. Pauline Komnenich's ethnographic retrospective of the evolution of advanced practice nursing (see Chapter 1), several themes echo from the past with a message to today's APNs:

- Times of change create opportunities for APNs to define and shape themselves.

- Forces outside the profession of nursing—often economic—have been the stimulus for this development.

- At the same time, the professional establishment—both in nursing and medicine—have at times erected barriers to independent advanced nursing practice.

A similar time of change exists for APNs in today's health care revolution. To position themselves as leaders in the reform movement, APNs must become sensitive to the various forces that have stimulated the movement toward health care restructuring. Health care reform is not only about who is going to pay for coverage—businesses, individuals, and families as taxpayers—but also about who is going to manage the plan—private companies, the government, and/or consumers themselves. To compete, APNs must better understand factors as they relate to payment and reimbursement mechanisms and the aggregate resources necessary for this new order.

This chapter provides a brief history of the evolution of health care financing and describes the current state of the American health care system. Strategies that can be used by APNs to gain entry into health care markets will be discussed.

THE AMERICAN HEALTH CARE SYSTEM

It is likely that the 1990s will be remembered as the decade in which the nation acknowledged, although grudgingly, that the demand for medical services is apparently unlimited, but that the capacity of the society to pay for such services is not.[2]

Excess and Deprivation

The 1990s was characterized as a paradox of excess and deprivation. Excess and deprivation refers to the observation that people with comprehensive health insurance may receive unnecessary and inappropriate health services while those without insurance, or with inadequate insurance, may be deprived of needed care.[2] Some patients receive too little care because they are uninsured or inadequately insured. Some patients receive too little care because they have Medicaid or Medicare coverage, which some health care providers do not accept.

The United States spent $1.4 trillion on health care in 2001, yet 41.2 million Americans lacked basic health coverage.[3] For most of the past 16 years, the number of people without health insurance has been on the rise. Many are victims of the changing economy. The economy has shifted from a manufacturing economy based on highly paid, full-time jobs with good fringe benefits to a service economy with lower-paid jobs that are often part-time and have no paid benefits. Two-thirds of the uninsured are in families with an employed adult. Although the number of uninsured declined between 1998 and 2000, that number is on the rise again because of a weakened economy and layoffs at many companies. Currently, some 41.2 million Americans lack health coverage, up 1.4 million from 2000.[3] This includes 8.5 million children.[3] Underinsurance is also an important issue. Medicare covers only 45 percent of the health care costs of the elderly.[2] Since Congress established the program, the benefits covered by Medicare have remained largely unchanged, with the exception of a few added preventive services. The benefits are inadequate by current medical standards. A major problem for many elderly is that prescription medications are not covered by Medicare. A new prescription drug provision signed into law December 2003 will address part of this problem.

While some people cannot access the care they need, others receive too much care that is costly and may be unneccessary or harmful. Most studies that have looked for overuse have discovered at least double-digit overuse. In extrapolating from the available literature, Brooke found one-fourth of hospital days, one-fourth of procedures, and two-fifths of medications could be done without.[4] A 1998 report estimated that 20 to 30 percent of patients were receiving care that was not appropriate.[5]

Managed Care

In the 1990s, the U.S. health care system experienced a paradigm shift. Managed care became the overarching concept describing and influencing the U.S. health care system, revolutionizing it. Managed care forged a new relationship among the purchasers, insurers, and providers of care. It is a concept that pervades all aspects of health care financing and organization. In the past, health care providers were able to make most health care decisions and determine their compensation with minimal intrusion. With managed care, health care providers had to share or give up decision-making to insurers and purchasers and accept financial risk. Medical practices that had been in business for decades went bankrupt. Health maintenance organizations (HMOs) are one type of managed care. HMOs cover approximately 80 million people in the United States. In 2002, the organizing principle of managed care was beginning to falter. Patients and health care providers expressed a growing concern over a conflict between the HMOs' desire to increase profits and their responsibility to provide necessary care.[6]

Public's View of System

Health care is now evolving from its prior structures. For people with private or public insurance who have access to health care services, the melding of high-quality primary care and preventive services with the appropriate specialty care can produce the best medical care in the world. Unfortunately, health care in the United States encompasses a wide spectrum, ranging from the highest-quality cutting-edge technology and most compassionate treatment of those with illness to turning away the very ill because of their lack of ability to pay; from well-designed practice guidelines for the prevention or treatment of disease to inappropriate or unnecessary surgical procedures performed on uninformed patients. Despite all the upheaval in the health care system over the past 15 years, the United States still has the least universal, most costly health care system in the industrialized world.[7] In 1998, only 17 percent of people in the United States thought that the health care system worked well. Almost 80 percent thought that the system needed fundamental changes or a complete overhaul. About 18 percent of Americans had difficulty paying medical bills during the previous year, compared with 5 percent of Canadians and 3 percent of Britishers.[8]

FINANCING HEALTH CARE

The United States operates a health care system that is unique among nations. It is the most expensive of systems, outstripping by over half again the health care expenditures of any other country. The problem of soaring health care costs is not a new one. From 1970 to 1990, health expenditures in the United States increased at a yearly rate of 12 percent.[6] Americans spent $42 billion on health care in 1965, representing 6 percent of the gross national product (GNP) for that year. In 1981, that figure rose to $287 billion, or 9.8 percent of the GNP. In 2000, that figure rose to 1.310 trillion, or 13.3 percent of the GNP. In 2001, the figure jumped to $1.424 trillion, or 14.1 percent of the GNP.[9]

Prescription drugs and hospitals were two of the fastest growing expenditures. U.S. per capita health spending was $4,631 in 2000, an increase of 6.3 percent over 1999. These expenditures far exceeded the overall inflation rates prevalent in the American economy at the time. The numbers mean health care spending averaged about $5,035 per person.[9] Prescription drug spending—which made up $140.6 billion of total health spending—continued to grow faster than all other areas. One of the other biggest increases was in hospital spending, which increased 8.3 percent—the fastest growth for that sector in a decade. Economists pointed to huge hospital consolidations that have given facilities more bargaining power with managed care plans for payments as the reason for the jump in hospital services.

Critics of the current system said the spending increases are proof that once-touted HMOs are losing their ability to control costs. Health insurance premiums grew 10.5 percent, while benefits grew only about 10.1 percent.[9] The system for financing health care services is a key factor that has shaped the delivery of health care in the United States. Unlike many European systems, which are largely publicly financed, the American system, as it has evolved during the past 30 years, involves a complex blend of private and public responsibilities.

What the Health Care Dollar Buys

To understand health care financing better, one must first understand what is being accomplished with the ever-increasing health care expenditures. As measured by the federal Centers for Medicare and Medicaid Services (CMS), the national health expenditures are grouped into two categories:

1. Research and medical facilities construction
2. Payments for health services and supplies

Five types of personal expenditures accounted for more than 75 percent of the 1998 total health care spending. Ranked in order of spending, the five are: hospital care, "physician" services, drugs and other medical nondurables, nursing home care, and dental services. Not included in the CMS figures were medical education costs, except insofar as they are inseparable from hospital expenditures and biomedical research. These personal health care expenditures (PHCEs) constituted the bulk of the national health care "bill"—more than $1,016,129 million in 1998.[9] According to the Department of Commerce, the figure for PHCEs is expected to grow by 12 to 15 percent annually during the next 5 years unless significant changes occur in the health care delivery system.[10]

Where the Health Care Dollar Comes From

In the early part of this century, people paid for medical care "out of their own pockets," much as they purchased any other service. Costs and utilization were kept at a minimum because there was little in the way of medical care that physicians or hospitals could offer and that money could buy. In the 1930s, with the introduction of ether as an anesthetic and with the advent of other advances in surgical technology, physicians and hospitals had more to sell. Consequently, resource utilization increased, and the price of medical care climbed. In response to this increased demand and escalated cost for medical services, the first health insurance plan, Blue Cross, was developed and offered jointly by a group of hospitals and surgeons. Although the plan limited coverage to inpatient care, with physician services and medications remaining available only to those who could afford to pay for them, the third-party reimbursement system, with its attendant insensitivity to economics, was established.[11]

Although it is said that health care monies come from different sources, what is really meant is that dollars take different routes on their way from consumers to providers. Close to 60 percent of total U.S. health spending in 1999 was financed through taxes.[12] Ultimately, the American people pay all health care costs, indirectly or directly, regardless of whether payment occurs via government, private insurance companies, or independent plans. Moreover, these third-party costs are paid in addition to the out-of-pocket payments. Out-of-pocket spending for health care consists of direct spending by consumers for all health care goods and services. Included in this estimate is the amount paid out-of-pocket for services not covered by insurance and the amount of coinsurance and deductibles required by private health insurance and by public programs such as Medicare and Medicaid (and not paid by some other third party).

Total public funding (which paid for 45 percent of all health care) continued to accelerate in 2001, increasing 9.4 percent and exceeding private funding growth by 1.2 percentage points. Medicare spending growth accelerated 2.8 percentage points in 2001 to 7.8 percent. Medicaid, the state-federal health insurance program for the poor, grew to $224.3 billion in 2001. Medicaid spending increased at double-digit rates for all services, except for nursing homes. Total Medicaid spending growth, excluding State Children's Health Insurance Program (SCHIP) expansions, accelerated two percentage points to 10.8 percent in 2001, the fastest growth since 1993.

Private health insurance premium growth accelerated for the fourth consecutive year, with benefits growing more slowly than premiums in the past 3 years. Premiums rose 10.5 percent in 2001 to $496.1 billion, while benefits grew 10.1 percent. Consumer out-of-pocket spending increased 5.6 percent. Hospitals spent a lot more money in 2001. Spending by hospitals rose 8.3 percent, totaling $451 billion. Spending on physician and other clinical services rose by 8.6 percent in 2001 to $314 billion. Prescription drugs accounted for $140.6 billion of the total health care budget.

Figure 3–1 shows a pie chart of the nation's health care spending for 2001 and where the money came from and where it went.[10]

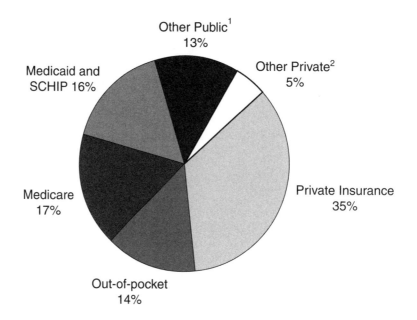

The Nation's Health Dollar: 2001

Where It Came From

SOURCE: Centers for Medicare & Medicaid Services, Office of the Actuary, National Health Statistics Group.

[1] "Other Public" includes programs such as workers' compensation, public health activity, Department of Defense, Department of Veterans Affairs, Indian Health Service, and state and local hospital subsidies and school health.
[2] "Other Private" includes industrial in-plant, privately funded construction, and non-patient revenues, including philanthropy.

FIGURE 3–1   The Nation's Health Dollar: 2001.

Where It Went

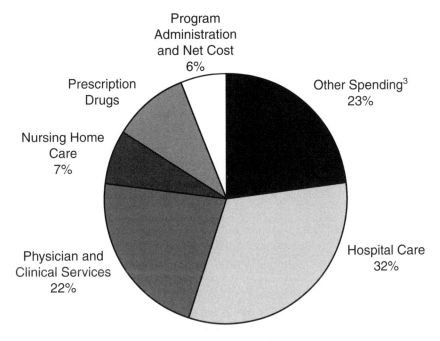

SOURCE: Centers for Medicare & Medicaid Services, Office of the Actuary, National Health Statistics Group.

[3] "Other Spending" includes dental services, other professional services, home health care, durable medical products, over-the-counter medicines and sundries, public health activities, research and construction.

FIGURE 3–1   *(Continued)*

Public Outlays

The significant rise in federal spending is accounted for by the Medicare, Medicaid, and SCHIP programs, Titles XVIII and XIX, respectively, of the Social Security Act.

Medicare

The Medicare program serves persons over the age of 65 years and many persons with disabilities.

The program was implemented in 1966, and the number of persons served has increased from 19 million to 40 million. Expenditures for Medicare have risen faster than those for any other major federal program. Medicare now insures one of every seven Americans. Medicare remains at the forefront of debate because of the aging of the baby-boom generation and the likelihood that health care expenditures will continue to increase. By 2030, the program is expected to serve

77 million people—more than one of every five Americans—and to account for about 4.4 percent of the gross domestic product. The increase in life expectancy in the United States since 1965 is undoubtedly attributable in part to Medicare.[13]

Medicare is a federally funded health insurance program created by Title XVIII of the Social Security Act of 1965; it was originally designed to protect people 65 years of age and older from the high cost of health care. The program also covers permanently disabled workers eligible for old age, survivor's, and disability insurance benefits and their dependents, as well as people with end-stage renal disease.

As currently structured, Medicare comprises two programs, each of which has its own trust fund[44]:

1. Part A, the hospital insurance program, is financed by payroll taxes collected under the Social Security system. It provides coverage for inpatient hospital services, post-hospitalization skilled nursing services, home health care services, and hospice care.

2. Part B, a voluntary supplemental medical-insurance (SMI) program, pays certain costs for physicians' services, outpatient hospital services and therapy, and other health expenses. The SMI program is financed by monthly premiums collected from elderly enrollees and by general tax revenues.

The Medicare Prescription Drug, Improvement, and Modernization Act of 2003 was signed into law on December 8, 2003. It creates a new drug benefit as Part D of Medicare. The drug benefit begins in January 2006. Starting in 2004, there is an interim Medicare-endorsed drug discount card and a transitional assistance program. The new law also includes other changes for beneficiaries, including increases in the Part B deductible, income-relating the Part B premium, and new preventive benefits.[46]

Medicaid

Medicaid was established by the federal government in 1965 to provide health care to the poor.[23]

This program was designed to ensure health care services to the aged poor, the blind, the disabled, and families with dependent children if one parent was absent, unemployed, or unable to work. Persons become eligible for Medicaid on the basis of their financial status and by fitting into one of these federally defined categories.

Unlike Medicare, which is solely a federal program, the Medicaid program is jointly funded and administered by federal and state governments. The name Medicaid is more or less a blanket label for 50 different state programs designed specifically to serve welfare recipients. Different states give their individual Medicaid programs different names. For example, in California, Medicaid is known as MediCal; in Arizona, the program is called Access, and in Tennessee, it is called TennCare. Medicaid provides federal funds to states on a cost-sharing basis according to each state's per capita income.

The Medicaid program represents a high degree of decentralization in that the federal government requirements are only minimally restrictive. States exercise significant control over Medicaid eligibility and benefit packages within federal guidelines. For the most part, Medicaid is available only to very-low-income persons. The program also has categorical restrictions; that is, only families with children; pregnant women; and those who are aged, blind, or disabled can qualify.

The basic set of services mandated by the federal government for Medicaid programs includes[45]:

- Inpatient and outpatient hospital care
- Other laboratory and x-ray services
- Physicians' services
- Nursing-facility care for persons older than 21 years
- Home health for those entitled to nursing-facility services
- Screening, diagnostic, and treatment services for persons younger than 21 years
- Family planning

Although states must provide the basic set of services, they can set their own rates based on how much they are willing to spend on their percentage of the cost. Generally, the federal government will reimburse states from 50 to 83 percent of what they spend. Because each state can determine how much it will pay for services under the Medicaid program, much variability exists. For instance, in Massachusetts, a physician might be reimbursed about $1,500 for delivering a baby, whereas in New Mexico a physician might only receive about $900 for the identical service.

Other Public Expenditures

Medicare and Medicaid account for more than 76 percent of public outlays for personal health care services. State and local government outlays represent the next largest expenditure category, but only account for about 10 percent of the total amount. The remaining four major personal health care categories for which government monies are spent include:

1. Federal outlays for hospital and medical services for veterans
2. Department of Defense provision of care for the armed forces and military dependents
3. Workers' compensation medical benefits
4. Other federal, state, and local expenditures for personal health care

Finally, public spending for research and facilities construction totaled approximately $52 billion in 2001. Of this amount, public outlays for research totaled $32.8 billion, with the federal government representing the primary source for most of the money spent.[13]

SCHIP

In 1997, Congress enacted the SCHIP, which provides coverage to 4.6 million children whose family incomes are too high to allow them to qualify for Medicaid but too low to afford private health insurance. The SCHIP law appropriated $40 billion in federal funds over 10 years to improve children's access to health coverage. Each state sets its own eligibility and process similar to the Medicaid plans.

The Current Challenge to Publicly Financed Health Care

Medicare has large deductibles, co-payments, and gaps in coverage. Sixty percent of Medicare beneficiaries carry supplemental private "Medigap" insurance, and an additional 13 percent are enrolled in a Medicare HMO plan. Medicare does not cover outpatient prescription medications. The average beneficiary pays more than $3,000 out of pocket each year for health care, excluding long-term care.[14] Limitations on the amount of coverage exist as well. For example, hospital benefits cease after 90 days if the patient has exhausted the lifetime reserve pool of 60 additional hospital days, and extended-care facility benefits terminate after 100 days. Medicare payments represent approximately 65 percent of the total annual national expenditure of hospital services and 27 percent of physicians' services. Because Medicare clarified its conditions for nursing home payment in 1988 with the Catastrophic Coverage Act, it seems likely that Medicare will maintain its current share of total spending for nursing home care at 4 to 5 percent.[15]

As of 2002, approximately 51 million people received some type of Medicaid benefit, with approximately $259 billion of combined federal and state funds being spent for personal health care. As a result of this accelerated growth, Medicaid's share of the nation's PHCEs has increased significantly. In 2002, the Medicaid program financed health care and social services for more than one of every seven Americans. In 2002, the federal governement provided 57 percent of all Medicaid expenditures, totaling $259 billion. Medicaid pays for more than one-third of all births. It is the nation's largest purchaser of long-term care services. It funds more than half of all nursing home expenditures. It is the largest payer of medical care for persons with HIV infection or AIDS. It provides major support to hospitals, which are "safety net" providers. Medicaid's expenditures are largely institutional, with more than 40 percent spent on hospital care and approximately 35 percent spent on nursing home care annually. Medicaid continues to be the largest third-party payer of long-term care expenditures, financing almost 50 percent of nursing home care annually.

Confronted with increasing numbers of recipients and recent legislative expansions to the Medicaid program in the face of limited revenues available to finance the program, states have been pressured to control their individual Medicaid costs. Strategies used or proposed by states include:

- Overall spending cuts
- Reallocation of available funds from high-cost services to lower-cost services
- Rationing high-technology services to selected recipients to provide lower-cost services to a broader group of recipients
- Provider-specific taxes
- "Voluntary donations" from physicians and hospitals

Private Outlays

Although the amount of public funding for health care is staggering, the predominant funding for the American health care system comes from private sources. The bulk is derived from individuals receiving treatment and from third-party insurers making payments on the behalf of individuals.

In 1929, private payment of PHCEs represented 88.4 percent of the total amount spent on PHCEs. In 1935, that figure dropped to 82.4 percent. In 1965, before the advent of Medicare and Medicaid, such private payments accounted for nearly 77 percent of the total. In 1998, private payment accounted for 56 percent of all PHCEs.[16]

The decline in the private share of PHCEs is primarily due to the sharp drop in out-of-pocket payments associated with federal spending. In 1965, 53 percent of personal health care expenditures was paid by the patient, and in 2001, 14 percent. Yet because of inflation and other factors, the per capita dollar amount paid directly by a patient has increased dramatically.[16]

Private Third-Party Administrators

Most Americans receive their health insurance as a tax-free benefit through their employers.[16] This employer-based financing of health care was started during World War II and has grown steadily ever since. The system relies predominantly on private, employment-based, insurance-type financing schemes that, at least until recently, divorced financing from the delivery of services.

Private health insurance companies constitute one of the largest sectors of the health industry. The United States has more than 1,000 for-profit, commercial health insurers and 85 not-for-profit Blue Cross and Blue Shield plans. These private insurance organizations, along with health maintenance organizations (HMOs), preferred provider organizations (PPOs), and other third-party payers, paid for 35 percent of the total health care expenditures in 2001.[17]

Employment is the foundation of the private health insurance system in the United States. In 1999, 83 percent of Americans under the age of 65 had some form of health insurance coverage; of these, 67 percent were covered by an employment-based plan. Employment enables many workers to obtain health coverage. Three out of every four workers (74 percent) are offered health insurance by their own employers, and six out of 10 (63 percent) receive employment-based coverage through their jobs.[18] In 2000, employer-based insurance covered some 172 million people, including 18 million retirees who have coverage that supplements Medicare, and about 22 million people purchased their own insurance. Overall, employer-based health insurance touches the lives of nearly two of every three Americans. PPOs enroll the largest proportion of workers (41 percent), followed by HMOs (29 percent) and point of service plans (22 percent). PPO enrollment has grown substantially in recent years, while HMO enrollment largely stagnated. Enrollment in conventional insurance plans constitutes only 8 percent of workers, down from 27 percent in 1996.[19]

Blue Cross and Blue Shield and the Rise of Indemnity Insurance

The term "insurance" originally meant, and often still refers to, the contribution by individuals to a fund to provide protection against financial loss following relatively unlikely but damaging events. Thus, there is insurance against fire, theft, and death at an early age. All of those events occur within a group of people within a predictable rate but are rare occurrences for any one individual in a group.[20]

Medical insurance was introduced in the mid-1800s to defray costs associated with unexpected disabilities. Essentially, it consisted of cash payments by some carriers to individuals to offset income losses attributed to accident-related disabilities. Medical insurance continued in this tradition until the 1930s when, coincident with the rise in available medical services, a number of prepayment plans that offered care at various hospitals were organized in several cities. These hospital insurance plans soon became known as Blue Cross.[21] Shortly thereafter, Blue Shield was developed independently as an insurer for physicians' services. With the organization of Blue Cross and Blue Shield, a new policy for reimbursing general health care costs started.

The "Blues" were established as nonprofit membership plans that served state and regional areas and offered both individual and group membership. For many years, the Blues were committed to community rating.[22] In exchange for offering coverage to anyone in the community, the Blues were able to secure significant discounts in costs by way of negotiations and through regulations known as the "most-favored-nation status," which ensured that the Blues would have the lowest rates given to any payer.

In recent years, this community-rating approach has placed the Blues at a disadvantage when competing with commercial insurers that have entered the health insurance field adhering to a policy of experience rating. Experience rating has allowed commercial insurers to charge different individuals and groups different premiums, based on individual risk and on the use of services. Low-risk groups could secure benefits at lower premiums because of the "healthy worker effect," whereas high-risk groups received commercial insurance coverage only at prohibitively high premium rates. Consequently, the Blues have been left as the insurers of last resort for those individuals who might have chronic illnesses and/or are unable to obtain employer-based group insurance coverage.

Commercial Insurance

Like the Blues, commercial insurance plans offer comprehensive coverage for hospital and physicians' services; however, they differ in that they also sell medical and cash-payment policies. The commercial portion of the industry has grown rapidly in this country, primarily because experience rating has allowed them to respond to consumer demand for reduced out-of-pocket costs for medical care and because of the "employer-based" model for financing health care that developed during World War II.

Initially, commercial insurance companies were slow to enter a market dominated by the Blues. However, during and after World War II, tax laws changed to permit employers to offer tax-free health coverage as part of employee benefit packages, allowing commercial companies that previously had offered limited coverage to individuals to offer hospital insurance to groups. Since that time, commercial insurance companies have acquired more than half of the health insurance market from Blue Cross and Blue Shield. Currently, there are more than 1,000 private insurance companies providing individual and group health coverage in the United States.[23]

Self-Insurance

To avoid high tax premiums, administrative overhead, and marketing expenses, a majority of large corporations have become self-insured. Commercial insurance companies have found themselves to be little more than transaction processors for these corporations, providing claims payment services to the self-insured on a cost-plus basis. Consequently, these insurance companies are experiencing operating losses due to the shrinking fully-insured market. To compete and survive, group insurance carriers have transformed themselves into managed care companies, thereby improving internal operating and marketing efficiencies. However, it is estimated that only 25 of the nearly 500 group health insurance carriers have the capability, financial support, management, and customer volume to accomplish this task.[24]

HMOs and the Rise of Nonindemnity Insurance

As health care costs escalated in the 1970s, Congress passed legislation that encouraged the formation of HMOs, or systems that would integrate the delivery and financing of health care. These operate differently from traditional indemnity insurance plans that reimbursed on a fee-for-service basis. HMOs provide comprehensive health "maintenance" care (and restorative care when necessary) for its enrollees at a flat prepaid fee. Although this "capitated" form of health insurance has been available for the past 20 years, it has recently reshaped the way many Americans relate to the health care arena.

Although several different types of prepaid plans are available, the basic notion of each is that an annual fixed payment is made by or for beneficiaries in exchange for the delivery of all necessary health care by a group of providers within the scope of their contracts. Distinctions among HMOs pertain to the ways in which fiscal agents or the financing organizations relate to groups of care providers.[25] Most prepaid plans contract with providers for scheduled reimbursement, capitated payments, discounted charges, or per-episode payments. Currently, there are four distinct HMO models in operation in the United States (Table 3–1).

Regardless of the type of plan, a capitated annual insurance premium is paid in exchange for all necessary care, including preventive and routine services not generally covered under indemnity plans. Presumably, HMOs reduce health care costs (owing, for the most part, to lower rates of hospitalization) while providing coverage that has fewer copayment features and uncovered services. These plans have grown popular with employers who are looking for ways to reduce health care benefits spending.

Between 1984 and 1993, the proportion of employees enrolled in HMOs increased from 5 percent to 50 percent. By 1998, 85 percent of employees with health insurance coverage were in some form of managed care plan, whereas 15 percent were in fee-for-service indemnity plans.[26] Currently managed care dominates health care in the United States. By 1999, only 8 percent of persons with employer-sponsored health insurance coverage had traditional indemnity insur-

TABLE 3–1.	Health Maintenance Organization Models in the United States
Model	**Description**
Staff model	In this traditional HMO system, the fiscal agent engages individual physicians who are paid a salary to deliver services to the HMO's enrollees.
Group model	This model is similar to the staff model; however, it varies in that a single group of physicians contracts with the fiscal agent to deliver services.
Network model	Fiscal agents contract with multiple groups of physicians to deliver services to enrollees. Physicians in this model do not have exclusive contracts with fiscal agents and generally provide services to non–HMO enrollees.
Independent	Fiscal agents contract with a range of independent physicians' practices or multispecialty group practices to deliver care to its enrollees.
IPA model	As in the network model, physicians in the IPA model provide services to HMO enrollees as well as to patients with other forms of insurance. Usually, HMO enrollees represent a small percentage of IPA physicians' practices.

ance.[27] Enrollment in managed care plans grew because managed care cost less than fee-for-service care. Managed care business practices, such as preauthorization of hospital and other services and restricted formularies for medications, reduced utilization and cost.[26]

PPOs

The success of the independent practice association (IPA) model of HMO increased experimentation with varying levels of consumer and physician choice, eventually leading to the introduction of PPOs. PPOs, like HMOs, offer the consumer a choice of full coverage for ambulatory and inpatient services provided by a selected panel of providers, combined with a limited range of coverage for out-of-plan use.[28] Frequently, PPOs are established by groups of physicians who are interested in maintaining patients and revenues in the face of competition from HMOs.

PPOs provide health care at a lower cost to those beneficiaries who use participating providers, who are paid on the basis of negotiated or discounted rates. Beneficiaries are usually given some type of incentive, such as lower insurance premiums or waivers of cost-sharing requirements, for selecting a preferred provider. PPOs are gaining popularity, especially in markets where there is significant competition among physicians and other health care providers.[29]

In such competitive areas, providers can be persuaded more easily to offer discounted services in exchange for a larger share of the patient volume. The enhancement in consumer choice afforded by PPOs mimics the freedom of choice found in traditional fee-for-service medicine.[30] Enrollment in PPO plans has been growing steadily since 1996, and PPOs now cover more than half of workers.[27] PPO enrollment remains highest in the South, where PPOs enroll 61 percent of workers.[27]

The Current Challenge to Privately Financed Health Care

Although private health insurance coverage for Americans is extensive, it is far from complete. More than 41 million Americans are uninsured, and their numbers are growing as the economy weakens. The problem of the uninsured is one of America's biggest health challenges. Too many families do not have access to affordable health insurance, and they live sicker and die younger as a result. And being uninsured is not primarily a problem for the unemployed. Eight of 10 uninsured Americans are in working families.[3] In 1999, 11 percent of whites were uninsured compared with 21 percent of African Americans, 21 percent of Asian Americans and 33 percent of Latinos. Nearly a quarter of individuals with annual household incomes of less than $25,000 were uninsured compared with 8 percent of individuals with incomes over $75,000.[31] These data support the notion that the proportion of the population that has insurance is directly related to income and ethnic membership. At the same time, employers are applying pressure on insurers to pare down premiums. This trend was most evident in a push by a consortium of 11 large employers in San Francisco that joined to negotiate premium reductions from 17 Bay Area HMOs.[27]

Premium increases affect all employees with health insurance coverage. Insurers, at the behest of employers, are also redesigning their benefit packages in ways that will have the greatest effect on workers who seek medical care. These packages generally feature fewer benefits, larger cost-sharing requirements at the point of service, or both, but also smaller premium increases than would have otherwise been the case. Structuring benefits in ways that subject patients to larger out-of-pocket expenditures is a reversal of a pattern that had been in place for decades, according to the CMS. The agency estimates that approximately 15 percent of personal health expenditures were borne by consumers in the form of out-of-pocket costs in 2000, down from 20 percent in 1990 and 48 percent in 1960. Cost-sharing by patients comes in a variety of forms: an annual deductible (an amount that a patient pays up front, before using health care services), a specific deductible for hospital admission, a copayment (an amount that a patient pays per unit of service, such as an office visit or a hospital stay), and various cost-sharing features for generic and brand-name drugs, all of which can be "mixed and matched to achieve whichever premium price point is desired by the purchaser."[32]

One of the newest cost-containment methods being used by insurers differentiates prescription drugs, hospitals, and, in California, medical groups and physicians on the basis of cost. This approach was first used with prescription drugs. According to a survey of employers published in 2002, 57 percent of workers with drug coverage had benefits that were based on a three-tier cost-sharing formula, as compared with 36 percent in 2001 and 28 percent in 2000.[32] Under such coverage, the lowest copayment is required if a generic drug is prescribed, a higher copayment is required for a brand-name drug when no generic equivalent is available, and the highest copayment is required for a brand-name drug when a generic drug is available. The most recent form of tiered benefits—different levels of copayments for hospital care that are based on costs—is being offered by some of the nation's largest insurers on either a trial or a permanent basis.

PacifiCare and Blue Shield of California are exploring ways to provide tiered benefits for physicians' services based on the fees they charge and possibly on selected indicators of the quality of care they provide. Blue Shield of California will evaluate hospitals not only on the basis of their costs but also on the basis of data on patient satisfaction and the quality of care, compiled by two independent organizations.

The basic change that many employers are considering, but that only a handful have thus far implemented, is to abandon the traditional approach of offering employees a defined set of insurance benefits and instead offer them a fixed amount of money to pay for coverage. Under this approach, the employee would pay for any costs that exceeded the employer's contribution, up to a maximal amount, beyond which insurance would cover the cost of a serious or catastrophic illness.

How the Money is Paid Out

The predominant manner of payment to hospitals and providers has been the retrospective fee-for-service method. However, with the spiraling costs associated with Medicare and Medicaid, the federal government began to exercise its prerogative in scrutinizing the value received for the health care dollars it reimbursed hospitals and physicians. Commercial health insurance companies were quick to follow the government's lead by adopting similar payment policies.

With the proliferation of HMOs and PPOs and with increased fee regulation by public programs, physicians and hospitals are now less able to set prices for their services freely. At this time, there are three basic approaches that insurers may use to pay physicians for their services:

1. Fee for service
2. The preferred-provider approach
3. Capitation and salary

Although there are many permutations within these hospital reimbursement categories, the two dominant approaches are retrospective and prospective payment. A description of these reimbursement methods and their development follows.

Federal Cost Control and its Effect on Hospital Reimbursement

Beginning in the 1970s, the related issues of the cost and the quality of the care delivered under federal entitlement programs were addressed by the passage of legislative amendments. Professional standards review organizations (PSROs) were established in an effort to monitor the quality and quantity of institutional services delivered to Medicare and Medicaid recipients. Subsequent amendments attempted to limit the growth in health care expenditures by changing the manner in which the amount to be reimbursed hospitals and physicians was calculated.

In 1982, Congress passed the Tax Equity and Fiscal Responsibility Act (TEFRA). Designed to provide incentives for institutional cost containment, it replaced the PSROs with a "utilization and quality-control peer review organization"

(PRO). The TEFRA legislation introduced the cost-per-case reimbursement system known as diagnoses-related groups (DRGs) and, simultaneously, placed limits on the rates of increase in hospital revenues. Additional legislation mandated that hospitals covered under Medicare's new case-based reimbursement system contract with a PRO by 1984.[33]

The 1983 amendments to the Social Security Act further refined the case payment system by establishing a prospective payment system. These amendments created a revolutionary method of reimbursing hospitals for inpatient care to Medicare patients based on DRGs. Under the prospective payment system, hospitals are paid a pre-fixed amount per case treated. Research exploring the impact of DRGs suggests that the utilization patterns of hospitals are changing as a result of the reimbursement system. Most notably, hospital admissions and length of hospital stays have significantly decreased, and a sharp increase in post-hospital care, including the use of home health services and nursing homes, has increased sharply.[34]

While prospective payment represents the most significant change in reimbursement methods in the past 20 years, it is not the exclusive means by which institutions are paid. Retrospective payment, or paying for services already provided, remains a mode by which some third-party payers reimburse hospitals. Most commercial insurers, such as Blue Cross, pay hospitals on the basis of submitted charges, or the prices set by hospitals for the care they provide. A more sophisticated retrospective repayment system is based on cost. In this system, third-party payers take a sum of total hospital costs and then, based on allowable items, reimburse hospitals on a per-patient-day basis.

Federal Cost Control and its Effect on Physician Payment

Physician reimbursement mechanisms were changed as a result of federal legislation, primarily under provisions in the Omnibus Budget Reconciliation Acts (OBRAs), especially OBRA 1989 and OBRA 1993.[35-39] Before the enactment of OBRA 1989, physicians were permitted wide discretion in establishing their own prices for each type of service they delivered. Once care was received, patients or their insurers paid the set price.

After OBRA 1989 was enacted, the amount that Medicare reimbursed and the amount that physicians were allowed to charge patients in excess of that amount were restricted to repayments in amounts equal to the "prevailing" fee (also known as "usual and customary rates") and by limiting the maximum payment allowed in communities for each type of physician's service. Many insurers have followed Medicare's approach by adopting a wide range of methods for establishing scales for covered services, limiting the ability of the physician to establish prices.

The resource-based relative value system (RBRVS) that went into effect in 1992 represents another attempt by the federal government to control physician-related costs. With its introduction, Medicare substantially changed its approach to paying physicians. Based on a national fee schedule, the RBRVS assigns cash values to services based on the time, skill, and intensity required to provide them. The relative values are then further adjusted for geographic variations in payment. The object of this new system was to rebalance reimbursement so that payment for cognitive services would be increased and payment for procedural services decreased relative to prices established in prior years. Unfortunately, evidence suggests that the RBRVS has not been as successful as expected.

In the private arena, the preferred provider approach to paying physicians used by PPOs offers a variation on the fee-for-service system. Using this approach, insurers pay physicians discounted amounts for care delivered to enrollees on a service-by-service basis. The discounted payment schedule is usually negotiated between the insurers and the physicians or by physician groups.

Salary and capitation are the two other forms of provider reimbursement. The use of salary arrangements as a payment mechanism for health professionals is widespread and needs little explanation. Generally, this arrangement proves satisfactory to both employer and provider. In a salaried arrangement, employers can generally enjoy administrative simplicity, while providers are usually assured a more protected income as compared with those being reimbursed through other arrangements.

The Need for Change

According to advocates of managed care and others who have studied health-spending trends, patients and physicians have grown insensitive to the rising cost of health care in this country. On average, insured patients pay very little directly for every dollar spent for hospital care and physicians' services. Most of the expense is borne by either employers or the government.

Because patients feel relatively little financial burden associated with their health care expenses, they have exerted little pressure on providers to keep costs low. Providers generally had no real incentive to seek and use medical services that would yield the same health care outcome at reduced cost. Rather, they were and, to a great extent, continue to be rewarded for delivering as many of the most expensive services as possible. Consequently, there has been little competition among providers to produce services efficiently and pass savings on to the consumers. In light of these perceptions, most proposed health care reform initiatives, regardless of their origin, are directed toward restraining medical inflation by sensitizing consumers and providers to the high cost of health care.

THE EVOLUTION OF MANAGED CARE

Managed Competition as a Solution

The health care delivery system built with such little regard for cost is one characterized by Alain Enthoven as the "paradox of excess and deprivation."[40,41] As a strategy for curbing health care costs, Enthoven advanced a proposal known as managed competition. According to the basic theory of managed competition, groups of purchasers could negotiate with large groups of providers to determine price and some other terms of services in advance of purchase.[42,43] Managed competition has been proposed as a strategy that can solve the problem of skyrocketing health care costs by restructuring the market to promote cost-conscious consumer choice among health plans. The market, as presented by Enthoven, involves three key groups of players:

1. The consumer
2. The health plan
3. The sponsors

Consumers include both the individual and the employer-employee dyad. In managed competition, individuals could choose from, and employers would be required to offer employees, a variety of health plans. Employees would be encouraged to select the most economical plan from among the options offered because managed competition (as originally conceived) limits the tax-free employer contributions to the cost of the lowest-priced plan. Individuals joining more costly plans would not receive extra subsidies, as they currently do, but would have to pay extra costs out of their own pockets. As a result, consumers would be more likely to obtain necessary information to make informed decisions in selecting plans that offer them the most value for their money.

Health plans in managed competition models are equivalent to accountable health partnerships that integrate financing and delivery of health care. HMOs, PPOs, and IPAs represent several examples of these health plans as they exist today. Although configurations vary, these plans, which integrate providers (physicians, nurses, laboratories, and so forth), insurers, and hospitals, would compete for subscribers and would be required to deliver value for money spent.

The structure of such health plans is significant to the organization's ability to manage a patient's care. Organizations that are able to improve quality while cutting costs would be most successful in attracting and maintaining subscribers. Strategies short of constituting all of the elements of managed competition that are being used by health plans to improve quality while limiting costs include:

- Closed- versus open-panel plans
- Prepaid group practices
- Economic credentialing
- Gatekeeping
- Utilization review
- Resource allocation
- Risk-sharing reimbursement
- Truncated treatment plans

Public sponsors are the third group of players identified as critical in managed competition. Sponsors would be recognized in each state and would act as the final guarantor of health coverage, acting as collective purchasing agents for employment groups of 100 or fewer employees and for the self-employed. State sponsors would be essential for those without employment-based coverage; these public sponsors would subsidize enrollment and contract with private sector health plans on behalf of potential subscribers. Sponsors would essentially act as brokers for groups of subscribers.

IMPLICATIONS FOR ADVANCED PRACTICE NURSING

APNs must be prepared for the substantial opportunities and considerable threats that are evolving in health care reform. For the first time, both delivery and receipt of health care are operating on a budget. In addition, the consumer, whether an elderly person selecting from among several health insurance plans to supplement Medicare coverage or a large corporation's employee benefits administrator deciding between a self-insured health plan or an HMO, is once again in a position to exercise control over what to buy and how much to pay.

This change to a value-driven consumer in a cost-conscious environment translates to an opportunity for APNs to be the value-conscious health care provider. This is an opportunity that should not be squandered. As reiterated by each of the leaders interviewed by Dr. Komnenich, there was in the past—and should be today—the commitment by APNs to promote themselves and the advanced practice roles as essential elements in the solution for health care reform.

Some of the concepts integral to managed care have permeated all of health care. APNs have strengh and expertise in all of these areas. APNs need to become familiar with the use of clinical practice guidelines, which can lead to improvements in health care delivery. The guidelines need to be well-designed, goal-oriented, specific, evidence-based, and adapted for local use with input from the health care providers who will use them. Utilization management has been portrayed as a drive toward cost containment at the expense of quality. The guiding principles of utilization management, however, are to minimize inappropriate variations in practice and promote cost-effective patient care, which should meet best practice standards and simultaneously reduce costs. Their goal is to enable health professionals to practice comfortably and effectively in a high-quality, cost-effective health care system.

APNs are challenged by a health care system that increasingly demands prevention and management of chronic diseases. Disease management for chronic diseases is a systems-based approach for improving patient outcomes to help achieve the best possible health outcomes through the use of evidence-based practice guidelines. Pressures on the U.S. health care system and greater focus on health promotion and prevention have opened up opportunities for APNs. A population-based approach to health care is being promoted as a solution to the spiraling costs. This is an approach taught and promoted at all levels of nursing education and one in which APNs have strength and expertise.

Another area APNs need to recognize is the focus on measuring quality of care delivered. Patient satisfaction as one measure of quality is now emphasized. This is an area where APNs have traditionally excelled. APNs are knowledgeable and aware of how quality is being measured at their institutions and by the insurers. Health Plan Employer Data and Information Set (HEDIS) measures are commonly used as well as practice profiling.

APNs must be knowledgeable about the business aspects of health care. Health care in the United States is, unfortunately, a business. APNs need to obtain their own provider identifcation numbers and bill directly for Medicare, Medicaid, and any private plans that permit it. Many plans will credential and reimburse APNs directly. Some plans will allow APNs to be PCPs for their patients. APNs need to query insurers continually regarding their policy on credentailing and reimbursement; and they must petition plans to recognize them as providers.

As Dr. Komnenich makes clear in Chapter 1, the APNs who brought advanced practice nursing to where it is today did so largely by the dint of their own initiative and by a commitment to excellence. They made their mark and thus made a place for today's APNs by collecting and disseminating data that promoted their value, by refusing to accede to organized nursing's and medicine's efforts to constrain their vision to some preconceived idea about what a nurse should be, and by actively seeking out and seizing opportunities for advancement presented by others outside the profession or occasioned by sociological, political, and/or economic events.

SUGGESTED EXERCISES

1. As a result of the health care revolution in America, medical care is evolving into health care. Develop a platform that illuminates the actual and potential effects or consequences of this transformation on advanced practice nursing.

2. Vast opportunities exist for APN entrepreneurs and entrepreneurs in today's competitively managed market. Create a business plan for the new health care environment that recharacterizes the APN identity, redefines APN role components, and relocates advanced practice nursing arenas.

3. Organize a portfolio that can be presented to prospective markets providing evidence to support the position that APNs are well suited to assume a variety of positions in integrated health care systems.

4. Debate whether APNs would be better advised to assume complementary (value-added) or substitution positions in managed care markets.

5. Design a master plan for an IPA that consists exclusively of APNs. Identify potential consumer groups to be served as well as insurers to be approached. Discuss strategies for reimbursement.

6. How would you "sell" or market the concept of an APN IPA to selected consumers and prospective insurers? Develop a marketing plan to accomplish that goal.

REFERENCES

1. Fox, JC: The role of nursing. J Psychosocial Nurs 31:9, 1993.
2. Bodenheimer, TS, and Grumbach, K: Understanding Health Policy A Clinical Approach, 3rd ed. Lange, New York, 2002.
3. Robert Wood Johnson Foundation: Covering the Uninsured. http://covertheuninsuredweek.org/ Accessed June 1, 2003.
4. Brooke, RH: Practice guidelines and practicing medicine. JAMA 262:3027, 1989.
5. Schuster, M, et al: How good is the quality of health care in the United States? Milbank Quarterly, 76:517; 1998.
6. Blendon, RJ, et al: Understanding the managed care backlash. Health Affairs 17:80, 1998.
7. Starfield, B: Is US health really the best in the world? JAMA 284:483 2000.
8. Donelan, K, et al: The cost of health system change: Public discontent in five nations. Health Affairs 18:206 1999.

9. Levit, K, et al: Trends in US health care spending 2001. Health Affairs 22:154, 2003.
10. Center for Medicare and Medicaid Services, Office of the Actuary, National Health Statistics Group NHE 2001.
11. Baldor, RA: Managed Care Made Simple. Blackwell Science, Cambridge, MA, 1996.
12. Anderson, G, et al: It's the prices, stupid: Why the United States is so different from other countries. Health Affairs 22:89, 2003.
13. Center for Medicare and Medicaid Services, Office of the Actuary, National Health Care Expenditure Projections 2002.
14. Moon, M: Health Policy 2001 Medicare. New Engl J Med 344:928, 2001.
15. Kaplan, RM: A look at solutions. In Kaplan, RM (ed): The Hippocratic Predicament. Academic Press, San Diego, 1993.
16. Iglehart, JK: The American health care system: Expenditures. N Engl J Med 340: 70, 1999.
17. Health Insurance Industry of America: Employment-Based Health Insurance Coverage. Health Insurance Association of America, Washington, DC, 2003.
18. Kaiser Family Foundation: Employer Health Benefits 2000; 1–190, 2001.
19. Kuttner, R: The American Health Care System. Employer Sponsored Health Insurance. N Engl J Med 340:240, 1999.
20. Jonas, S, and Kovner, A: Health Care Delivery in the United States. Springer, New York, 1999.
21. Blue Cross/Blue Shield Corporate Report: Blue Cross/Blue Shield of Massachusetts, Boston, May 1990.
22. State initiatives in health care reform: New York adopts pure community rating: Other states take incremental approach. Robert Wood Johnson Foundation, Alpha Center 7:1, 1994.
23. Harris, JS: Strategic Health Care Management. Jossey-Bass, San Francisco, 1994.
24. Abramowitz, KS: The Future of Health Care Delivery in the United States. Sanford C Bernstein & Co, New York, 1993.
25. Group Health Association of America: National Directory of HMOs: 1991. Group Health Association of America, Washington, DC, 1991.
26. Dudley, RA: Managed care in transition. N Engl J Med 344:1087, 2001.
27. Gabel, J et al: Job-based health benefits in 2002: Some important trends. Health Affairs 21:143, 2002.
28. Morrison, EM, and Luft, HS: Health maintenance organization environments in the 1980s and beyond. In Harrington, C, and Estes, CL (eds): Health Policy and Nursing: Crisis and Reform in the U.S. Health Care Delivery System. Jones and Bartlett, Boston, 1994.
29. Loeppke, RR: Restructuring the American health care system. Managed Care J 2:30, 1993.
30. Kassler, J: Bitter Medicine: Greed and Chaos in the American Health Care System. Birch Lane Press, New York, 1994.
31. US Census Bureau, Health Insurance Coverage 1999, 2000.
32. Iglehart, J: Changing health insurance trends. N Engl J Med 347: 956, 2002.
33. Relman, AS: What market values are doing to medicine. In Harrington, C, and Estes, CL (eds): Health Policy and Nursing: Crisis and Reform in the U.S. Health Care Delivery System. Jones and Bartlett, Boston, 1994.
34. Harrington, C: Quality, access, and costs: Public policy and home care. In Harrington, C, and Estes, CL (eds): Health Policy and Nursing: Crisis and Reform in the U.S. Health Care Delivery System. Jones and Bartlett, Boston, 1994.
35. Omnibus Budget Reconciliation Act of 1989, Public Law No. 101–239.
36. Omnibus Budget Reconciliation Act of 1990, Public Law No. 101–508.
37. Omnibus Budget Reconciliation Act of 1987, Public Law No. 100–203.
38. Omnibus Budget Reconciliation Act of 1980, Public Law No. 96–499.
39. Omnibus Budget Reconciliation Act of 1986, Public Law No. 99–509.
40. Enthoven, AC: Health tax policy mismatch. Health Aff (Millwood) 4:5, 1985.
41. Enthoven, AC: Theory and Practice of Managed Competition in Health Care Finance. Amsterdam Publishing, North Holland, 1988.
42. Enthoven, AC, and Kronick, R: A consumer-choice health plan for the 1990s: Universal health insurance in a system designed to promote quality and economy. N Engl J Med 320:29, 1989.
43. Enthoven, AC, and Kronick, R: A consumer-choice health plan for the 1990s: Universal health insurance in a system designed to promote quality and economy. N Engl J Med 320:94, 1989.
44. Kronenfeld, JJ: Controversial Issues in Health Care Policy. Sage Publications, Newbury Park, CA, 1993.
45. Thorpe, KE: Health care cost containment. In Kovner, AR (ed.): Jonas's Health Care Delivery in the United States, 5th ed. Springer, New York, 1995.
46. The Henry J. Kaiser Family Foundation. March 2004 Medicare Fact Sheet. The Medicare Prescription Drug Law. From www.Kff.org Retrieved March 2004.

CHAPTER 4

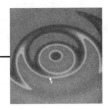

Selected Theories and Models for Advanced Practice Nursing

CHAPTER 4

Michelle Walsh, PhD, RN, CPNP
Linda A. Bernhard, PhD, RN

Michelle Walsh, PhD, RN, CPNP, is a pediatric nurse practitioner certified by the Pediatric Nursing Certification Board. She has provided primary care to children of all ages in pediatric practices in Columbus, Ohio. She has also served as a clinical preceptor for pediatric nurse practitioner students. Before becoming a nurse practitioner, she taught pediatric nursing, research, and nursing leadership to baccalaureate, master's, and doctoral students. She is coauthor of *Leadership: The Key to the Professionalization of Nursing.*

Linda A. Bernhard, PhD, RN, is Associate Professor of Nursing and Women's Studies at The Ohio State University in Columbus, Ohio. She is also Associate Dean of Academic Affairs in the College of Nursing. Her specialty is women's health. She has taught nursing leadership for many years and is coauthor of *Leadership: The Key to the Professionalization of Nursing.*

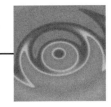

Selected Theories and Models for Advanced Practice Nursing

CHAPTER OBJECTIVES

After completing this chapter, the reader will be able to:

1 Select a theory of leadership appropriate to an area of advanced practice.

2 Explain the research utilization process in the context of planned change.

3 Apply theories of health promotion to all types of advanced practice nursing.

4 Summarize a variety of advanced nursing practice and other related nursing models.

5 Evaluate a conceptual model of collaborative nurse-physician interaction for usefulness in advanced practice nursing.

This chapter provides an introduction to a variety of theories and models that can be used in advanced practice nursing. Theories provide a framework and may lead to new ways of thinking about practice situations. Advanced practice nurses (APNs) have to think more broadly and perform at a higher level and within a broader scope of practice than other nurses. APNs may be more successful, for example, when they examine the familiar nursing process and apply concepts from various leadership or change theories in the assessment and management of clients. Theories of leadership will be presented as well as related theories and models of change, health promotion, and advanced practice nursing.

THEORIES OF LEADERSHIP

Leadership is a process that is used to move a group toward goal setting and goal achievement.[1] The components of leadership are the leader and group, the theory of leadership, and the organization. Leadership can be used by any nurse but is especially important for APNs. APNs use leadership skills to promote the health of clients and families.

Leadership theories are presented in an historical manner, demonstrating how the theories have built on each other. Although other theories can be used, the Tridimensional Leadership Model/Situational Theory[2] is the most comprehensive and is recommended. However, if the APN is conducting research on leadership, Fiedler's Contingency Theory[3] is recommended because it has been used extensively in research.

Theory X and Theory Y

Assumptions about motivation are the basis for McGregor's[4] theories of leadership. Theory X reflects the traditional view of direction and control, whereas Theory Y includes an integration of individual and organizational goals. McGregor was careful to indicate that X and Y are not opposite but separate philosophies. Theory X is the basis of managerial theory; Theory Y is operationalized through a strategy commonly referred to as management by objectives.

In Theory X, the assumption is that people dislike work and avoid it whenever possible. Because of the dislike of work, people must be controlled and directed to engage in goal-directed activity. Further, according to McGregor, people wish to avoid responsibility and prefer direction to feel secure.

A different view of people is proposed in Theory Y, which states that work is as natural as play. People are self-directed and engage freely in goal-directed activity as long as they are in agreement with the goals. It is the commitment to the goals, as well as goal attainment, that is fulfilling, making external direction unnecessary. Because all individuals have the potential to succeed, the creation of conditions that allow the individual to pursue goals is essential. By creating conditions that enable goal-setting, the leader fosters participation and creative problem-solving.

Consideration and Initiating Structure

The two constructs of consideration and initiating structure were identified through investigations to determine which behaviors used by a leader had a positive influence on group satisfaction and productivity.[5] Consideration encompasses those behaviors of the leader that emphasize concern for the individual or group. Consideration includes trust, respect, warmth, and rapport and thus encourages communication.[6] Initiating structure includes the behaviors of the leader that focus on the task to be accomplished or on the organizational goals. Initiating structure includes defining roles, assigning tasks, planning, and encouraging production.[6]

Researchers found that group productivity is more closely associated with initiating structure, whereas individual satisfaction is more dependent on consideration. However, individuals seem to be more secure when they know what is expected of them; thus, both behaviors are important for success at individual and organizational levels. Moreover, group cohesiveness is fostered by both consideration and initiating structure.

While reviewers of leadership theory indicate that the most effective leaders use consideration and initiate structure,[7] the measures and, consequently, the validity of the measurement of these two behaviors have been questioned.[8] Inconsistent findings among the studies have led to further investigation of missing variables that could explain effective leader behavior.

Path–Goal Theory

The path-goal theory was an attempt to identify the missing variables by specifying the conditions in which the leader's behavior affects member satisfaction.[9] The extent to which the leader exhibits consideration determines the members' perceptions of available rewards, whereas the extent to which the leader initiates structure determines the members' perceptions of the paths that will ultimately lead them to their goals.[7]

Using the path-goal theory, the leader initiates structure to demonstrate to members how their actions will result in goal attainment. The leader also exhibits consideration by helping to remove barriers, thereby making the path to the goal easier.[10] Both consideration and initiating structure enhance members' motivation and satisfaction to the extent that such leadership behaviors clarify the path to the goal.

Fiedler's Contingency Model and Cognitive Resource Theory

Using similar variables to develop a model of leadership effectiveness, Fiedler[11] created the contingency approach, or contingency theory. Fiedler's model measures leadership effectiveness by examining group productivity. According to Fiedler, leadership is an interpersonal relation in which power and influence are unevenly distributed so that one person is able to direct and control the actions and behaviors of others to a greater extent than they direct and control the leader's. In this model, the leader has the primary responsibility for completion of the group task.

Because leadership is a relationship based on power and influence, the leader must classify each situation based on the amount of power and influence that the group members allow the leader. In any given situation, the amount of power and influence depends on a combination of three variables, which yields a favorable or unfavorable situation for the leader.

The first variable that determines a favorable situation for the leader is the relationship between the leader and group members. The notion that the leader-member relationship is the single most important variable determining the leader's power and influence is well supported in the literature.[12] The extent to which group members accept the leader determines whether leader-member relationships are classified as good or poor.

The second variable is task structure. Routine or predictable tasks are classified as structured, whereas tasks that require analysis of multiple possibilities are classified as unstructured. The third variable, position power, refers to the leader's place within the organization and the amount of authority given to the leader by virtue of that position. Position power is not a personality characteristic; rather, it measures the leader's status in the organization. Position power is classified as strong or weak.

According to Fiedler, these three variables create eight different situations that can be ranked from "most favorable" to "least favorable." Each possible situation is numbered and termed a cell, with cell 1 characterized as the most favorable situation and cell 8 the least favorable.

On the basis of his earliest research, Fiedler predicted that cells 1, 2, and 3 were the very favorable situations and that cell 8 was the least favorable situation. Thus, using a task-centered, controlling behavior would be most effective. Cells 4, 5, 6, and 7 were intermediate situations. Thus, a more effective approach for the leader is a permissive, relationship-centered one (Table 4–1).

Fiedler continued to predict that with cells 1, 2, 3, and 8, the leader should use a more controlling or task-oriented behavior. However, he eventually determined that only cells 4 and 5 represented situations of intermediate or moderate favorableness, requiring a permissive or relationship-oriented approach.[13] Cells 6 and 7 were defined as unfavorable to the leader, and Fiedler predicted that little difference would occur in outcome, whether permissive or controlling behavior was used. Even though the model is predictive, only two conclusions are specified:

1. Task-oriented leaders will perform best in groups in which the situation is either very favorable or very unfavorable.

2. Relationship-oriented leaders will perform best in groups in which the situation is either of moderate or intermediate favorableness.

Considerable research supports the validity of the contingency model of a leader's effectiveness. Although only three variables are evaluated to determine the favorableness of a situation, these variables are the most significant in a given situation. Nonetheless, the model has been criticized because it fails to explain the underlying processes that result in a leader's effective performance.

Cell	Leader–Member Relationship	Task Structure	Position Power	Situation Rating	Preferred Behavior
1	Good	Structured	Strong	Very favorable	Controlling
2	Good	Structured	Weak	Very favorable	Controlling
3	Good	Unstructured	Strong	Very favorable	Controlling
4	Good	Unstructured	Weak	Intermediate favorableness	Permissive
5	Poor	Structured	Strong	Intermediate favorableness	Permissive
6	Poor	Structured	Weak	Intermediate favorableness	Permissive
7	Poor	Unstructured	Strong	Intermediate favorableness	Permissive
8	Poor	Unstructured	Weak	Very favorable	Controlling

TABLE 4–1. Fiedler's Contingency Table

From Fiedler, FE: A Theory of Leadership Effectiveness. McGraw-Hill, New York, 1967, p. 142, with permission.

Fiedler addressed the limitations of the contingency model by developing the cognitive resource theory.[14] Cognitive resources include the intellectual abilities, technological competencies, and job-relevant knowledge of a leader. Cognitive resources are acquired during formal education and through experience.

Cognitive resource theory is depicted in Figure 4–1. The cognitive resource theory attends to task accomplishment and the role that the group members play in task accomplishment. Task accomplishment is often the outcome of the leader's effectiveness. The leader's behavior results from both the situation and the leader's personality, as measured by the Least Preferred Coworker Scale.[14]

The most important idea from cognitive resource theory is that the situation is the most important variable. Only under certain conditions do the leader's and the members' abilities contribute positively to group performance.[14]

Tridimensional Leadership-Effectiveness Model

Hersey and Blanchard[15] used Fiedler's[11,13] early work and the consideration and initiating structure theories to propose another way of viewing leadership. They believed that no single leadership style or behavior could be effective in every situation. Combining the variables of task orientation and relationship orientation with effectiveness, Hersey and Blanchard created the tridimensional leadership-effectiveness model, in which the leader's behavior is integrated with situational dimensions. Leadership style is defined as the behavior pattern that a leader exhibits when attempting to influence the activities of others as perceived by those others.[15]

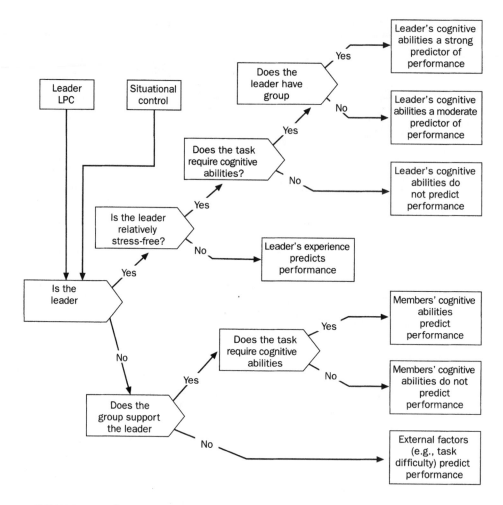

FIGURE 4–1 Fiedler's cognitive resource theory. (From Fiedler and Garcia,[14] p. 9, with permission.)

According to Hersey and Blanchard, task behaviors include organizing and defining roles of group members and directing activities. Task behaviors focus on production. Relationship behaviors include facilitating, supporting, and maintaining personal relationships through open communication. The four basic leadership styles in the model are arranged in quadrant style, with high and low combinations of relationship and task behavior, i.e., high relationship/low task, high task/high relationship, low relationship/low task, and high task/low relationship.

In addition to the task and relationship behavioral dimensions, a third dimension, effectiveness, is added. Effectiveness depends on appropriateness to the situation and is conceptualized as a continuum from effective to ineffective. The four basic styles are effective or ineffective depending on their appropriateness for the situation as seen by the group members; hence the model has been expanded as the Situational Leadership model (Fig. 4–2).

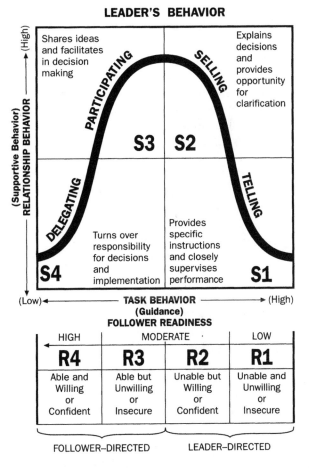

LEADER'S BEHAVIOR

FIGURE 4–2   Situational leadership model. (From Hersey and Blanchard,[15] p. 171, reprinted with permission from Paul Hersey, Escondido, CA: The Center for Leadership Studies. All rights reserved.)

Hersey and Blanchard developed an instrument, the Leader Effectiveness and Adaptability Description (LEAD), to be used with their model. The LEAD instrument measures leadership style, style range or flexibility, and style adaptability or effectiveness. Style range and adaptability are particularly important, because the more flexible a leader can be, the more likely the leader is to be effective in any situation. There are two forms of the LEAD, one for leaders to evaluate themselves (LEAD-self) and a second for group members to rate their perceptions of the leader (LEAD-other).

Certain predictions are possible without using the LEAD instruments. An indication of group members' willingness or motivation in relation to a given task, in addition to their ability or competence, gives an indication of readiness (see Fig. 4–2). Four classifications of readiness can be determined[15]:

1. R4 Member is both willing and able to accept this responsibility.

2. R3 Member is unwilling or insecure to accept this responsibility.

3. R2 Member is willing but unable to accept this responsibility.

4. R1 Member is both unwilling or insecure and unable to accept this responsibility.

After determining which level of readiness members represent, the leader can select an appropriate style.

Research results demonstrate a curvilinear relationship within the quadrants. The low-relationship, low-task quadrant style is called delegating; the high-relationship, low-task quadrant style is participating; the high-task, high-relationship quadrant style is called selling; and the high-task, low-relationship quadrant style is called telling.[15] The relationships between style and readiness are depicted in Figure 4–2. The telling style is best used with group members who have the lowest level of readiness. Members with the second lowest level of readiness respond better to the selling style. For members in the third level of readiness, participating is the most effective style. Finally, delegating, or allowing a maximum amount of freedom, is most effective for members with the highest level of readiness.[15]

Another prediction that should help the leader become more effective is based on the readiness of the group as reflected in its actual performance.[15] The leader style should shift to the left on the curvilinear line (see Fig. 4–2) when performance in the group increases and should shift to the right when performance declines.

APNs can use Situational Leadership theory by assessing their followers' readiness. Followers could be clients and families or other staff members. In the Situational Leadership theory, it is the followers who determine the appropriate leader behavior.[2] Thus, it is the needs and characteristics of clients or others that dictate the leadership behavior that will be most effective. The APN needs to be able to use a variety of leadership styles to fit each situation: persuading those who are willing while clarifying their abilities, guiding with specific clear instruction, empowering those with greater ability, and delegating.

Followers are not always in the same place on the continuum of readiness, thus the leader must use different strategies, as appropriate. When the follower/family caregiver is unable and insecure, the APN gives information in small amounts, with step-by-step guidelines, helps overcome insecurity by focusing on instructions and not overwhelming the caregiver with too much information at one time.

Health care colleagues usually may be perceived by the leader as competent, willing, and able, but they are not always. Sometimes followers are viewed as more ready, such as in an emergency, when one APN takes the leadership and directs other staff in tasks needed in priority order. Thus, the APN assesses their readiness and acts according to their readiness, moving from strategy to strategy as the situation changes.

THEORIES OF CHANGE

Change is inevitable in nursing and in society. APNs must be able to accept the changes they face as well as function as change agents to foster change in individuals and groups. Integration of the theories and models of change into the knowledge base of APNs will facilitate APNs' relationship to change.

The Freezing Model

Planned change occurs in a three-step process[16]:

1. Unfreezing
2. Moving
3. Refreezing

The freezing theory derives from field theory, a method of analyzing causal relationships. In field theory, change is due to certain forces within the field. Forces are directional entities that work in opposition to each other to maintain a dynamic equilibrium. For every force, there is an opposite force. Positive, or driving, forces indicate the likelihood of moving a system toward a desired goal. Negative, or restraining, forces indicate obstacles that decrease the likelihood of a system moving toward a desired goal.

Three possible situations result from an analysis of the forces within a field:

1. A state of dynamic equilibrium exists when the sum of the driving forces is equal to the sum of the restraining forces.
2. Change occurs in the desired direction when the sum of the driving forces is greater than the sum of the restraining forces.
3. A change in the undesired direction, or away from the desired goal, occurs when the sum of the driving forces is less than the sum of the restraining forces (Fig. 4–3). Change occurs whenever the forces in a given field are unequal.

Change involves three stages[16]:

1. Unfreezing the present level of equilibrium
2. Moving to a new level of equilibrium
3. Refreezing the new level so that it is relatively permanent

The three stages occur sequentially, with the moving phase dependent on the outcome of the unfreezing phase and with the refreezing phase dependent on the outcome of the moving phase.

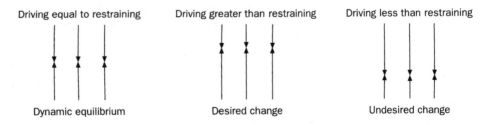

FIGURE 4–3 Driving and restraining forces. (From Bernhard and Walsh,[1] p. 169, with permission.)

Unfreezing

During unfreezing, conditions are viewed as stable, or "frozen." Change begins with a felt need, a desired goal that has not been achieved. When one individual shares a felt need with another individual, unfreezing has begun. During the unfreezing phase, the current condition is analyzed critically.

The goal of the unfreezing phase is to clarify the present situation and make persons aware of the need for change by creating dissatisfaction with the situation. The target of change can be attitudes, knowledge, and/or behaviors. A change agent encourages group members to raise questions and explore their feelings and attitudes about present conditions. When group members acknowledge their dissatisfaction with the present situation, they begin to commit themselves to the change process. For change to occur, a plan that maximizes driving forces and minimizes restraining forces is made.

Moving

The goal of the moving phase is to achieve the desired change. The moving phase is also known as the changing phase because it is during this phase that the change is implemented. The moving phase depends on the outcome of the unfreezing phase. If the equilibrium has been upset in a favorable fashion—driving forces exceed restraining forces—then the desired change can occur. Moving ends when the change has been fully implemented; that is, the desired change in knowledge, attitude, or behavior has occurred. When the target has been changed, refreezing can occur.

Refreezing

The goal of the refreezing phase is stabilization of the change. The new knowledge, attitude, or behavior learned during the moving phase must continue to be practiced until it becomes as familiar as the one that preceded it. The change agent can help the group to refreeze by actions that help to legitimate the change, such as providing articles for the group to read about others who have made the same or a similar change.

Refreezing represents the end point in the change process and indicates that the change has been fully accepted and internalized. The change agent knows that refreezing has occurred when group members consistently demonstrate the new attitude or behavior and talk positively about it, their words and actions being congruent. Once it has been determined that refreezing has occurred, the group's performance should be evaluated periodically to confirm that the planned change is indeed refrozen.

Strategies for Changing

Chin and Benne[17] presented a model of strategies for changing. Strategies are approaches used by the change agent to influence a group to adopt a proposed change. The three strategies, which may be used individually or in combination, are:

1. Empirical-rational
2. Normative-reeducative
3. Power-coercive

The empirical-rational strategy is based on the closely related assumptions that human beings are rational and that they follow a pattern of self-interest. From these basic assumptions, it follows that people will change when they understand that a proposed change is rationally justified and is beneficial to them. The empirical-rational strategy is the oldest and most frequently used strategy. It is based on reason and intelligence.

The normative-reeducative strategy is a more active strategy. People do what they do because of held norms and commitment to those norms. Norms come from society, culture, religion, and family or from other sources. Change occurs when commitment to some present norm decreases to a point where a new norm can be adopted. Thus, change resulting from the normative-reeducative strategy is a modification of values and attitudes as well as of behavior.

The normative-reeducative strategy requires direct intervention by a change agent to aid in the unlearning and relearning process. The individual and change agent actively work together to produce the change. Behavioral science techniques, such as consciousness-raising, may be used to help individuals become aware of their values and norms so that they may change to new ones.

The power-coercive strategy requires some type of legitimate power to force compliance with change. Very simply, those with greater power influence and control those with lesser power. The power-coercive strategy may be used by persons in top-level positions of an organization to effect change that they believe is needed. The group affected by the change is forced to comply, without having any input. Because of its approach, there are many disadvantages to the power-coercive strategy; however, combined with another strategy, it may be used to promote acceptance by group members.

With any strategy, the change agent must allow time for the group to accept and/or practice the change. Practice time serves as a trial period that allows the group to adjust to and experience the benefits of a new condition. The group is then able to evaluate its new knowledge, attitude, or behavior. When group members see that their new knowledge, attitude, or behavior meets their desired goal, they will be reluctant to return to their former ways of thinking and acting.

When selecting a strategy, change agents must take into account both their relationship with the group and the target of change. Change agents will be most effective when the strategy used is consistent with the overall goals of the planned change and does not jeopardize the relationship with group members.

Change in Practice by the APN

In addition to the theories of Lewin[16] and Chin and Benne,[17] the APN should be familiar with the process of research utilization. Research utilization or evidence-based practice is a planned change process. Research utilization is important to improve clinical practice, providing a link between problem identification and problem-solving that incorporates current research-based knowledge.

The research utilization process involves reviewing existing research-based knowledge to determine whether substantive investigations have been conducted that address the practice problem to be solved. Elements of traditional research critique are used in identifying and summarizing the research base. In Stetler's model[18] of research utilization, at least three phases must occur before the decision is made to use research in practice:

1. Preparation
2. Validation
3. Comparative evaluation

When data are insufficient or when no research base to guide the APN exists, an original research approach may be needed. The research process and the research utilization process are quite similar (Table 4–2). When a sufficiently strong research base exists, the change or "innovation" can be introduced by the APN. The innovation should first be introduced on a trial basis to allow group modification and acceptance of the innovation. The APN should incorporate a sufficient evaluation plan—often a replication study in one's own setting to determine the effectiveness of the innovation to solve the identified practice problem.

TABLE 4–2. The Research Process Compared with the Research Utilization Process

Research ← Interdependent processes →	Research utilization
Purpose: To identify and refine solutions to problems through the generation of new knowledge	*Purpose:* To get the new solutions used for the good of society: to identify need for refinement
Delimit problem.	Identify patient-care problem.
Review related literature. Develop conceptual framework.	Identify and assess research-based knowledge to solve problem.
Identify variables.	Design nursing practice innovation and patient outcomes based on research knowledge.
Select design. Formulate hypothesis.	Compare patient outcomes produced by innovation with those of existing practice.
Specify population. Select sample.	Choose patient sample representative of those in original research.
Develop or select instruments.	Use instruments identified in original research.
Collect data.	Conduct clinical trials.
Analyze data.	Analyze data.
Interpret results.	Decide to adopt, alter, or reject full-scale implementation of innovation.
Communicate findings.	Develop a means to extend (diffuse) the new practice and maintain it over time.

From: Firlit, S, Kemp, MG, and Walsh, M: Preparing master's students to develop clinical trials to confirm research findings. West J Nurs Res 8:108. Copyright 1986 by Sage Publications, Inc. Reprinted by permission of Sage Publications, Inc.

The process of research utilization includes the following phases or steps[19]:

1. Identify the patient care problem.
2. Identify and assess relevant research-based knowledge.
3. Conduct a trial of the innovation.
4. Decide whether to adopt, modify, or reject the innovation.
5. Develop the means to extend or diffuse the adopted innovation.
6. Develop mechanisms to maintain the innovation over time.

As guidelines or standards of practice change, the APN can use change theory to move a group to accepting and using the new standard of care. Many clinical areas are using needle-less systems and changing to newer safety needles to decrease needlestick injuries among health providers. The APN can facilitate such changes by introducing the new needle-less systems or demonstrating the safety needles to other health professionals. The APN may involve other health professionals in comparative evaluation of the available products and, when feasible, include them in final decision-making.

MODELS OF HEALTH PROMOTION

Advanced practice nursing consists of a variety of skills, but one of the most important for all APNs is health promotion. Health promotion is a goal of all nurses, but for many APNs it is their principal goal. If the best method for predicting people's participation in health behaviors can be identified, APNs can intervene in the most effective ways with their clients. These are some of the models and theories that the APN might use for health education, anticipatory guidance, and health promotion.

Health Belief Model

The health belief model (HBM) was developed in the 1950s to explain people's actions (or lack of actions) regarding preventive health behavior.[20] Through considerable research over the years, the HBM has been clarified and modified, and it is now used to explain or predict people's use of a broad range of health actions.[21]

The underlying assumption of the HBM is that behavior is determined more by a person's perceived reality than by the physical environment. People take actions to screen for or prevent a disease or health problem but only to the extent that the disease exists in their perception. Further, people must have incentives for action and feel themselves capable before undertaking a given health action.[22] The HBM is represented in Figure 4–4. Sociodemographic variables, such as age or race, are assumed to influence behavior indirectly, through effects on the other components.

The likelihood of action is based on individual perceptions of the threat of disease, modifying factors including cues to action, and perceived benefits minus barriers. Threat consists of the perceived susceptibility, that is, people's subjective beliefs about their own vulnerability to develop a disease or their ability to accept the

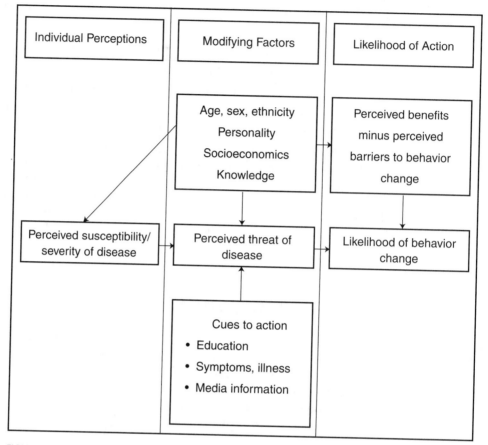

FIGURE 4–4   Health belief model. (From Strecher and Rosenstock,[21] p. 48. Health Behavior and Health Education, Glanz, K, Lewis, FM, and Riner BK (eds.). Copyright 1997 Jossey-Bass. Reprinted by permission of John Wiley & Sons, Inc.)

diagnosis of a disease, and their perception of the seriousness or severity of the disease and the (medical or social) consequences of the disease should it develop.

Demographic characteristics, e.g., sex, socioeconomic status, influence how an individual perceives threat as well as benefits and barriers. Cues to action are triggers that may promote action. Cues may be internal, such as physical symptoms, or external, such as the media or discussion with someone who has the disease. Cues to action apparently influence how individuals perceive threat, but they have not been studied systematically.

Peoples' perceived benefits to action minus the barriers of taking the action directly affect the likelihood of action. Both benefits and barriers are beliefs, rather than objective facts; that is, they are individual perceptions.

Self-efficacy, the belief that a person can actually perform the necessary behavior to achieve the desired outcome,[23] has become an important concept in its own right. Although some have tried to incorporate self-efficacy into the HBM, the originators of the model consider self-efficacy, or the lack thereof, to be a barrier to action.[21]

The most common criticism of the HBM is that the relationship between beliefs and behavior has never been established clearly. Many studies have been conducted using the HBM to explain or predict actions as diverse as having a Pap smear, maintaining a diet, and writing a living will. The amount of variance explained differs considerably, suggesting that other factors are involved. Still, until other factors are identified specifically, many researchers and APNs will continue to use the HBM in research and to guide practice.

Health Promotion Model

In an attempt to define additional variables that might explain preventive health behavior, Pender[24] took the HBM, added a number of cognitive variables, and applied it to nursing practice. As she expanded and clarified her thinking, she created the health promotion model (HPM).[25] Pender views the HPM as an organizing framework for theory development and research and acknowledges that it is continually subject to change.

The HPM is shown in Figure 4–5. The HPM shows the great complexity involved in explaining the performance of health behaviors, and the model has increased in complexity as it has developed. Most simply, the model shows that an individual's personal biological, psychological, and sociocultural characteristics, as well as certain behavioral and cognitive processes, are responsible for health behaviors. The boxes and arrows in the model demonstrate that the cognitive processes are interrelated and that personal characteristics and cognitive processes may, both directly and indirectly, result in health behavior.

New variables were added to this revision of the model. Perhaps the most important is commitment to a plan of action, as researchers have long questioned whether deciding to perform a behavior and actually performing a behavior are the same or different processes. Pender apparently has joined the forces of those who believe that they are unique.

To facilitate their health promotion research, Pender and her colleagues[26] developed the Health-Promoting Lifestyle Profile (HPLP), to be used in research as a predictor variable that represents health action. The original HPLP was used in large numbers of research studies, but it too has been revised. The HPLP-II is a 52-item questionnaire that has been analyzed to include six factors[27]:

1. Health responsibility
2. Physical activity
3. Nutrition
4. Interpersonal relations
5. Spiritual growth
6. Stress management

Together, these factors represent a balanced and positive approach to healthful living and wellness potential.

Researchers and APNs can use the HPM and the HPLP-II. Researchers may use the HPLP-II as either a dependent or an independent variable. APNs can use the HPM as a framework for thinking about health behavior. APNs can use results

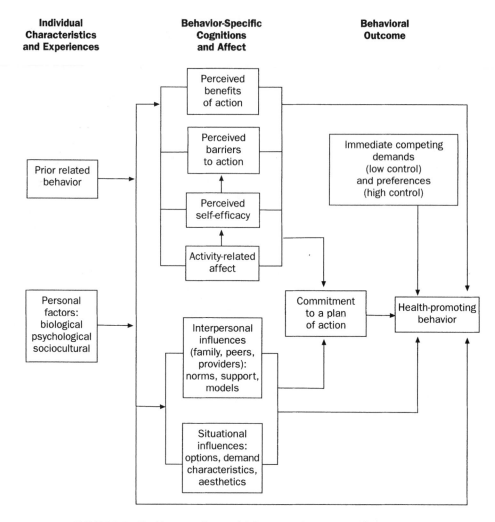

FIGURE 4–5   Health promotion model. (From Pender,[27] p. 67, with permission.)

of the HPLP-II to communicate specifically with clients about aspects of their health.

PRECEDE-PROCEED Model

The PRECEDE-PROCEED model is used for comprehensive planning in health education and health promotion with individuals and communities.[28-30] The acronym stands for predisposing, reinforcing, and enabling causes in educational diagnosis and evaluation (PRECEDE) and policy, regulatory, and organizational constructs in educational and environmental development (PROCEED). Although PRECEDE was developed and used before PROCEED was added, both are integrated into a single model.

The PRECEDE portion of the model is the diagnostic phase that assists the APN in considering the many factors that influence health status and in choosing a highly focused subset of factors as the target for a health intervention.[28-30] The PROCEED phase provides steps for developing policy and for initiating the implementation and evaluation processes of health intervention.[29]

A unique feature of the model is the concept of "beginning at the end." Instead of planning an intervention that promotes outcomes, the APN looks first at extant outcomes or the quality of life of the designated population or individual. The APN must ask "why" before "how" and, by thinking deductively, identify consequences before seeking causes. As seen in Figure 4–6, the process is ultimately circular.

In the initial social diagnosis phase, the APN considers the general hopes or problems of the target population by having them engage in a self-assessment, which, in itself, can be an educational process. In phase 2, epidemiological diagnosis, specific health goals or problems that contribute to the issues or problems identified in phase 1 are identified. During phase 3, specific behavioral or environmental factors that could be linked with the problems established as most important

Precede

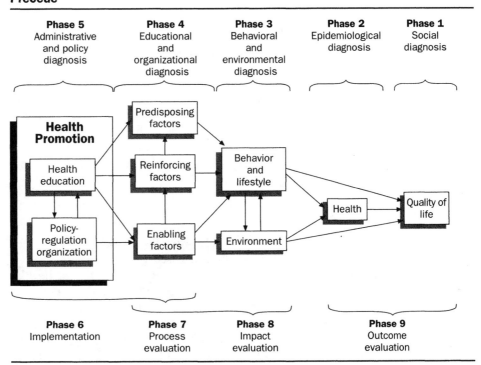

Proceed

FIGURE 4–6   PRECEDE-PROCEED model. (From Green and Kreuter,[29] p. 24, with permission.)

in phase 2 are identified. Because these problems will be the focus of the intervention, they must be described as specifically as possible.

Phase 4 is termed the educational and organizational diagnosis. The large number of potential factors that could influence a given health behavior are identified, sorted, and categorized into three classes:

1. Predisposing factors
2. Enabling factors
3. Reinforcing factors

Predisposing factors are those attitudes, values, perceptions, and knowledge that foster or inhibit motivation for change. Enabling factors are those skills and resources that make possible behavioral or environmental changes. Barriers to change must also be considered, because some resources (e.g., laws) may either foster or inhibit changes. Reinforcing factors include the rewards, feedback, and support received after adoption of a change. As with enabling factors, there are some reinforcing factors (e.g., weight gain) that can encourage or discourage continuation of a change.

In phase 5, the APN assesses the resources, policies, abilities, and constraints of the situation or organization, then selects the best combination of methods and strategies to be implemented in phase 6. Although various types of evaluation are noted for phases 7 through 9, evaluation is a continuous process throughout the model.

PRECEDE-PROCEED can be used in a variety of community, workplace, and health care settings. PRECEDE has been used for health education programs of many types and in numerous settings. PRECEDE-PROCEED has been used in programs to decrease blood pressure and to stop smoking. Green and Kreuter[29] suggested that using the whole model makes planning and evaluation of health promotion programs more efficient and effective. For example, women who quit smoking cigarettes when pregnant tend to believe that smoking cessation will benefit their babies. The APN who wants to foster continued smoking cessation after delivery might place more emphasis on teaching the mother about the effects of second-hand smoke on infants.

Theory of Care-Seeking Behavior

A more recent theory for health promotion is the theory of care-seeking behavior (CSB) developed by Lauver[31] and based on the concepts from Triandis's theory of behavior. According to the CSB theory, engaging in health care behavior is a function of the psychosocial variables of affect, utility, norms, and habits, which may be influenced by facilitating conditions (e.g., insurance and having a regular health provider). Clinical and sociodemographic variables, such as the presence of symptoms or age, do not influence behavior directly but may influence the psychosocial variables (Fig. 4–7). Affect refers to feelings; utility (i.e., expectations and values about outcomes of care) refers to one's own beliefs; norms refer to others' beliefs; and habits refer to one's usual actions concerning a proposed health behavior.[32]

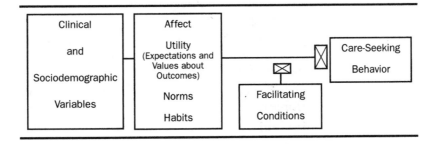

FIGURE 4–7   Care-seeking behavior model. (From Lauver,[31] p. 281, with permission.)

Empirical research findings from a number of studies support the individual relationships proposed in the CSB theory for secondary prevention, such as cancer screening.[31,32] For example, the APN who wants to teach young adult men about the importance of testicular self-examination must consider the man's feelings and beliefs about developing testicular cancer and what he hears from his buddies about it as well as the risk because of his age.

The CSB theory is similar to HBM and HPM theories, although it uses fewer variables to explain behavior, which can be an advantage for both research and practice if the CSB can be shown to predict behavior. Still, like HBM and HPM, there are very few studies that have examined all the possible variables and all the relationships within a single study. If APNs use CSB, HBM, or HPM, their clinical experiences can give support for the theory, which can then be further developed in research.

MODELS OF ADVANCED PRACTICE NURSING

Models and theories of advanced practice nursing describe primarily who an APN is and/or what an APN does. In comparison with leadership and change theories, the models of advanced practice are relatively new and are more descriptive than predictive theories.

Novice to Expert

Benner's novice-to-expert theory[33] may be the most familiar theory of advanced practice nursing. However, what Benner really describes is expert nursing[33] rather than advanced practice nursing. Nonetheless, the expert nurse may very well be an APN.

Benner's theory was based on Dreyfus's model of skill acquisition, in which increments of change occur with increases in skilled performance, based on education and experience. Three kinds of changes occur with increasing levels of proficiency:

1. There is movement from reliance on abstract principles to use of past concrete experiences as paradigms.

2. Perception of situation changes so that a situation is seen less as a compilation of equally relevant bits and more as a complete whole in which only certain parts are relevant.

3. The person changes from a detached observer to an engaged and involved performer.

Benner identified five levels of performance for nursing:

1. Novice

2. Advanced beginner

3. Competent

4. Proficient

5. Expert

Novices, with no experience in situations in which they are expected to perform, are focused only on rules and are unable to use discretionary judgment. Advanced beginners demonstrate marginally acceptable performance. Advanced beginners have had enough experience to recognize (or to see when pointed out by a mentor or instructor) the recurrent characteristics of a situation, but cannot make those characteristics objective nor differentiate importance among them. Advanced beginners operate on general guidelines or standards of care and are beginning to recognize recurrent patterns in clinical practice.

Competent nurses begin to see their actions in terms of long-range goals or plans. Competent nurses establish plans using considerable conscious, abstract, and analytic consideration of problems. However, their use of plans also limits awareness of the situation because they are focused on the plan rather than on the whole situation. Competent nurses feel a sense of mastery and the ability to cope with and manage the many contingencies of clinical nursing. They become efficient and organized. This level of competence is often viewed as ideal.

Proficient nurses continue to move forward with a vision of what is possible. Proficient nurses perceive situations as wholes rather than as parts, and their performance is guided by maxims, which are developed over time through a deep understanding of the situation. Proficient nurses know what to expect from a given situation, quickly recognize when a situation is different, and know how to modify plans when a situation varies from the expected. They acquire a perspective about the important attributes and characteristics of a situation and use fewer options while developing focus for the most important aspects of situations.

Proficiency marks the transition from competence to expertise.[34] A transformation occurs between the level of the competent nurse and the next two higher levels of performance. Proficient (and expert) nurses use past concrete experiences to guide their analyses of present situations in a way that competent nurses do not.

Expert nurses do not rely on analytic principles to connect their understanding of a situation to an appropriate action. Experts use their vast background of experience and intuitive grasp of situations to focus immediately on the accurate range of problems without wasting effort and time on a large range of unlikely possible solutions. Experts see what needs to be accomplished and how to accomplish it. They operate from a deep understanding of situations and often cannot clearly describe the rationale for their actions. What experts can describe with clarity are the goals established and the outcomes achieved.

From the descriptions of nurses about their practices, Benner[33] identified seven domains of nursing practice:

1. The helping role
2. The teaching-coaching function
3. The diagnostic and patient-monitoring function
4. The effective management of rapidly changing situations
5. The administration and monitoring of therapeutic interventions and regimens
6. The monitoring and assuring of quality of health care practices
7. The implementation of organizational and work-role competencies

In their continuing research and development of the novice-to-expert theory, Benner and her colleagues explore the complexity of clinical judgment and caring practices.[34] A limitation of Benner's work for use by APNs is the fact that the research has been limited to hospital nurses, and particularly critical care nurses.

Brykczynski, one of Benner's students, studied how experienced nurse practitioners make clinical judgments.[35] She identified the same domains in nurse practitioner practice that Benner had identified in hospital nurse practice, with one exception: the diagnostic and patient monitoring function (3 above) and the administering and monitoring of therapeutic interventions (5 above) were combined into a single "management of patient health and illness" function.

After Brykczynski presented her results to the National Organization of Nurse Practitioner Faculties (NONPF), educators began to use the domains in their teaching of nurse practitioners, and NONPF used them in revising their curriculum guidelines.[36,37] Hence, Benner's model, at least indirectly, has become the framework for education, and thus the practice, of many nurse practitioners.

Advanced Nursing Practice

Calkin[38] described a model of advanced nursing practice, defining advanced practice as that enacted by nurses with master's degrees. Calkin used the 1980 American Nurses Association definition of nursing, the "diagnosis and treatment of human responses to actual or potential health problems," as the basis for differentiating advanced practice from other levels of practice.

Calkin describes three levels of practice:

1. Novice
2. Expert-by-experience
3. Advanced

Novices, or beginning nurses, can manage only a narrow range of usual or average human responses. Because of the knowledge they bring to the clinical situation from their educational programs, Calkin suggested that novices have greater knowledge than skill. That is, they are more comfortable with the science of nursing than with the art of nursing.

Experts-by-experience are those nurses who have excelled in their ability to diagnose and treat human responses. They are able to identify and intervene in a much wider range of human responses than novices. Calkin said experts-by-experience may intuit much of their skill and may be unable to explain their actions. Nonetheless, they provide skillful care, having developed skill greater than knowledge.

Advanced practice nurses are those able to manage the fullest range of human responses that is closest to the actual range of potential responses. This ability develops as a result of the specialized knowledge and skills they acquired through education and experience. They can identify and intervene in the extremes of responses and in unpredictable as well as in predictable situations.

Calkin suggested that APNs use deliberation and reasoning more than intuition when diagnosing and treating. She argued that APNs articulate about nursing, use reasoning to deal with practice innovations, and develop or contribute to newer forms of practice. They do not focus on tasks and skills.

Differentiated Practice

Differentiated practice is another approach to describing the differences between levels of nursing practice. Koerner[39] described three levels of practice based on education:

1. Associate degree
2. Baccalaureate degree
3. Master's degree

In her integrated model, competency can be achieved at each level of nursing practice, as long as the differentiated roles and functions are clear.

The associate-degreed nurse provides care for a specified time and/or in structured settings with established policies and procedures. Care is focused primarily on the client and family. The baccalaureate-degreed nurse provides integrated health care from preadmission through post-discharge in structured and unstructured settings and/or in environments that may not have established policies and procedures. This nurse also collaborates with members of the interdisciplinary health care team for a total plan of care. The master's-degreed APN provides leadership that promotes holistic patient outcomes, functions in a variety of dynamic settings across the entire continuum of care, and uses independent nursing judgment based on theory, research, and specialized knowledge.[40] When all providers function as a team and assume equal accountability for client outcomes, quality of care can improve to a higher level.

Koerner[39] discussed the importance of mutual valuing, partnerships, and collegiality among nurses at all levels and suggested that at each level, the nurse can be an expert. Koerner further suggested that APNs support professional development by focusing on contextual and environmental issues more than do the other levels of nurses and that APNs have more career options.

Comparison of Advanced Practice Models

Advanced practice models for nursing practice consider two factors:

1. Education

2. Experience

Advanced practice requires a minimum of a master's degree. Both Koerner[39] and Calkin[38] base their models on educational preparation and define advanced practice as master's preparation. Advanced practice also requires experience in nursing, beyond that of newly graduated RNs, even if the experience is limited to that required for completion of the master's program. There is no novice APN.

Advanced practice nursing is not the same as expert nursing practice. Although Calkin[38] equated her expert level with that of Benner,[33] we believe that any nurse at any level can be an expert practitioner, but APNs are distinguished by the master's degree. Benner's model[33] was developed through research with practicing clinical nurses and reveals much about what nursing practice includes. Nurses practicing in any setting for a long enough period may become expert in that role. It is our contention that Benner's model can be applied to any nurse in any kind of practice, regardless of educational level. The level of expertise develops with experience as well as with education.

Leadership is not explicitly described by either Benner[33] or Calkin.[38] It is implicit in Benner's domains of nursing practice, especially those dealing with teaching, managing, monitoring, and organizing. Leadership is also inherent in Calkin's advanced nursing practice, because it is based on deliberative action that requires specialized skill and rationale. Leadership is an explicit part of the role of Koerner's APN.[39] APNs use leadership in all of their actions by making judgments based on theory, research, and specialized knowledge.

Collaborative Practice

Much has been published about collaboration in advanced nursing practice, even that collaborative practice by APNs and physicians (or others) is the "ideal" form of implementing the role.[41] Working together, APNs and other health care professionals create a synergism that can result in "a product that is greater than can be produced by the [individual] professionals alone."[42] Roberts[43] described a continuum of interdisciplinary practice, from parallel practice to collaborative practice. She notes that as collaboration increases, the level of professional autonomy decreases.

Parallel practice is the least collaborative, although the most familiar.[43] Communication and functions of the providers are separate; for example, the APN, physical therapist, and physician are all working with the patient on the patient's pain but do not communicate their plans except in separate medical records that may or may not be reviewed periodically by other team members. They never see the patient together.

Coordinated practice is the next level on the continuum.[43] There is a structure in place to minimize duplication of effort and to maximize use of client and provider time and resources. Consultation is common in this type of practice, but a primary provider maintains responsibility for care delivery. This type of care is usually the one preferred by third-party payers because the primary provider acts as a gatekeeper to eliminate unnecessary costs and duplication of services.

The collaborative practice model reflects increased interaction among providers. There is direct, usually face-to-face, communication and shared responsibility or comanagement for patient care. Usually, one provider seeks the expertise of another; for example, a primary care physician may ask the APN who is a diabetes educator to comanage the care of a client newly diagnosed with diabetes.

Most of what is written about collaborative practice simply lists components of collaboration and barriers to collaboration, and before any model of collaborative practice can be developed, these elements must be identified. Components of collaborative practice include: open communication, mutual trust, professional competence, shared power, joint responsibility and accountability, shared goals and vision, understanding of each other's practice style and scope of practice, and frank discussion of financial issues.[44,45] Barriers tend to be the absence or opposites of these factors, as well as gender issues, reimbursement issues, and lack of understanding by clients and families.[46]

One comprehensive model of collaborative practice is the Conceptual Model of Collaborative Nurse-Physician Interactions[44] (Fig. 4–8). Although we believe that the model can apply to any health professional collaborators, Corser developed the model for APN and physician collaboration. Central to the model is the collabora-

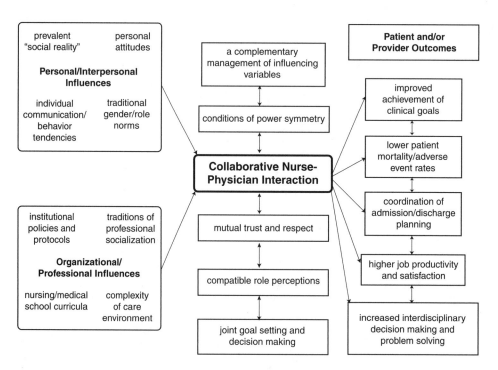

FIGURE 4–8   Conceptual model of collaborative nurse-physician interactions. (From Corser, WD: A conceptual model of collaborative nurse-physician interactions. Sch Inq Nurs Pract 12:325, 1998. Copyright. Springer Publishing Company, Inc., New York, 10012, used by permission.)

tive interaction between APN and physician. This interaction consists of many of the factors described earlier, which are affected by personal/interpersonal and organizational/professional influences that are experienced by APN and physician. Finally, this model is the only collaborative practice model that includes outcomes—for both patients and providers—as the purpose or result of collaborative practice.

SUMMARY

In each of the leadership and change models and theories, assessment of the group members is key to choosing the specific approach or style the APN would use. Assessment of the situation or organization is also necessary so that the APN can focus on goals appropriate for individuals in that setting. Finally, the relationship between the APN and the group members is critical to achieving any desired goal, such as health promotion.

The models of advanced practice nursing show the importance of education and experience of the APN. The model of collaborative practice extends beyond nursing to include interacting with other health care professionals for the improvement of client outcomes and greater job satisfaction of the professionals.

SUGGESTED EXERCISES

1. Select one of the theories of leadership presented in this chapter. Specify the variables that you would assess to determine an effective style of leadership to enact in your practice.

2. Analyze a change that occurred in your organization. Was the change planned or unplanned? Who was the change agent? What strategies were used by the change agent? Evaluate the effectiveness of the strategies, and suggest alternatives.

3. Identify a needed change in your organization. What are the driving and restraining forces that will enable or prevent the change? Develop a prospectus for planned change that takes into account the identified forces. Role-play with student colleagues, and present your prospectus to them; convince them of the soundness of your plan.

4. Discuss a problem in clinical practice. Plan a course of action to determine if a research base exists that could be used to solve the problem. Propose a clinical trial of the research-based solution.

5. Form teams. Create a health promotion clinical scenario or describe one in which you were involved. Detail all important factors in one of the health promotion models, and describe a plan for implementation. Present your work to your student colleagues, and have them critique your interpretation.

6. Analyze the similarities and differences between the Calkin and Benner models. Are these models sequential, and of what importance is this? Describe how one might apply the models to your practice situation.

7. Consider how the Calkin and Benner models relate to the concept of leadership described in this chapter. Sketch the parallels among key ideas. Again, how do the models relate to those of change presented in this chapter? Create a comparison chart.

8 Calkin described the APN role and compared it with other levels of nursing practice. A nurse colleague declares to you that "there is little or no difference between you and me in the way you practice and what you can capably perform. Just compare my 15 years of practice and experience to your education and credentials." Respond as Calkin would by identifying major characteristics of advanced nursing practice, and relate Calkin's ideas to the need and justification for your role.

9 Analyze a practice situation. Determine where the practice is on the continuum of inter-disciplinary practice. What characteristics of collaborative practice are present? What barriers to collaborative practice exist? How can you use change theory to minimize barriers?

REFERENCES

1. Bernhard, LA, and Walsh, M: Leadership: The Key to the Professionalization of Nursing, 3rd ed. Mosby, St. Louis, 1995.
2. Hersey, P, Blanchard, KH, and Johnson, DE: Management of Organizational Behavior: Utilizing Human Resources, 7th ed. Prentice-Hall, Upper Saddle River, NJ, 1996.
3. Ayman, R, Chemers, MM, and Fiedler, F: The contingency model of leadership effectiveness: Its levels of analysis. In Vecchio, RP (ed): Leadership: Understanding the Dynamics of Power and Influence in Organizations. University of Notre Dame Press, Notre Dame, IN, 1997.
4. McGregor, D: The Human Side of Enterprise. McGraw-Hill, New York, 1960.
5. Fleishman, EA: Twenty years of consideration and structure. In Fleishman, EA, and Hunt, JG (eds): Current Developments in the Study of Leadership. Southern Illinois University Press, Carbondale, IL, 1973.
6. Fleishman, EA, and Harris, EF: Patterns of leadership behavior related to employee grievances and turnover. Personnel Psychol 15:43, 1962.
7. Stogdill, RN: Handbook of Leadership: A Survey of Theory and Research. Free Press, New York, 1974.
8. Korman, AK: "Consideration," "initiating structure," and organizational criteria: A review. Personnel Psychol 19:349, 1966.
9. Evans, MG: The effects of supervisory behavior on the path-goal relationship. Organizational Behav Hum Performance 5:277, 1970.
10. Davis, K, and Newstrom, JW: Human Behavior at Work: Organizational Behavior, 7th ed. McGraw-Hill, New York, 1985.
11. Fiedler, FE: A Theory of Leadership Effectiveness. McGraw-Hill, New York, 1967.
12. Fiedler, FE, and Chemers, MM: Leadership and Effective Management. Scott, Foresman, Glenview, IL, 1974.
13. Fiedler, FE: The trouble with leadership training is that it doesn't train leaders. Psychol Today 6:23, 1973.
14. Fiedler, FE, and Garcia, JE: New Approaches to Effective Leadership: Cognitive Resources and Organizational Performance. John Wiley & Sons, New York, 1987.
15. Hersey, P, and Blanchard, KH: Management of Organizational Behavior: Utilizing Human Resources, 5th ed. Prentice-Hall, Englewood Cliffs, NJ, 1988.
16. Lewin, K: Field Theory in Social Science. Harper, New York, 1951.
17. Chin, R, and Benne, KD: General strategies for effecting change in human systems. In Bennis, WG, Benne, KD, and Chin R (eds): The Planning of Change, 4th ed. Holt, Rinehart, and Winston, New York, 1985.
18. Stetler, CB: Refinement of the Stetler/Marram Model for application of research findings to practice. Nurs Outlook 42:15, 1994.
19. Horsley, J, et al: Using Research to Improve Nursing Practice: A Guide. Grune and Stratton, Orlando, FL, 1983.
20. Rosenstock, IM: Why people use health services. Milbank Memorial Fund Quarterly 44:94, 1966.
21. Strecher, VJ, and Rosenstock, IM: The health belief model. In Glanz, K, Lewis, FM, and Riner, BK (eds): Health Behavior and Health Education, 2nd ed. Jossey-Bass, San Francisco, 1997.
22. Rosenstock, IM, Strecher, VJ, and Becker, MH: Social learning theory and the Health Belief Model. Health Educ Q 15:175, 1988.
23. Bandura, A: Self-Efficacy: The Exercise of Control. Freeman, New York, 1997.

24. Pender, N: A conceptual model for preventive health behavior. Nurs Outlook 23:385, 1975.
25. Pender, NJ, Murdaugh, CL, and Parsons, MA: Health Promotion in Nursing Practice, 4th ed. Pearson Education, Upper Saddle River, NJ, 2002.
26. Walker, SN, Sechrist, KR, and Pender, NJ: The health-promoting lifestyle profile: Development and psychometric characteristics. Nurs Res 36:76, 1987.
27. Pender, NJ: Health Promotion in Nursing Practice, 3rd ed. Appleton & Lange, Stamford, CT, 1996.
28. Green, LW, et al: Health Education Planning: A Diagnostic Approach. Mayfield, Palo Alto, CA, 1980.
29. Green, LW, and Kreuter, MW: Health promotion planning: An educational and environmental approach, 2nd ed. Mayfield, Mountain View, CA, 1991.
30. Green, LW, and Kreuter, MW: Health Promotion Planning: An Educational and Ecological Approach, 3rd ed. Mayfield, Mountain View, CA, 1999.
31. Lauver, D: A theory of care-seeking behavior. Image J Nurs Sch 24:281, 1992.
32. Lauver, D: Psychosocial variables, race, and intention to seek care for breast cancer symptoms. Nurs Res 41:236, 1992.
33. Benner, P: From Novice to Expert: Excellence and Power in Clinical Nursing Practice, Commemorative Edition. Addison-Wesley, Menlo Park, CA, 2001.
34. Benner, PA, Tanner, CA, and Chesla, CA: Expertise in Nursing Practice. Springer, New York, 1996.
35. Brykczynski, KA: Reflections on clinical judgment of nurse practitioners. Sch Inq Nurs Pract 13:175, 1999.
36. National Organization of Nurse Practitioner Faculties: Curriculum Guidelines and Program Standards for Nurse Practitioner Education, 2nd ed. NONPF, Washington, DC, 1995.
37. Price, MJ, Martin, AC, Newberry, YG, et al: Developing national guidelines for nurse practitioner education: An overview of the product and process. J Nurs Educ 31:10, 1992.
38. Calkin, JD: A model for advanced nursing practice. J Nurs Adm 14:24, 1984.
39. Koerner, J: Differentiated practice: The evolution of professional nursing. J Prof Nurs 8:335, 1992.
40. Nelson, RJ, and Koerner, JG: Context. In Koerner, JG, and Karpiuk, KL (eds): Implementing Differentiated Nursing Practice: Transformation by Design. Aspen, Gaithersburg, MD, 1994, pp. 1–21.
41. Bush, NJ, and Watters, T: The emerging role of the oncology nurse practitioner: A collaborative model within the private practice setting. Oncol Nurs Forum 28:1425, 2001.
42. Waldman, R: Collaborative practice—balancing the future. Obstet Gynecol Surv 57:1, 2002.
43. Roberts, J: Educational approaches that promote interdisciplinary collaborative practice within academic health centers. Womens Health Issues 7:323, 1997.
44. Corser, WD: A conceptual model of collaborative nurse-physician interactions: The management of traditional influences and personal tendencies. Sch Inq Nurs Pract 12:325, 1998.
45. Stapleton, SR: Team-building: Making collaborative practice work. J Nurse Midwifery 43:12, 1998.
46. Neale, J: Nurse practitioners and physicians: A collaborative practice. Clin Nurs Spec 13:252, 1999.

CHAPTER 5

Primary Care and Advanced Practice Nursing: Past, Present, and Future

Catherine L. Gilliss, DNSc, RN, FAAN

Linda Lindsey Davis, PhD, RN

Catherine L. Gilliss, DNSc, RN, FAAN, is Dean and Professor of Nursing at Yale University. She was formerly Professor and Chair of the Department of Family Health Care Nursing at the University of California, San Francisco (UCSF), where she coordinated the UCSF's Primary Care Nurse Practitioner Program, the largest graduate primary care nurse practitioner program in the nation. In 1995, the Pew Health Professions Commission recognized that program as the winner of the Excellence in Primary Care Education Award. Dr. Gilliss received her undergraduate nursing education at Duke University and has been honored by Duke's School of Nursing as a distinguished alumna. She earned her master's degree in psychiatric–mental health nursing from The Catholic University of America and an adult nurse practitioner certificate from the University of Rochester. She completed her doctoral and postdoctoral work at the UCSF's School of Nursing. Her research interests include families and chronic illness and the development of the primary care work force. Currently, she serves as Principal Investigator of the NIH/NINR–funded Exploratory Center to Eliminate Health Disparities at Yale. Dr. Gilliss has served on the boards of numerous professional societies and journals. She was the President of the Interdisciplinary Primary Care Fellowship Society, the President of the National Organization of Nurse Practitioner Faculties, and a Regent at the University of Portland (Oregon). She now serves on the Board of the American Academy of Nursing.

Linda Lindsey Davis, PhD, RN, is a Professor of Nursing at the University of Alabama at Birmingham (UAB) and senior scientist in the UAB Center for Aging. Dr. Davis is an adult nurse practitioner who holds a doctorate in nursing from the University of Maryland at Baltimore, a master's of science in nursing from the University of North Carolina at Chapel Hill, and a bachelor's in nursing from Old Dominion University in Norfolk, Virginia. Her work is in primary and long-term health care for families and family care-giving for the aged. Dr. Davis was a Robert Wood Johnson Nurse Fellow in Primary Care and has published numerous papers on family health and well-being around chronic illness issues. She has served as a scientific review group member for the TriServices Group, the American Nurses Foundation, the National Alzheimer's Association, and The National Institute of Nursing Research. Dr. Davis currently is principal investigator for a 5-year randomized trial funded by the National Institute of Nursing Research on care-giver skill training around home care for an aged family member with Alzheimer's disease or Parkinson's disease.

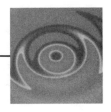

Primary Care and Advanced Practice Nursing: Past, Present, and Future

CHAPTER OBJECTIVES

After completing this chapter, the reader will be able to:

1 Analyze socioeconomic and political forces contributing to the continued emphasis on primary care systems in the United States.

2 Synthesize the implications of various health care work force projections for emerging primary care systems in the first half of the twenty-first century.

3 Weigh the advantages and disadvantages of using the following methods for evaluating advanced practice nursing in primary care settings: (a) classification of patient encounters, (b) comparison in standards of care, and (c) documentation of functions of primary care.

4 Explore facilitating and inhibiting factors influencing advanced practice nursing in emerging primary care systems.

5 Articulate a personal philosophy on the nature and scope of advanced practice nursing skills and primary care services.

Although governmental efforts in the mid-1990s failed to bring about health care reform, the American health care system implemented many of the proposed changes. While problems with health care access, quality, and service fragmentation continue to influence health care delivery models in some areas of the United States, the focus on reducing health care system expenditures through managed-care delivery has fueled continued interest in primary care systems. This chapter provides an overview of the social, political, and economic issues that have influenced primary care over the past decade and the factors that facilitate and inhibit the participation of advanced practice nurses (APNs) in primary care systems for the next two decades.

HEALTH CARE IN THE TWENTIETH CENTURY

In hierarchical health care systems, primary care has been the term used to describe basic services on which other, more specialized services are built. Presumably, primary care systems can handle as much as 99 percent of the health problems in a community.[1] In 1978, the World Health Organization proposed that primary health care, designed to bring accessible, economical care into communities where people live and work, should be a basic component of every country's health care system.[2] Primary care has been accepted as the necessary foundation for health care in the majority of industrialized nations, with the United States being a notable exception. The U.S. health care system has been described as a pluralistic, overlapping collection of practitioners providing different aspects of care in a variety of settings.[3] The late twentieth century witnessed continued dissatisfaction with U.S. health care, described by many as:

- Disease-focused, concerned more with the technology of medical diagnosis and treatment of specific diseases, rather than with holistic health care
- Fragmented, so that patients and their families receive uncoordinated, episodic treatment from various specialists for their health problems
- Inaccessible, in that services and providers are located primarily in urban population centers, creating pockets of unserved or underserved areas in rural towns and inner cities
- Costly, in that many people, particularly elderly persons, minorities, and the poor, are unable to afford needed health care services, creating growing numbers of underinsured and uninsured Americans

HEALTH CARE IN THE TWENTY-FIRST CENTURY

Because health care costs continue to account for more than 20 percent of the gross national product, solutions to the problems in the American health care system continue to be defined in economic terms.[4] Because of the promised cost savings of managed care, the numbers of individuals, families, and communities enrolled in health maintenance organizations (HMOs) have stimulated competition between large and small, public and private health care organizations to develop and offer various primary care plans. In part, as a result of these trends, changes in the system that contributed to these trends over the past decade have included the following[5-9]:

- Downsizing or closure of many hospitals nationwide
- Increased emphasis on disease prevention and health promotion, both for cost savings to the system as well as for quality-of-life benefits to consumers
- Development of health care partnerships between medical centers and corporate and business entities to deliver the most economical health care for enrolled and prepaid populations
- Utilization of health outcome data as justification for spending health care dollars
- Significant expansion of primary care in ambulatory and community-based settings
- Sweeping changes in the education and practice of health professionals to staff these emerging primary care systems

For more than 30 years, health care providers, educators, and policy makers in the United States have described primary care as an economical strategy for increasing consumer access to a broad range of holistic and humanistic services. To many, continued investment in primary care systems in the United States represents a logical solution to long-standing problems that have troubled the American health care delivery system in the past: unequal access, rising costs, fragmentation, and overemphasis on medical technology.

THE NATURE OF PRIMARY CARE

Definitions of Primary Care

Definitions of primary care have evolved. White[10] defined primary care as first-contact care. Alpert and Charney[11] added that primary care medicine involves longitudinal responsibility for a patient, including integration of both health and disease services. In 1978, the Institute of Medicine[12] (IOM) defined primary care as having the functions of improved accessibility, continuity, comprehensiveness, coordination, and accountability. Golden[13] reported that primary care is characterized by long-term, close relationships between practitioner and patient and family, in which the primary care provider treats common and acute illnesses, with referral to specialists of patients with less frequently occurring and more complex problems. Starfield[14] summarized the four key functions of primary care:

1. First contact, in which services are timely, accessible, and available at the point of entry into the system
2. Longitudinal, in that services, organized to focus on the patient and not the illness, are provided to the patient by the same provider over time

3. Comprehensive, in that a broad range of services are offered by the provider

4. Coordinated, in that a single provider organizes information related to patient referral, procedures, and therapies to improve the continuity and quality of care

The IOM[15] reexamined early definitions of primary care as a first step toward projecting the future of health care in the United States. The revised IOM definition includes many of the elements originally introduced but added a focus on the family and community contexts in which care should be provided:

> Primary care is the provision of integrated, accessible health care services by clinicians who are accountable for addressing a large majority of personal health care needs, developing a sustained partnership with patients, and practicing in the context of family and community. (p. 16)

In fact, there is mounting concern that the very definition of primary care must be challenged.[50] A recent proposal suggests seven core principles to support the renaissance of primary care[51]:

- Health care must be organized to serve the needs of patients.
- The goal of primary care systems should be the delivery of the highest quality care as documented by measurable outcomes.
- Information and information systems are the backbone of the primary care process.
- Current health care systems must be reconstructed.
- The health care financing systems must support excellent primary care practice.
- Primary care education must be revitalized, with an emphasis on the new delivery models and training sites that deliver excellent primary care.
- The value of primary care practice must be continually improved, documented, and communicated.

Content of Primary Care

Based on the IOM definition, a number of assumptions can be made about the nature of primary care. Integrated primary care must include consideration of the total person—body and mind—as well as the context in which care occurs. Accessible care must be personalized according to the needs of individuals within their communities. The majority of primary care includes both episodic and ongoing services. A sustained partnership between primary care provider and patient over the life cycle implies the provider's need for knowledge about biomedical health problems, social sciences (including personal, interpersonal, and larger social systems), and the way to work successfully with other providers in interdisciplinary practice teams. Given the socioeconomic and political contexts in which primary care is practiced today, providers also need to understand expected and desired outcomes of care based on normative evidence and the particular client's situation. The sophistication required to accomplish these expectations cannot be overestimated.

Generalist Versus Specialist Care

The more recent IOM definition of primary care suggests that there are significant distinctions to be made between generalist and specialist care. Primary care involves the delivery of health care services by generalist practitioners, with referral of patients to specialists for complex health problems. Table 5–1 shows examples of generalist services delivered by primary care providers. The characteristics, processes, and goals of generalist and specialist care are not the same. The goal of specialty practice is to cure or treat a specific problem, disease, or illness. The goal of generalist care is health promotion, prevention of disease or illness, and amelioration of symptoms.[13] Table 5–2 compares generalist with specialist care.

According to Starfield,[14] the nature of hospital-based education and practice makes it difficult for specialists to provide the key components of primary care described earlier. First-contact primary care typically occurs early in the natural history of a health problem, when evolving signs and symptoms cannot easily be tied to a specific disease or illness. In addition, because many of the presenting problems seen in primary care settings can be traced to stressful personal, familial, or environmental factors, counseling and affective support are often the major treatment components. Hospital-based training and practice do not provide experiences and skills necessary for managing the physical, psychological, or social problems that are commonly presented in primary care settings (e.g., individual patient problems such as stress reaction, vague anxiety and confusion, family turmoil

---

TABLE 5–1. Examples of Primary Care Services

- Preventive care and screening
- Health and nutrition education and counseling
- History-taking
- Physical examination
- Diagnostic testing
- Prescription and management of drug therapy
- Prenatal care and delivery of normal pregnancies
- Well-baby care
- Diagnosis and treatment of common health problems and minor injuries
- Diagnosis and treatment of chronic conditions
- Minor surgery
- Coordination of services and referral for specialty care when needed

Adapted from The Alliance for Health Reform: A Primary Care Primer, The Alliance for Health Reform, Washington, DC, 1993, p 14, with permission.

TABLE 5–2. Specialist Versus Generalist Services

Service Characteristic	Specialist Care	Generalist Care
Nature of service	**Scope of services:** Management of specific, complex problems	**Scope of services:** Management of varied problems, needs
Focus of service	Problem-focused, short-term, episodic service for diagnosis and treatment of specific problem	Patient-focused, long-term, continuous delivery of services
Role of service provider	Direct-care provider	Direct-care provider, plus plan and coordinate service delivery provided by others

relating to marital conflict or adolescent crises, alcohol or other substance use, divorce or death or dying of a family member). Because of the time spent in developing and implementing successful interventions for managing these and similar primary care problems, specialist providers often have less time to see specialty patients and less time to stay current on new knowledge and discoveries in their specialties. Finally, primary care delivery is difficult for a specialist because few specialists have the educational preparation, background experiences, or skills to perform the time-consuming but necessary function of coordinating services provided by others.

Evaluation of Primary Care

There are numerous approaches to evaluating clinical services. Three methods that have potential for documenting the nature and scope of advanced nursing practice in primary care systems are:

1. Classification of patient encounters
2. Comparison in standards of care
3. Documentation of functions of primary care

A brief description of the three methods and an example of a recent study using each method demonstrate their usefulness for evaluating advanced nursing practice in primary care settings.

Classification of Patient Encounters

Patient encounters are classified according to whether visits are first encounters; encounters for continuing care by the same provider; encounters for ongoing, nonspecialized services; or encounters for consultation and referral to a specialist. Alternatively, visits are classified according to whether they are primarily for health screening or prevention, for health promotion, for management of a specific illness (acute or chronic), or for referrals to specialized services not available in the primary care setting.

Most of the information on patient encounters in primary care settings comes from data collected through the periodic National Ambulatory Care Survey (NACS).[16] The NACS is an ongoing survey of community-based physicians stratified by specialty and by geographic regions in the United States. Conducted annually since 1990, the survey data continue to demonstrate that the majority of visits to U.S. physicians by individuals in all age groups is for management of specific symptoms, the most common being that of colds. Screening or preventive services continue to rank below symptom management as the common reason for patient encounters with a primary care physician.[16] The NACS's exclusive focus on physicians does not permit characterization of patient encounters with non-physician providers. A more widely defined focus would be useful in classifying APN encounters with patients in primary care settings.

Classification of encounters provides a typology of service needs and of services delivered. Classification of the purposes of patient encounters allows providers and administrators to identify individual and family service needs within a target population. Classification of patient encounters according to the predominant focus of each encounter also enables evaluators in multidisciplinary settings to determine which member of the multidisciplinary team is providing those services. By classifying the encounter, evaluators are able to determine whether physicians are providing most of the illness management services and/or whether nurse practitioners (NPs) are providing most of the health screening procedures.

This method also enables evaluators to analyze the nature of service referrals. For example, the evaluator may wish to know whether providers are referring emotional or social problems outside the primary care setting, even though competent care providers are available in that setting. Finally, a frequency count of the types of services offered can assist in determining whether staff continuing education is needed. However, classification of patient encounters by service need and service frequency does not assess quality of care.

Comparison in Standards of Care

With the standards-of-care method, patient encounters are analyzed to determine whether they meet commonly accepted standards for quality of care, such as the appropriate use of diagnostic tests, the accurate recognition of the patient problems, selection and implementation of an acceptable regimen for treatment, documentation of plans for patient education, and follow-up care. Given the current emphasis on patient outcome data, this evaluation method enables evaluators to compare actual patient outcomes with expected patient outcomes.

A good example of a study of compliance with commonly accepted standards of care in primary care practice may be found in the work of Avorn, Everitt, and Baker.[17] These investigators compared 501 practicing physicians and 298 practicing NPs in their approach to a patient presenting with epigastric pain. Using a case vignette of a patient presenting with a history of aspirin, coffee, cigarette, and alcohol use plus severe psychological stress and the negative results of an endoscopy, the investigators compared the reported treatment decisions of the two types of providers. An analysis of the reported practices of the two provider groups indicated that nearly half of the physician sample recommended immediate treatment of the hypothetical patient with medication, whereas only 20 percent of the NPs recommended immediate medication as the desirable action. Investigators found that the physician sample more often omitted the standard practice of collecting an adequate medical history. In contrast, the NP group more often recommended a more extensive medical history before making a treatment choice and, when making treatment choices, more frequently began with nonpharmacological interventions. These findings led investigators to conclude that the medical providers were less likely to comply with standard history-taking procedures. Although this study relied on the responses of two types of providers regarding their actual practice activities, the results indicate a significant difference in physician and NP practice activities. This method has great potential for further exploration of APN adherence to quality-of-care standards.

Comparing practice activities with commonly accepted standards of care is a useful assessment of the quality of patient care. Evaluation of compliance with quality-of-care studies is also useful to identify continuing education needs among providers. The Avorn, Everitt, and Baker[17] study recommended enhanced physician continuing education about the importance of extensive history-taking before initiating a treatment regimen.

The standards-of-care method would be particularly useful for documenting the quality of care delivered by APNs in primary care settings. However, this evaluation method does not document whether desirable primary care functions, as described earlier, are present in the practices of providers.

Documentation of Functions of Primary Care

Documentation of functions of primary care assesses whether selected primary care characteristics are present in the care delivered. For example, patient encounters might be analyzed and given a score based on whether the encounters are longitudinal, comprehensive, and coordinated. As managed care models continue to proliferate, evaluation studies that document the existence of functions believed to demonstrate the advantages of primary care will likely become more commonplace. An example of a study of how provider characteristics can influence care delivery demonstrates the potential of this method for documenting the advantages of advanced nursing practice in primary care.

As part of a larger study of medical outcomes in the United States, Safran, Tarlov, and Rogers[18] documented primary care characteristics in the care provided to 1208 patients by physicians. The physicians practiced in either traditional fee-for-service care plans or were employed by HMOs or independent practice associations (IPAs). Patients with one of four conditions—hypertension, diabetes, congestive heart failure, or recent myocardial infarction—were asked to complete a series of questionnaires about whether the care they received over a 2-year period had the characteristics of:

- Accountability (interpersonal and technical)
- Accessibility (financial and organizational)

- Continuity and comprehensiveness
- Coordination

Patients who received care through the HMO or IPA model reported greater financial accessibility and better coordination of care. However, those patients who received care through a traditional fee-for-service (private practice) model reported greater continuity and better organizational access and provider accountability. Investigators concluded from these mixed findings that the orientation of individual practitioners influences the characteristic nature of the services provided.

The documented-characteristics evaluation method can also be used to identify the presence of other functions considered to be exemplary of high quality primary care (e.g., the family-centered nature of a patient encounter, the use of existing community-based resources for referrals, and so forth). This method also would be useful in determining whether advanced practice in primary care settings demonstrates the desired function of primary care contacts. Table 5–3 outlines the three different approaches to evaluation of primary care. Because each of these common approaches to primary care evaluation has both strengths and limitations, some combination of the three would likely provide the best assessment of the nature, scope, and quality of care and of the unique characteristics of advanced nursing practice in primary care settings.

PRIMARY CARE PROVIDERS IN THE TWENTY-FIRST CENTURY

The rapid and successful growth of managed care plans in the last decade has stimulated considerable discussion about who will provide care in the emerging health care delivery systems. Successful efforts in building a primary health care delivery system, to a great extent, depend on the number and types of health care generalists needed for delivery of services; the availability and ideal mix of providers; and the incentives for, benefits of, and barriers to practice.

Physicians as Primary Care Providers

Although the need for primary care physicians (i.e., generalist practitioners in family practice, internal medicine, or pediatrics) by the year 2000 was estimated to be as high as 50 percent of practicing physicians, medical practice continues to focus largely on specialty care.[19] A recent report on the physician work force projects that medical and surgical specialists will continue to increase in states where personal income levels are greater. Conversely, general practitioners are in shorter supply in the "richer" states.[20] In December 1999, there were 797,634 physicians in the United States, only 11 percent of whom self-identified as family or general practitioners.[60] These data run counter to the Council on Graduate Medical Education projection set forth in a 1999 report,[61] forecasting an increase in the numbers of generalist physicians. In fact, changes in health care economics have worked in favor of increasing the numbers of non-physician clinicians and decreasing the

TABLE 5–3. Three Approaches to Evaluating Primary-Care Services

Method	Purpose of Evaluation	Examples of Evaluation Data	Strengths/ Limitations of Methods
Classification of patient encounters	Determine the nature and scope of services provided.	Classification of patient visits according to a purpose such as screening, management of disease, or consultation	• Helpful for determining needs of target population • Useful for determining staffing needs • Useful for staff continuing education • Not useful in assessing quality of services provided • Useful in assessing quality of specific services
Comparision of standards of care	Compare services provided against accepted standards for quality of care.	Comparison of encounter against known standards of care for problem such as: • Problem identification • Use of diagnostic tests • Treatment regimen • Patient education	• Useful for staff continuing education • Not helpful in considering the unique characteristics of primary care
Documentation of functions of primary care	Document the presence or absence of functional characteristics of high-quality primary care.	• Use of setting for first contact • Length of relationship with one care provider for longitudinality • Documentation of results of referrals in patient records for coordination • Evidence that a variety of patient problems are managed for comprehensiveness	• Useful in assessing whether key primary care functions are present in patient encounters • Not useful in assessing quality of care

numbers of physicians entering primary care. There are two competing predictions about the supply of primary care physicians for the next decade: there will be either a deficit or an adequate supply of primary care physicians.

The Physician Supply-Deficit Prediction

Critics have identified several organizational factors that discourage the rapid shift of medical education and practice from hospital-based specialty care to community-based generalist care. First, as secondary and tertiary settings, hospitals and health science centers provide the necessary technological support for medical-specialist education and practice. Second, existing mechanisms for medical-student education funding continue to favor specialty practice. Most medical student education occurs traditionally in hospitals, with more than 80 percent of the cost of medical resident training covered by the provision of in-patient clinical services. Last, because primary care residencies typically generate less clinical revenue than specialty residencies, many teaching hospitals have been reluctant to reduce specialty residencies in exchange for an increase in the number of generalist care residencies.[21]

Efforts to increase the number of medical primary care providers in the United States have concentrated on providing incentives for medical schools to establish more family practice training and residency programs and to encourage more new physicians to choose the generalist practice option.[11,14,19] Despite incentives that favor medical school applicants with a stated interest in generalist practice, which increases medical students' exposure to primary care and generalist practice by way of more community-based education and residency training, and despite offering student loan forgiveness for those choosing primary care, the number of new graduates entering specialty practice has remained constant.[22] Levinsky[23] speculated that primary care practice will continue to be unattractive to physicians for several reasons:

- Lack of financial incentives, because the annual income of generalist physicians is typically 40 to 60 percent less than that of specialists
- Reduced satisfaction with the physician-patient relationship, which many physicians relate to the loss of practice autonomy as physicians become employees of managed-care practices
- The large number of "unsatisfying" patients seen in primary care settings (i.e., elderly, poor, HIV-positive, and substance-use patients and others for whom medical treatment options are limited and long-term and for whom successful medical outcomes are unlikely)

In the early 1990s, the growth of managed care was hailed as an impetus for growth in the number of primary care physicians in the United States. However the opposite has occurred, with graduating medical student interest in primary care declining an estimated 8 percent between 1997 and 2000.[52] In a widely cited paper published in the Harvard Business Review,[53] the reasons given for decline in new medical school graduates interested in primary care were defined as the era of "disruptive" innovation that resulted from increased production of nurse practitioners and physician assistants who perform many primary care services faster, better, and (most importantly in the managed-care marketplace) cheaper.

The Adequate Physician Supply Prediction

More optimistic forecasters predict that the same market issues catalyzing change in the health care system during the last decade will ultimately bring about the necessary refocusing of medical education and practice. Iglehart[24] has noted that, as academic health science centers find themselves increasingly in competition with HMOs and other providers of comprehensive services, attempts to recast medical education and service delivery programs into community-based models will accelerate. The resulting adjustment in medical education and practice will produce the necessary numbers of generalist (primary care) physicians well into the twenty-first century. These two competing predictions—for a deficit of primary care physicians and an adequate supply of primary care physicians—complicate drawing conclusions about the supply of primary care physicians for the next decades.

Physician Assistants in Primary Care

Since the passage of Medicare and Medicaid laws in the 1960s, federal efforts in primary care have focused on increasing the numbers of both non-physician and physician generalists. Early efforts to build a cadre of primary care providers in the United States occurred in the 1960s, when physician shortage and maldistribution stimulated the development of various non-physician primary care provider programs, primarily to provide physician substitutes for rural and underserved areas.[25]

The physician assistant (PA) program at Duke University and the Medex programs at the University of Washington and University of Utah are early examples of non-physician provider education programs. The first PA program opened at Duke University under the direction of Eugene Stead, MD. Interestingly, Stead had originally planned to develop this role in conjunction with his nursing colleague, Thelma Ingeles. However, the nursing community reacted strongly against the development of a nursing role that appeared to take on medical tasks. Consequently, Stead initiated this first PA program by drawing from the large pool of military corpsmen returning from the Vietnam War. In 2003, the American Academy of Physician Assistants reported that approximately 42,000 individuals were in practice as PAs. This number has almost doubled since 1992.[54] The content of PA practice, as described by Jones and Cawley,[26] includes evaluation, monitoring, diagnostic testing, therapy, counseling, and referral. The scope of PA practice is regulated under state medical practice acts and, thus, the activities of PAs in primary care practice vary from state to state. However, PAs are generally licensed as dependent to physicians, in contrast to NPs whose practices are more independent.

The majority of PA programs in the United States are based in medical schools or have strong relationships with medical schools. Numerous studies have documented the PA's ability to provide medical services with a high level of patient satisfaction.[27] PAs are reported to see patient populations similar to those of physicians and are considered capable of providing approximately 75 percent of physician-specific services.[28] Regan and Harbert[29] reported that, depending on their particular use in a practice, a PA can reduce overhead and increase the financial productivity of a physician by a total of $72,077 to $332,200 annually. Reports have suggested that managed-care organizations are using PAs and APNs to control costs; roughly two-thirds of all sampled groups reported employment of APNs and PAs.[39]

APNs as Primary Care Providers

To date, APNs in primary care settings have practiced as NPs or certified nurse midwives (CNMs). The introduction of the NP occurred simultaneously with that of the PA. Conceived as a primary care generalist, the NP role (initially called a pediatric associate) was originally developed by Loretta Ford, Ed.D., a nurse, and Henry Silver, MD, a pediatrician, both practicing in Colorado.[30] The role developed over time and extended into adult health, family health, and gerontological health.

In 2000, there were over 102,000 NPs and over 9,000 CNMs in the United States,[55] with an estimated 325 graduate nursing programs or post-master's nursing programs preparing NPs for a variety of specialist roles.[56] The greatest numbers of programs offer preparation for family NPs (38 percent), followed by adult NPs (18 percent), pediatric NPs (16 percent), and all other types of NP programs (28 percent).[59] According to the National Organization of Nurse Practitioner Faculties (NONPF), NPs are educated to practice independently and interdependently in collaborative practice arrangements.[62] As primary care generalists, NPs employ a population-based perspective to care for individuals, families, and communities. Clinical decision-making, based on critical thinking, is essential to the work of the NP, who must synthesize theoretical, scientific, clinical, and practical knowledge to diagnose and manage actual and potential health problems. Central to the role of the NP is the promotion and maintenance of health. NPs have major roles in health promotion, disease prevention, service coordination, and acute and chronic disease monitoring.[32] Although NPs are expected to use short-term encounters to address the restoration of health, long-term contact and teaching encounters are viewed as more meaningful opportunities to contribute to the long-term health of the patient. Strategies of NP care include patient advocacy, therapy and health education, counseling, service coordination, and treatment evaluation. According to NONPF, NP practice is not setting-specific but, rather, is focused on the primary care needs of patients, wherever they may occur.[32] More recently, NPs have begun to move into acute care settings, taking the place of medical residents in hospitals.[33, 34, 55] In addition to NPs or, more specifically, women's health nurse practitioners, CNMs provide primary care services to women across the lifespan.

Research on Advanced Nursing Practice

An extensive body of literature is available documenting the effectiveness of APNs (in particular NPs). Three reviews of APN practice in primary care are considered definitive. The first, a study commissioned by the U.S. Congress and conducted by the Office of Technology Assessment (OTA),[35] reviewed the published reports of NP practice. The OTA study findings demonstrated that NP care is of a quality equal to that of physicians in the areas of history-taking; diagnosing of minor, acute illnesses; and managing stable, chronic diseases and of a superior quality in the areas of communication and preventive care.[35]

In the second literature synthesis, Crosby, Ventura, and Feldman[36] reviewed 248 published reports on NP practice from 1963 to 1983. The review included 187 reports judged to be methodologically sound and summarized findings in relation to

NP utilization, delivery of patient care services, short-term patient outcomes, and long-term patient outcomes. On the basis of their analysis of the reports, Crosby, Ventura, and Feldman concluded that NPs:

- Work primarily in ambulatory settings and physicians' offices
- Perform a range of services, including physician-substitute services (history-taking, physical and diagnostic examinations, and management of chronic illnesses) and complementary services (patient teaching and counseling) comparable or superior to that of other providers
- Have positive, short-term patient outcomes (patient knowledge, compliance, return for health maintenance and follow-up visits) equal to, or better than, those of other providers

Long-term patient outcomes were described in only 14 percent of the reports and, therefore, were not analyzed.[36]

Brown and Grimes[37] provided a synopsis of both NP and CNM practice. The strength of their report is found in its use of rigorous statistical techniques that combined the probability values (P values) and arrived at standard mean differences across statistical comparison studies of APN providers (experimenting groups) and physicians (control group). To be included in the review, the report had to describe:

- Practice in American or Canadian settings
- An intervention provided by an NP-CNM or an NP-CNM-physician team
- Data on a control group of patients managed by a physician
- Outcomes related to process of care, clinical (patient) outcomes, or utilization and cost-effectiveness
- Use of a traditional research design (i.e., experimental, quasi-experimental, or ex post facto)
- Statistical data sufficient to compare the experimental and control groups

More than 900 reports were reviewed; 38 NP and 15 CNM studies met the methodological requirements for inclusion. From the review of the 38 NP studies, the investigators concluded that NPs:

- Provided more health promotion care and ordered more diagnostic tests than the physician group
- Had comparable scores on patient knowledge but higher scores than their physician counterparts on patient compliance, functional outcomes, resolution of pathological conditions, and satisfaction with care
- Spent more time with patients and had lower laboratory costs and fewer hospitalizations than their physician counterparts

While costs per NP visit were lower, the investigators noted this finding was confounded by salary differentials between NPs and physicians. Statistically significant findings indicated that, for the variables listed, NP care was comparable to or better than physician care.

CNMs, individuals educated in both nursing and midwifery, are considered to be well qualified primary care providers for women and newborns.[38] In the CNM studies reported by Brown and Grimes,[37] only those in which CNMs and physicians had patients with comparable risks were compared. These nine studies demonstrated that CNMs:

- Used less analgesia and intravenous fluids and performed less fetal monitoring, episiotomies, and forceps deliveries
- Induced labor less frequently than physicians
- Had patients who more often delivered in sites other than delivery rooms (process of care)
- Had infant outcomes (incidence of low birth weight, fetal distress, 1-minute Apgar scores, and neonatal mortality) comparable to their physician counterparts (clinical outcomes)
- Had shorter hospital lengths of stay and more postpartum visits than their physician counterparts

CNMs and physicians differed most in the process-of-care variables, reflecting the midwives' tendency to provide less technology-oriented care.

Critics of these three reports cite lack of control for differences in the complexity of patients managed by physicians and NPs-CNMs. However, Brown and Grimes,[37] who selected for analysis only those randomized clinical trials where patient complexity was comparable for NPs and physicians, still found results indicating that NP-CNM care is comparable or superior to that of physicians.

NPs can provide 80 to 90 percent of the services provided by physicians. Because the cost of educating NPs and CNMs is approximately 20 to 25 percent less than the cost of educating physicians, these two types of APNs are considered economical sources for primary care providers.[35]

In a more recent study of NP and physician practice, Mundinger[57] reported outcomes from a study of NPs in primary care settings. Patients who received care from either a physician or an NP reported the same level of satisfaction and had the same health outcomes. This study is important because it was a prospective study of NP outcomes in a practice where NPs had the same authority, responsibility, and type of patient population as physicians in comparable practice settings.

POLICY ISSUES INFLUENCING ADVANCED PRACTICE IN EMERGING PRIMARY CARE SYSTEMS

Barriers to Advanced Practice in Primary Care

Given that NP and CNM outcomes are comparable to physician outcomes, the lower health care education and delivery costs associated with APNs should result in more APNs in primary care settings. Yet professional barriers continue to influence APN practice. Despite the increased number of nurses completing programs preparing them for primary care practice, the number of APNs actively involved in practice is far smaller. Safriet[4] identified three major barriers to advanced nursing practice in primary care settings:

1. Regulation of advanced nursing practice
2. Prescriptive authority for APNs
3. Reimbursement for APNs' services

Regulation of Advanced Nursing Practice

Every state has licensing laws designed to protect the public. State practice acts govern the nature and scope of the practices of physicians, nurses, and other health professionals. Physicians were the first practitioners to receive legislative approval for their practice activities, and state medical practice acts are all-encompassing in reserving for physicians the legal right to diagnose, prescribe, treat, and cure health problems. Because medical practice acts deny these functions to anyone not licensed as a physician, other health professionals seeking to perform these functions are compelled to negotiate changes in their own practice acts to include diagnosis, prescriptive, and curative functions.

Prescriptive Authority for APNs

The ability to prescribe drugs and therapeutic agents is a second requisite for comprehensive primary care. Numerous strategies have been used by APNs to prescribe medications in primary care settings, even in the absence of legal authority. These include choosing a medication for a patient and then having a physician write and sign a prescription for that medication, using a physician's name to call a prescription to a pharmacy, cosigning (with a physician) a prescription, and using written protocols to allow the nurse to prescribe medications with the type and dosage determined by formulary. Although these strategies have enabled APNs to manage medication regimens, they often result in APNs being "hidden" providers of this important primary care service.

Reimbursement for APN Services

Perhaps the greatest barrier to advanced nursing practice in primary care settings has been the uneven success nurses have experienced in receiving reimbursement for their services. Because reimbursement decisions rest almost exclusively with states (where third-party insurers are regulated), the issue of reimbursement for APNs' services depends on state statutes. Where they do permit reimbursement for APNs' services, Medicaid-approved nurse provider rates range from 60 to 100 percent of what physicians are paid for the same services.[40] Progress on resolving these three barriers to primary practice by APNs has been slow. Using economic projection techniques, Nichols[41] estimated that barriers to practice preventing APNs from providing the full range of services that they are educated to provide cost the nation $9 billion annually, or much more in today's economy. Progress by APNs to achieve legislative authority in all 50 states and the District of Columbia to perform these functions has been slow but successful.[58]

In a study of practice barriers among a sample of practicing California NPs,[42] those reporting the greatest barriers were NPs whose practices addressed the needs of unserved populations (prisons, psychiatric patients, rural communities), thus documenting the fact that advanced nursing practice barriers continue to limit access for those groups who can least afford denial of primary health care. Removal of practice barriers is necessary if APNs are to be major providers of primary care in the future. In a 1994 report, the Pew Health Professions Commission[43] specifically called for removal of barriers to the expansion of NP practice. In its 1995 report, the Commission called for changes in the health professions' regulatory system to permit standardized regulation, where appropriate, to support optimal access to a competent work force.[44]

The Mix of Providers for Primary Care Systems

Health care over the lifespan requires services ranging from health promotion and disease prevention to management of chronic or life-threatening illness to end-stage, palliative care. This broad range of services cannot likely be delivered by a single health professional. Thus, a major issue for future primary health care systems is creating an ideal mix of interdisciplinary service providers to provide the broadest range of needed services with the greatest economy.

The value of interdisciplinary provider teams is often praised in the literature.[45-47] According to the Pew Commission,[45] interdisciplinary collaborative practice is necessary for integrated clinical care. It requires providers conversant in team concepts who can respectfully engage in open communication with other team members. Practice situations that favor collaborative teamwork are those characterized by situational complexity requiring more than one set of skills, clinical knowledge too great for one clinician to possess, and team members willing to sacrifice some degree of autonomy in order to achieve the best quality of care.

Despite the philosophical support for team practice, there is little literature on organizing the most efficient and effective team of health care clinicians. At least three factors will likely influence the mix of team providers for emerging primary care systems:

1. The needs of the target population
2. The provider's skills and services
3. Incentives for interdisciplinary practice teams

The Needs of the Target Population

The target population's characteristics to be served by a primary care system is a decisive factor in developing a mix of providers. For example, communities with a high proportion of families with school-age children will need a group of primary care providers with a set of skills and services different from those of communities with a large proportion of retired senior citizens. Primary care systems that serve homeless people need to have providers with skills in managing chronic and infectious diseases and in finding and using social services. Farm communities require a primary care system of providers skilled in accident prevention and management and controlling occupational toxic exposures. The skill base and expertise of providers in a primary care setting must vary depending on the target population's needs.

The Provider's Skills and Services

There are three approaches to multidisciplinary service delivery that have implications for APNs who seek to practice in primary care systems. Under a provider substitution model, all providers in the setting offer the same set of services. Thus, APNs, physicians, and PAs in the setting offer the same diagnostic, disease prevention, health promotion, and disease management services.

With a supplemental model, multidisciplinary providers offer a core set of services, with each team member also offering supplemental services. In this model, all APNs, physicians, and PAs in a setting might provide first-contact services (taking a health history, performing diagnostic tests, and identifying the priority health problem). However, only the physician would manage patients diagnosed with chronic illnesses. The PA would manage acute illnesses and trauma, and the APN would provide disease prevention and/or health promotion services.

Finally, in a complementary model, providers in a setting offer only those services for which they are uniquely prepared by education, experience, or legal statute. Using the complementary model for primary care services, the PA might do all initial first-contact patient encounters, the physician might see patients with illnesses, and the APN might provide health screening and disease prevention programs for individuals and families.

The decision to use a substitute, supplemental, or complementary model of provider practice in a setting will influence recruiting and employment decisions. In a substitution model, the decision to employ APNs, physicians, PAs, or other service providers would be influenced only by the availability and costs of employing those different types of providers. If there is an adequate and economical supply of physician generalists during the next decade, exclusive focus on a physician substitution model may have negative connotations for APNs who want to work in primary care settings.

In the provider supplement model, each provider offers the same core set of services plus a skill-specific service. However, in a system increasingly concerned with costs, the connotation that any provider's services are supplemental in nature could have negative implications for APNs, unless the need for and cost justification of those services are marketed successfully to consumers. Settings driven by economical concerns may elect not to offer supplemental services.

Exclusive emphasis on complementary services, such as those offered by physicians or by APNs, increases the risk of fragmentation of services in a system already criticized for lack of service articulation. However, if complementary interdisciplinary practice is implemented thoughtfully, it can result in each provider offering those services for which they are qualified. Complementary interdependent team practice has great promise for primary care settings.

Because the broad range of needed primary care services cannot likely be provided by a single professional, the manner in which primary care systems conceptualize and implement service delivery has great implications for new APNs who will enter practice in the next decade. Table 5–4 summarizes advantages and disadvantages of each method of skill and services division among providers. Although proponents of emerging primary care systems emphasize the need for collaboration and service coordination, little attention has been given to mechanisms for articulating the services of multidisciplinary providers. Given the forecasts of a crowded health care system, APNs must be clear when marketing their services whether their skills and services substitute, supplement, or complement those services offered by other providers.

Incentives for Interdisciplinary Practice Teams

Gatekeeping, patient ownership, and control of service delivery by selected professionals have been identified as deterrents to the delivery of economical primary care services. Efforts to limit patient access to the services of other providers are often seen in the "turf battles" regularly played between medical specialists and generalists, between physicians and nurses, and between nurses and PAs. In its recommendations for the future education of all health professionals, the Pew Commission[44] concluded that future health care systems must have practitioners who are able to work effectively as team members in settings that emphasize "integrated services."

However, current organizational and service reimbursement characteristics serve as strong disincentives to the development of interdisciplinary teams. Academic health centers, considered by many health policy planners to represent

TABLE 5–4. Advantages and Disadvantages of Substitutive, Supplemental, and Complementary Service Delivery in Primary Care		
Provider Services	**Potential Advantages**	**Potential Disadvantages**
Substitutive: multidisciplinary providers who offer the same services	• Standardization of services offered • Reimbursement tied to *services*, not to discipline of provider	• Provider competition • Little or no collaborative, interdependent team practice
Supplemental: multidisciplinary providers who offer a *core* set of services, plus additional, or supplemental, services	• Standardization of core set of services offered • Utilization of unique practice strengths of multidisciplinary providers for supplemental services	• Services of some providers considered supplemental "extras" • Collaborative, interdependent team practice around supplemental services only
Complementary: multidisciplinary providers who offer different services	• Utilization of interdependent collaborative practice to offer coordinated, comprehensive services • Utilization of unique practice strengths of multidisciplinary providers	• Potential fragmentation in service delivery • Lack of service coordination

the best hope for the practice education of future primary care providers, continue to emphasize separate education of physicians, nurses, pharmacists, and other health professionals.[48] Health care delivery models continue to emphasize the compartmentalization of services, organized around the single provider-patient encounter. Existing reimbursement patterns continue to factor reimbursement of a single provider without considering the unique skills and services of different providers or the specific health needs of individuals and families.[49]

Because existing professional education models continue to favor one-on-one provider-patient relationships, the development of productive interdisciplinary team practices for primary care will require the redesign of health-professional education as well as service delivery and reimbursement models. A novel approach to changing the behavior of practicing clinicians is one proposed by Scheffler, an economist.[47] He suggests that financial incentives be offered to primary care teams that will work together to enhance the quality of care. Changes in reimbursement patterns that promote team-practice reimbursement must occur as well. To offset the educational elitism of health professionals, the Pew Commission[44] published a sample curriculum guide for interdisciplinary education for primary care and a reference guide to assist educators in accomplishing this goal.

SUMMARY

High-quality health care systems are those that provide accessible, economical, and effective services to specific target populations. Spiraling health care costs and consumer dissatisfaction with unequal access and fragmented services have generated renewed interest in primary care systems and primary care providers. The most recent IOM definition of primary care manifests the wide-ranging expectation that the primary care system of the future must be staffed by generalists who are capable of providing comprehensive, holistic care that addresses a wide range of individual and family health problems. Because no single provider can be expected to possess the knowledge and skills to address the complete range of episodic and chronic health problems commonly experienced across the lifespan, multidisciplinary team practice will be a necessity. Whether future primary care systems will achieve their expected goals of first-contact, longitudinal, and coordinated and comprehensive care will depend, to a great extent, on whether multidisciplinary practice teams successfully collaborate in balancing substitutive, supplemental, and complementary services for target populations. The purpose of this chapter has been to explore the social, political, and economic issues that will facilitate or inhibit the participation of APNs in these types of primary care practice endeavors.

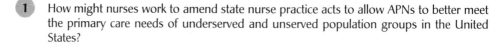

SUGGESTED EXERCISES

1. How might nurses work to amend state nurse practice acts to allow APNs to better meet the primary care needs of underserved and unserved population groups in the United States?

2 Which model of practice do you believe offers the greatest opportunity for APNs in primary care settings: the physician substitute model, the physician supplement model, or the physician complement model? Justify your answer.

3 What do you believe is the ideal provider mix for a multidisciplinary practice team in primary care? Design an interdisciplinary team to meet the primary care needs in your community.

4 Discuss incentives for developing and supporting multidisciplinary practice teams in primary care.

5 How might health policy planners ensure an adequate supply of primary care providers for the next decade?

REFERENCES

1. Starfield, B: Roles and functions of non-physician practitioners in primary care. In Clawson, D, and Osterweis, M (eds): The Role of Physician Assistants and Nurse Practitioners in Primary Care. Association of Academic Health Centers, Washington, DC, 1993.
2. World Health Organization: Primary Health Care. Geneva, Switzerland, 1978.
3. Franks, P, Nutting, P, and Clancy, C: Health care reform, primary care, and the need for research. Acad Med 270:1449, 1993.
4. Safriet, B: Health care dollars and regulatory sense: The role of advanced practice nursing. Yale J Regul 9:417, 1992.
5. American Nurses Association: Nursing's Agenda for Health Care Reform. American Nurses Association, Washington, DC, 1991.
6. Pew Health Professions Commission: Healthy America: Practitioners for 2005. Pew Health Professions Commission, San Francisco, 1991.
7. Council on Graduate Medical Education: Third Report: Improving Access to Health Care through Physician Workforce Reform: Directions for the 21st Century. US Department of Health and Human Services, Washington, DC, 1992.
8. Public Health Service, Health Professions Report. US Department of Health and Human Services, Washington, DC, 1993.
9. The Alliance for Health Reform: A Primary Care Primer. The Alliance for Health Reform, Washington, DC, 1993.
10. White, K: Primary medical care for families. N Engl J Med 277:847, 1967.
11. Alpert, J, and Charney, E: The Education of Physicians for Primary Care. US Department of Health, Education and Welfare, Public Health Service, Health Resources Administration, Rockville, MD, 1973. HRA Publication 74–3113.
12. Institute of Medicine: Report of a Study: A Manpower Policy for Primary Health Care. National Academy of Science, Washington, DC, May 1978.
13. Golden, A: A definition of primary care for educational purposes. In Golden, A, Carlson, D, and Hagan, J (eds): The Art of Teaching Primary Care. Springer, New York, 1982.
14. Starfield, B: Primary Care: Concept, Evaluation and Policy. Oxford University Press, New York, 1992.
15. Institute of Medicine: Defining Primary Care: An Interim Report. National Academy Press, Washington, DC, 1994.
16. National Medical Care Survey Data (2000). http://www.cdc.gov/nchs/about/major/ahcd/ambucare.htm Accessed June 2003.
17. Avorn, J, Everitt, D, and Baker, M: The neglected medical history and therapeutic choices for abdominal pain. Arch Intern Med 151:694, 1991.
18. Safran, D, Tarlov, A, and Rogers, W: Primary care performance in fee-for-service and prepaid health care systems. JAMA 271:1579, 1994.
19. Rivo, M, and Satcher, D: Improving access to health care through physician workforce reform. JAMA 270:1074, 1993.
20. Cooper, R, Getzen, T, McKee, H, and Laud, P: Economic and demographic trends signal an impending physician shortage. Health Aff 21:140, 2002.
21. Barnett, P, and Midtling, J: Public policy and the supply of primary care physicians. JAMA 262:2864, 1989.

22. Kassebaum, D, Szenas, P, and Ruffin, A: The declining interest of medical school graduates in generalist specialties: Students' abandonment of earlier inclinations. Acad Med 68:278, 1993.
23. Levinsky, N: Recruiting for primary care. N Engl J Med 328:656, 1993.
24. Iglehart, J: Health policy report: II. Rapid changes for academic medical centers. N Engl J Med 332:407, 1995.
25. Fowkes, V: Meeting the needs of the underserved: The roles of physician assistant and nurse practitioners. In Clawson, D, and Osterweis, M (eds): The Role of Physician Assistants and Nurse Practitioners in Primary Care. Association of Academic Health Centers, Washington, DC, 1993.
26. Jones, P, and Cawley, J: Physician assistants and health system reform: Clinical capabilities, practice activities, and potential roles. JAMA 272:725, 1994.
27. Hooker, R: The role of physician assistants and nurse practitioners in a managed organization. In Clawson, D, and Osterweis, M (eds): The Role of Physician Assistants and Nurse Practitioners in Primary Care. Association of Academic Health Centers, Washington, DC, 1993.
28. Cawley, J: Physician assistants in the health care workforce. In Clawson, D, and Osterweis, M (eds): The Role of Physician Assistants and Nurse Practitioners in Primary Care. Association of Academic Health Centers, Washington, DC, 1993.
29. Regan, D, and Harbert, K: Measuring the financial productivity of physician assistants. Med Group Manage J, November/December 1991, p 46.
30. Ford, L: Practice perspectives in primary care nursing. In Miller, R (ed): Primary Health Care: More than Medicine. Prentice-Hall, Englewood Cliffs, NJ, 1983.
31. National Organization of Nurse Practitioner Faculties: Curriculum Guidelines and Program Standards for Nurse Practitioner Education. Washington, DC, National Organization of Nurse Practitioner Faculties, 1995.
32. Booth, R: Leadership challenges for nurse practitioner faculty. Keynote address presented at the Twentieth Annual Conference of the National Organization of Nurse Practitioner Faculties, Portland, OR, 1994.
33. Genet, C, et al: Nurse practitioners in a teaching hospital. Nurse Pract 20:47, 1995.
34. Goskel, D, Harrison, C, Morrison, R, and Miller, S: Description of a nurse practitioner inpatient service in a public teaching hospital. J Gen Intern Med 8:29, 1993.
35. Congress and Office of Technology Assessment: Nurse Practitioners, Physician Assistants and Certified Nurse Midwives: A Policy Analysis. US Government Printing Office, Washington, DC, 1986. OTA-HCS Publication 37.
36. Crosby, F, Ventura, M, and Feldman, M: Future research recommendations for establishing NP effectiveness. Nurse Pract 12:75, 1987.
37. Brown, S, and Grimes, D: Executive Summary: A Meta-Analysis of Process of Care, Clinical Outcomes and Cost-Effectiveness of Nurses in Primary Care Roles: Nurse Practitioners and Nurse-Midwives. University of Texas, Houston, 1992.
38. American College of Nurse-Midwives: Position Statement. American College of Nurse-Midwives, Washington, DC, 1992.
39. Dial, T, Palsbo, S, Bergsten, C, Gabel, J, and Weiner, J: Clinical Staffing in Staff- and Group-Model HMOs. Health Aff (Millwood) 14:168, 1995.
40. Pearson, L: Fifteenth annual legislative update: How each state stands on legislative issues affecting advanced nursing practice. Nurse Pract 28:1, 2003.
41. Nichols, L: Estimating costs of underusing advanced practice nurses. Nurs Economics 10:343, 1992.
42. Anderson, A, Gilliss, C, and Yoder, L: Practice environment for nurse practitioners in California: Identifying barriers. West J Med 165:209, 1996.
43. Pew Health Professions Commission: Nurse practitioners: Doubling the graduates by the year 2000. In Commission Policy Papers. Pew Health Professions Commission, San Francisco, 1994.
44. Pew Health Professions Commission: Critical Challenges: Revitalizing the Health Professions for the Twenty-First Century. Pew Health Professions Commission, San Francisco, 1995.
45. Pew Health Professions Commission: Interdisciplinary Collaborative Teams in Primary Care: A Model Curriculum and Resource Guide. The UCSF Center for the Health Professions, San Francisco, 1995.
46. Baldwin, D: The Role of Interdisciplinary Education and Teamwork in Primary Care and Health Care Reform. Department of Health and Human Services, Public Health Service, Bureau of Health Professions, Office of Research and Planning, Rockville, MD, 1994.
47. Scheffler, R: Life in the kaleidoscope: The impact of managed care on the US health care work force and a new model for the delivery of primary care. In Donaldson, M, Yordy, K, Lohr, K, and Vanselow, N (eds): Institute of Medicine: Primary Care: America's Health in a New Era. National Academy Press, Washington, DC, 1996, pp 312–340.

48. Low, D: Commentary. In Larson, P, Osterweis, M, and Rubin, E (eds): Health Workforce Issues in the 21st Century. Association of Academic Health Centers, Washington, DC, 1994.
49. Pestronk, R, et al: Managed outcomes. J Am Acad Nurse Pract 63:121, 1994.
50. Showstack, J, Rothman, A, and Hassmiller, S: Primary care at a crossroads. Ann Intern Med 138:242, 2003.
51. Showstack, J, Lurie, N, Larson, E, Rothman, A, and Hassmiller, S: Primary care: The next renaissance. Ann Intern Med 138:268, 2003.
52. Sandy, L, and Schroeder, S: Primary care in a new era: Disillusion and dissolution? Ann Intern Med 138:262, 2003.
53. Christensen, CM, Bohmer, R, and Kenagy, J: Will disruptive innovations cure health care? Harvard Business Rev 78:102, 2002.
54. American Academy of Physician Assistants: www.aapa.org/research Accessed June 2003.
55. National Sample Survey of Registered Nurses: March 2000. ftp://ftp.hrsa.gov/bhpr/nursing/sampsurvpre.pdf Accessed June 2003.
56. Berlin, L, Stennet, J, Bednawh, G: 2002–2003 Enrollment and Graduations in Baccalaureate and Graduate Programs in Nursing. Washington, DC: Author, 2003.
57. Mundinger M: Primary care outcomes in patients treated by nurse practitioners or physicians: A randomized trial. JAMA 283: 2000, 59–68.
58. State Nurse Practice Acts: Administrative Rules (2002). www.Ncsbn.Org/Public/Regulation/Nursing_Practice_Model_Administrative_Rules.htm Accessed June 2003.
59. Berlin, L, Harper, D, Werner, K, and Stennett, J: Master's-Level Nurse Practitioner Education Programs Findings from the 2000–2001 Collaborative Curriculum Survey. American Association of Colleges of Nursing & National Organization of Nurse Practitioner Faculties, Washington, DC, 2002.
60. American Association of Family Physicians. Www.Aafp.Org Accessed June 2003.
61. Council on Graduate Medical Education (1999): COGME Physician Workforce Policies: Recent Developments and Remaining Challenges in Meeting National Goals. Www.Cogme.Gov/14.Pdf Accessed June 2003.
62. National Organization of Nurse Practitioner Faculties Curriculum Guidelines Task Force (1995). Advanced Nursing Practice : Curriculum Guidelines and Program Standards for Nurse Practitioner Education. NONPF, Washington, DC.

CHAPTER 6

Advanced Practice Nurses in Non-Primary Care Roles: The Evolution of Specialty and Acute Care Practices

Dennis J. Cheek, PhD, RN, FAHA
Karol S. Harshaw-Ellis, MSN, RN, A/GNP, ACNP-CS

Dennis J. Cheek, PhD, RN, FAHA, is Professor at Texas Christian University in the Harris School of Nursing, with a joint appointment in the School of Nurse Anesthesia. Dr. Cheek has previously been an assistant professor at the University of North Carolina at Chapel Hill, with a joint appointment in the Carolina Center for Genome Sciences. Dr. Cheek is also a Fellow of the American Heart Association and Council on Cardiovascular Nursing. He holds a doctorate in cellular molecular pharmacology and physiology from the University of Nevada, Reno; a master's of science from the University of California, San Francisco, as a critical care clinical nurse specialist, with a minor in education and curriculum development, as well as a bachelor's of science in nursing from California State University, Fresno. Dr. Cheek was the past director of Duke University School of Nursing Acute Care Nurse Practitioner Program. He is currently teaching undergraduate and graduate pathophysiology and pharmacology at Texas Christian University, Harris School of Nursing and School of Nurse Anesthesia.

Karol S. Harshaw-Ellis, MSN, RN, A/GNP, ACNP-CS, is a consulting clinical associate at Duke University School of Nursing. She also holds a clinical appointment at the Durham Regional Hospital. She holds a master's nursing degree from the Duke University School of Nursing, with a dual major in adult and gerontological nursing, and a bachelor of science in nursing from The University of North Carolina at Chapel Hill School of Nursing. She was one the first advanced practice nurses in North Carolina to practice as an acute care nurse practitioner in a collaborative practice model with Duke University Affiliated Practice and Durham Regional Hospital. She is currently practicing full time in the Heart Failure Clinic as well as team-teaching in the Duke University School of Nursing Acute Care Nurse Practitioner Program.

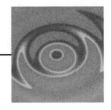

Advanced Practice Nurses in Non-Primary Care Roles: The Evolution of Specialty and Acute Care Practices

CHAPTER OBJECTIVES

After completing this chapter, the reader will be able to:

1 Describe the recent development of advanced practice nursing in non-primary care roles.
2 Identify acute care practice settings of the non-primary care advanced practice nurse (APN).
3 Discuss the implications of various health care projections for the developing acute care systems for the 21st century.
4 Explore the factors influencing advanced practice nursing in acute care systems and other non-primary care settings.

The American Nurses Association has identified four advanced practice nursing specialty areas: nurse anesthetist, nurse midwifery, clinical nurse specialist, and nurse practitioner.[1] The certified registered nurse anesthetist (CRNA) provides anesthesia and anesthesia-related care. The certified nurse midwife (CMW) is a clinical expert who has knowledge, skills, and expertise for the care and management of women and newborns. The clinical nurse specialist (CNS) is an expert clinician who provides comprehensive practice activities in the areas of indirect/direct patient care, education, consultation, and research utilization. The nurse practitioner (NP) provides comprehensive health assessments; determines diagnoses; plans and prescribes treatment; and manages health care regimens in a variety of settings for individuals, families, and communities. The NP role includes promotion of wellness, prevention of illness, and management of acute and chronic conditions.[1] Early in its evolution, the NP delivered health care from ambulatory care settings or established practices or clinics. This chapter focuses on advanced practice nursing in non-primary roles in the specialty and acute care setting.

ADVANCED PRACTICE NURSING ROOTS IN ACUTE CARE

Acute care roles are not new to advanced practice nursing. Advanced practice nursing roles and practice evolved almost exclusively within the context of an acute care delivery system. Even when the APN role, i.e., the CNM and NP, was created to provide health care services in community-based settings, this occurred within an acute care focused delivery system.

In Chapter 1, Dr. Komnenich provides a comprehensive review of the evolution of APN roles. Modern nurse anesthesia traces its roots to the last two decades of the 1800s, when records indicate that nurses were often asked to administer anesthesia. The first nurse anesthetist was Sister Mary Bernard at St. Vincent's Hospital in Erie, Pennsylvania, in 1877.[2] Anesthesia practice was so common that in her 1893 textbook, entitled *Nursing: Its Principles and Practices for Hospital and Private Use*, Isabel Adams Hampton Robb included a chapter on the administration of anesthesia.

In 1925, Mary Breckenridge established the Frontier Nursing Service in Kentucky and was the first nurse to practice as a nurse-midwife in the United States. She received her midwifery education in England and returned to the United States with other British nurse-midwives to set up a system of care similar to that which she had observed in Scotland.[4]

APNs have also been successful in creating roles that assisted in solving social, financial, and political health care problems for over 50 years. After World War II, nurse educators developed the CNS role to improve the quality of care in hospitals. This was the first advanced practice role in nursing that was not to provide direct patient care but rather to support nursing services through education. Initially, specialization for nurses was limited to administration and education. Reiter has been credited with the first use of the term "nurse clinician" in 1943 to designate a specialist in nursing practice.[5] The development of the first master's program in a clinical nursing specialty is attributed to Hildegarde Peplau at Rutgers University in 1954 to prepare nurses for the role of psychiatric clinical nurse specialist.[3]

The NP movement began at the University of Colorado. In 1965, Dr. Loretta Ford, a public health nurse, collaborated with Dr. Henry Silver, a pediatrician, to develop the first pediatric nurse practitioner post-baccalaureate program to prepare nurses for an expanded role in the care of children.[6,7] The purpose of the first NP project was to implement a new role for nurses and to evaluate the effectiveness of this role in improving the safety, efficacy, and quality of health care for children and families.

EVOLUTION OF NPs IN NEONATAL AND ACUTE CARE

Neonatal Nurse Practitioner

In the 1970s, the neonatal nurse practitioner (NNP) role evolved as a way to rectify health care delivery problems for this at-risk population. Pediatric residency slots were being eliminated as a result of an overabundance and uneven geographic distribution of pediatricians.[8] At the same time, neonates were demanding a higher acuity and complexity of care. In 1973, a group of interested physicians and nurses formed an ad hoc committee to discuss educational programs that would prepare nurses to function in intensive perinatal care settings. The Blue Ribbon Commission, with representation from a variety of professional organizations including nursing, grew out of this committee. Funded by the March of Dimes, the Commission met in 1974 to examine information reported by five consulting task forces. The result of this process was the development of *Guidelines for Short-Term Continuing Education Programs for the Nurse Clinician in Intensive Neonatal Care and the Nurse Clinician in Intensive Maternal-Fetal Care.*[9] The expectation was that the neonatal nurse clinician (NNC) would function primarily in the neonatal intensive care unit and that any reassignment tasks would be a collaborative effort between physicians and nurses, requiring reassessment of the functional roles of both professions.[8]

In 1974, the University of Wisconsin launched the first short-term continuing education program to prepare NNCs. The program was modeled after the design, content, and title recommendations of the still-unpublished Blue Ribbon guidelines. The University of Wisconsin program was the first of several to be funded by the March of Dimes.[8] The University of Arizona also launched a program in 1974 that was no different in design or content from the Blue Ribbon guidelines; this program, however, was called an NNP program.[8] Most of the original NNC/NNP programs were 4 to 9 months long and were hospital-based. It was not until the 1980s that hospital-based NNP certificate programs began to close as the trend toward university-based continuing education programs and graduate programs with NNP content integrated into the curricula were beginning to open.

In 1982, a group of NNCs and NNPs met during the American Academy of Pediatrics district meeting to discuss their future role. The first Neonatal Nurse

Clinician, Practitioner and Specialist (NNCPS) Conference was held in April 1983 with the primary purpose of promoting the NNC/NNP role.[8] In June 1984, the National Association of Neonatal Nurses (NANN) was established. In spring 1985, the NNCPS joined the newly established NANN. The NANN has provided the organizational support to move the advanced practice NNP forward. A survey conducted by NANN in 1993 demonstrated that most of the practicing NNPs have graduate degrees and most are working in Level III nurseries.[8] The NNP model has continued to evolve for the last 30 years. The NNP diagnoses and treats in collaboration with neonatologists and other pediatric physicians. The NNP makes independent and interdependent decisions in the assessment, diagnosis, management, and evaluation of the health care needs of neonates and infants. In addition, the NNP selects and performs clinically indicated advanced diagnostic and therapeutic invasive procedures.[10] This established role has provided some of the foundation and groundwork for the newer acute care nurse practitioner (ACNP) role.

Acute Care Nurse Practitioner

In the 1990s, the ACNP began to establish a presence within hospitals. However, as early as the 1970s, the title of ACNP was being used and roles described. The ACNP evolved as a direct result of blending the CNS and primary care NP roles. This role blending most likely stemmed from the similar educational preparations of the NP and the CNS. The core classes of most ACNP programs parallel those of the CNS programs,[11,12] but CNSs focus on leadership and research. The ACNP's primary focus is patient care.[11,12] ACNPs have more in-depth education in the areas of pharmacology, pathophysiology, health assessment, and history/physical–taking. [11-13]

The ACNPs in the 1970s and 1980s were adult primary care NPs who were recruited and employed in acute care settings. One such early role was the use of an ACNP within the department of cardiac surgery at the University of Rochester Strong Memorial Hospital. This was a collaborative practice model that incorporated both direct patient care and advanced practice nursing scholarly activities.[14] The role that was depicted in 1979 at Strong Memorial Hospital continues to be a prototype for APN roles in acute and critical care in the new millennium.[11,14] Spisso and colleagues[15] reported in 1990 the use of NPs at the University of California, Davis, Medical Center in their trauma service. These APNs were prepared as primary care NPs with experience in surgical, critical, or acute care. During the 1980s, residency hours were being reduced, so trauma NPs were recruited to decrease the patient burden.[16, 17] These NPs were successful in improving quality of care and patient satisfaction and decreasing length of stay.[15,16]

In the 1990s, as ACNP educational programs began to emerge, some of the first descriptions of ACNP roles came from the University of Pittsburgh, University of Pennsylvania, and Case Western Reserve University. The University of Pittsburgh Medical Center began using ACNPs in the neurological intensive care unit and liver transplant intensive care units. The ACNPs started by overseeing the care of two to three ICU patients, but as the physicians developed trust and confidence in their decision-making their responsibilities increased. Over time, the ACNPs were permitted to provide care to an increasing number of complex critically ill patients, interpret diagnostic studies, and perform procedures such as central line placement.[18]

It did not take long for health care leaders to realize that the acute care setting in the current health care delivery system required changes. As a result, the role of the ACNP began to gather support among physicians and administrators within tertiary health care centers across the country.[16,19-22] In 1995, the American Nurses Association (ANA) and the American Association of Critical Care Nurses (AACN) drafted the document *Standards of Clinical Practice and Scope of Practice for the Acute Care Nurse Practitioner.*[13]

The scope of practice for ACNPs is broad-based and involves providing advanced nursing care to patients who are acutely and critically ill. This includes providing direct patient care management by performing in-depth physical assessments, interpreting laboratory and diagnostic tests, and performing therapeutic treatments such as examining and cleaning wounds, inserting arterial or central venous catheters, and ordering pharmacological agents.[18]

The role of the ACNP represents an evolving career opportunity for critical care nurses. Currently, the ACNP examination, administered by the American Nurses Credentialing Center (ANCC), is the only certification for NPs who care for acutely ill patients. A pediatric acute NP examination will be launched by the Pediatric Nursing Certification Board (PNCB) in early 2005. This role in advanced practice nursing will continue to expand as a result of changes in acute care settings, including increased acuity of hospitalized patients, demands of managed care to reduce length of stay and better coordinate patient care, and decreases in the number of medical residency programs. [12, 16–18, 23,24]

University Hospital of Cleveland, an affiliate of Case Western Reserve University, selected four units in which to place their initial ACNP graduates. These units were the neuroscience unit, general oncology service, medical intensive care, and adult internal medicine ACNP practice, or the Collaborative Clinical Service. In each of these acute/critical care units, the ACNP performed the history and physical and some procedures such as arterial line insertion, lumbar punctures, insertion and removal of feeding tubes, and removal of pulmonary artery catheters. The neurology, oncology, and medical intensive care units were staffed with residents and/or fellows and attending physicians on a rotating basis. The ACNP, however, was based in a specific unit for continuity of care. Although the role and responsibilities of the ACNP differed among hospitals and units, there were commonalities, including patient management, leadership, teaching/mentoring, research, and professional development, activities common to the role of most ACNPs today.[25-27]

The University of Missouri Hospital and Clinics Columbia began to use NPs in the areas of general surgery, nephrology, and otolaryngology due to changes in their residency programs. The University of Missouri model was unique because these NPs provided both inpatient and outpatient care. Initially, the NPs provided care to patients with common problems frequently encountered in these specialty practices. Later, the NPs were allowed to follow more complex hospitalized patients. Urban gave an in-depth description of APN roles in cardiovascular surgery.[28] The two key functions of the ACNP were "case management" and "care coordination," which are also considered important components of the CNS role. Some of the highlights of the ACNP role were performing presurgical assessments, communicating with families and other health care team members, providing patient education, and discharge planning. In contrast, the CNS role has centered around expert clinician, consultant, educator, researcher, administrator and, in the 1990s, case and outcomes manager.[11] The new CNS role conceptualized by the National Association of Clinical Nurse Specialists centers around three spheres of influence: client (direct care), nursing personnel (advancing the practice of nursing), and organization (interdisciplinary).[32] The ACNP role focus has been direct comprehensive care, which includes conducting histories and physicals, diagnosing, and treating.[11]

Sole and colleagues[29] described the role of an ACNP and physician assistant (PA) in the care of stable trauma patients in a level I trauma center. The model of care delivery at this particular institution was a collaborative practice model.[29-31] The patients under the care of the ACNP and PA were assigned to an intermediate care service (ICS). The ACNP and PA managed four to six patients each on a daily basis. The trauma surgeon or surgical intensivist rounded on a weekly basis but were available at any time for urgent issues. The role of the ACNP included reviewing prior progress notes, diagnostic studies, and laboratory data and developing the plan of care for these patients with specialized needs. The ACNP and PA performed history and physicals, wrote orders, and educated staff and families. To evaluate the effectiveness of the ICS, a retrospective chart review of 93 patients was performed. The findings revealed that a quarter of the patients were discharged to a skilled nursing facility, rehabilitation center, or other hospital. All of the patients in the ICS survived, and none required a higher level of care.

Martin and Coniglio described using an ACNP in caring for patients with head and neck cancer.[31] Responsibilities included in the ACNP role were performing history and physicals, ordering and interpreting laboratory and diagnostic data, teaching and counseling, and coordinating referrals and consults to other disciplines and specialties. Martin and Coniglio provide an overview of the ACNP role for this population both in an inpatient and outpatient setting. The expansion of the ACNP role across inpatient and outpatient settings is quickly becoming a common ACNP role expectation. Martin outlined the use of the ACNP to provide seamless comprehensive care across the spectrum of health care to complex transplant patients.[33]

HOSPITALIST/ACUTE CARE NURSE PRACTITIONER MODEL

While the ACNP continues to forge into many areas of the health care delivery system, the future holds promise for yet another model of practice for the ACNP. This model involves working with a hospitalist team. Hospitalists are internists who specialize in inpatient medicine and work in academic and nonacademic health care settings. The hospitalist movement emerged out of California as a way to deal with the demands of managed care and decreased funding of residents.[17,34] This new health care provider evolved for many of the same reasons as the ACNP, and both the ACNP and hospitalist are being used as solutions to address many of the problems that plague the current health care system. As a result, ACNPs and hospitalists are establishing yet another model of health care delivery—the ACNP/ Hospitalist Model. Howie and Erickson[35] described the implementation of an ACNP/Hospitalist Model at the University of San Francisco Medical Center. Job opportunities and role descriptions for ACNPs working with hospitalists are becoming much more common.[36,37]

ACNP Hospitalist in Practice

In one practice, an ACNP, Harshaw-Ellis, was employed by a group of 12 internists to assist them in delivering care to their hospitalized patients. Prior to hiring the ACNP, each internist was responsible for rounding on his or her own hospitalized patients. Each internist had a primary care patient panel of at least 2,500 patients and was responsible for the total spectrum of care for each patient. Traditionally, about 25 percent of the patients in the practice were hospitalized for a variety of reasons at some time. As one solution, it had been decided that each physician would rotate independently on a weekly basis in the hospital. As patients became more complex, it was no longer cost-effective or efficient to continue this traditional care model. In addition, patients were experiencing longer lengths of stay, duplication of services, and dissatisfaction. At this point the physician group decided to hire an ACNP.

The ACNP was brought into the practice to provide care for the patients hospitalized at a 400-bed community hospital owned by a large teaching medical center. The physicians, through their insight, sought an NP to provide continuity of care for their hospitalized patients. The ACNP worked four 10-hour days with no weekends or holidays. Nights, weekends, and holidays were rotated among the internists. The ACNP/internist team covered an average census of 5 to 30 patients per week. Patients generally were admitted to the general medicine service but could be admitted to the medical intensive care, surgical intensive care, coronary intensive care, telemetry, or surgical units. The ACNP also evaluated and admitted patients through the emergency department.

Duties of the ACNP included performing histories and physicals, writing orders, prescribing pharmacological and nonpharmacological treatment modalities, interpreting laboratory and diagnostic data, family counseling and teaching, performing medical procedures and consults, consulting with specialists, planning discharge, preparing discharge or transfer summaries, communicating with managed care companies and case managers, and serving as a consultant to the hospital nursing staff. In addition to these responsibilities, the ACNP team taught in the ACNP program at the local university.

A typical day for the ACNP would begin with discharging appropriate patients and then completing daily rounds on other hospitalized patients. If admissions arose before rounds were completed, the internist and ACNP would decide who would do the admissions and who would continue rounding. Most of the time the ACNP was called to address any urgent or emergency patient needs. The ACNP also was frequently called to calm a distraught family member or provide needed counseling or education regarding a loved one's condition. Throughout the day, the

ACNP was also careful to review each patient's chart to ensure that all needed tests, consults, and procedures were completed in a timely manner.

After the first year, administrators verbalized satisfaction with the ACNP's role in helping to decrease admission and discharge times. Staff nurses expressed satisfaction as the ACNP extended and eased their own roles by assisting with procedures, starting intravenous lines, and coordinating and completing discharge planning and paperwork. The patients and families were very satisfied, evidenced by frequent letters sent to the CEO regarding the care provided, mentioning the ACNP and the role she played in the hospitalization. Finally, other medical specialties were so impressed with the model they hired NPs in their services as well, including neurosurgery, cardiology, and nephrology.

NON-PRIMARY CARE ROLES: GROWING SPECIALTIES

In 2003, schools of nursing reported having 277 APN programs (CNS and NP programs only) with an acute or critical care focus. [38,39] The number and type of acute and critical care programs are shown in Table 6–1.

Fifty-nine schools reported having an adult ACNP master's program, and 51 schools reported having a post-master's adult ACNP program.[38] In addition, 44 schools reported having a master's NNP program, and 35 schools reported having a post-master's NNP program. Six schools even reported having a master's pediatric ACNP program and six schools a post-master's pediatric ACNP program.[39] Fifty-two acute and critical CNS-Adult programs and nine acute and critical care CNS-Pediatric programs were reported. Finally, 15 schools reported having an acute or critical care CNS-Neonatal program.[38]

National certifying examinations are offered by the ANCC, the National

TABLE 6–1. Acute Care NP and CNS Education Programs, 2003[38]	
Number of Schools	**Programs**
59	Master's Adult Acute Care NP
6	Master's Pediatric Acute Care NP[39]*
51	Post-Master's Adult Acute Care NP
6	Post-Master's Pediatric Acute Care NP[39]*
44	Master's Neonatal NP
35	Post-Master's Neonatal NP
52	Acute and Critical Care CNS-Adult
9	Acute and Critical Care CNS-Pediatric
15	Acute and Critical Care CNS-Neonatal

*Number of Master's Pediatric Acute Care NP programs. Unpublished data from the American Association of Colleges of Nursing, Research Institutional Data System, 2003.

Certification Corporation, and the American Association of Critical Care Nurses (AACN) for all of these acute or critical care roles, except for the pediatric ACNP. A national certification examination for the pediatric ACNP is under development by the Pediatric Nursing Certification Board.

SUMMARY

The continuing turmoil in health care, sweeping changes in funding and reimbursement, growing dissatisfaction and crisis in managed care, and decreasing number of available physician residency positions have led to growing opportunities for APNs.[14,15,17] These opportunities have led to the emergence and resurgence of APN roles in acute and critical care settings, including the NNP, adult ACNP, pediatric ACNP, and pediatric and adult acute care CNS. The future for these acute care NP and CNS roles holds tremendous potential for addressing many of the current problems that plague the health care delivery system.

The ability to provide high-quality, hospital-based care by a permanent team of health care members who view the patient, family, and community in a holistic manner will be the task undertaken by this evolving APN cohort. As the population ages, ACNPs and CNSs will play even larger roles in the care of patients across the lifespan with multiple, complex problems. Improving quality of care, patient outcomes, and patient satisfaction are key aspects of APN care in all settings, including the acute care setting. Therefore, future opportunities for APNs in specialty and acute care settings are filled with potential for unlimited growth as we meet the patient care challenges of today's health care system.

SUGGESTED EXERCISES

1 Which model of practice do you believe offers the greatest opportunity for the APN in non-primary care settings? Justify your answer.

2 Design a hospitalist, interdisciplinary team for one service in a community hospital. Explain your rationale.

3 Discuss the differences in the ACNP and critical care CNS roles.

4 Describe the primary factors that contributed to the development of APN roles in acute care settings.

5 Prepare a presentation to be made to a physician group practice explaining the positive impact an ACNP can have on patient care outcomes and the practice as a whole.

REFERENCES

1. American Nurses Association: Scope and standards of advanced practice nursing. Washington, DC, 1996.
2. Bankert, M: Watchful Care: A History of America's Nurse Anesthetists. Continuum, New York, 1989.
3. Sheehy, CM, and McCarthy, MC: Advanced Practice Nursing: Emphasizing Common Roles. F.A Davis, Philadelphia, 1998.
4. Varney, H: Varney's Midwifery, 3rd ed. Jones and Bartlett, Sudbury, MA, 1997.

5. Reiter, F: The nurse-clinician. Am J Nurs 66:274, 1966.
6. Ford, LC, and Silver, HK: The expanded role of the nurse in child care. Nurs Outlook 15:43, 1967.
7. Ford, LC: A nurse for all settings: The nurse practitioner. Nurs Outlook 27:516, 1979.
8. Johnson, PJ: The history of the neonatal nurse practitioner: Reflections from "under the looking glass." Neonatal Network 21:51, 2002.
9. American Nurses Association: Guidelines for short-term continuing education programs for the nurse clinician in intensive neonatal care and the nurse clinician in intensive maternal-fetal care. Kansas City, MO, 1975.
10. National Association of Neonatal Nurses: Position statement on advanced practice neonatal nurse role. NANN, Petaluma, CA, 2001.
11. Mick, D, and Ackerman, M: Advance practice nursing role delineation in acute and critical care: Application of the strong model of advanced practice. Heart Lung: J Acute Crit Care 29:210, 2000.
12. Daly, BJ: Acute Care Nurse Practitioner. Springer Publishing Co., New York, 1997.
13. American Nurses Association and the American Association of Critical Care Nurses: Standards of clinical practice and scope of practice for the acute care nurse practitioner. Washington, DC, 1995.
14. Parinello, K: Advanced practice nursing. Crit Care Nurs Clin North Am 7:9, 1995.
15. Spisso, J, O'Callaghan, C, McKennan, M, and Holcroft, JW: Improved quality care and reduction of housestaff workload using trauma nurse practitioners. J Trauma 30:660, 1990.
16. Ingersoll, G: Evaluation of the advanced practice nurse role in acute and specialty care. Crit Care Nurs Clin North Am 7:25, 1995.
17. Kindig, D, and Libby, D: How will graduate medical education reform affect specialities and geographic areas? JAMA 272:37, 1994.
18. Kelso, LA, and Massaro, LM: Implementation of the acute care nurse practitioner role. AACN Clin Issues 5:404, 1994.
19. Kleinpell, RM: The acute care nurse practitioner: An expanding opportunity for critical care nurses. Crit Care Nurse 17:66, 1997.
20. Knaus, VL, Felton, S, Burton, SM, Fobes, P, and Davis, K: The use of nurse practitioners in acute care settings. J Nurs Admin 27:20, 1997.
21. Hicks, GL: Cardiac surgery and the acute care nurse practitioner—"the perfect link". Heart Lung: J Acute Crit Care 27:283, 1998.
22. Shah, SH, Bruttomesso, KA, Sullivan, DT, and Lattanzio, J: An evaluation of the role and practices of the acute-care nurse practitioner. AACN Clin Issues 8:147, 1997.
23. Rudisill, P: Unit-based advanced practice nurse in critical care. Crit Care Nurse Clin North Am 7:1, 1995.
24. Whitcomb, R., Wilson, S, Chang-Dawkins, S, Durand, J, Pitcher, D, et al: Advanced practice nursing: Acute care model in progress. J Nurs Admin 32:123, 2002.
25. Kleinpell, RM: Reports of role descriptions of acute care nurse practitioners. AACN Clin Issues 9:290, 1998.
26. Richmond, TS, and Keane, A: The nurse practitioner in tertiary care. J Nurs Admin 22:11, 1992.
27. Gates, SJ: Continuity of care: The orthopaedic nurse practitioner in tertiary care. Orthop Nurs 12:48, 1993.
28. Urban, N: Managed care challenges and opportunities for cardiovascular advanced practice nurses. AACN Clin Issues 8:78, 1997.
29. Sole, ML, Hunkar-Huie, AM, Schille, JS, and Cheatham, ML: Comprehensive trauma patient care by nonphysician providers. AACN Clin Issues 12:438, 2001.
30. Buchanan, L: The acute care nurse practitioner in collaborative practice. J Acad Nurse Pract 8:13, 1996.
31. Martin, B, and Coniglio, JU: The acute care nurse practitioner in collaborative practice. AACN Clin Issues 7:309, 1996.
32. National Association of Clinical Nurse Specialists: NACNS position paper: Regulatory credentialing of clinical nurse specialists. Clin Nurse Specialist 17:3, 2003.
33. Martin, R: Organ transplantation: The role of the acute care nurse practitioner across the spectrum of health care. AACN Clin Isssues 10:285, 1999.
34. Wachter, RM, and Goldman, L: The emerging role of "hospitalist" in the American hospital system. New Engl J Med 335:7, 1996.
35. Howie, JN, and Erickson, M: Acute care nurse practitioners: Creating and implementing a model of care for an inpatient general medicine service. Am J Crit Care 11:448, 2002.
36. Wolfe, S: Good news or bad news for nurses? RN 63:3, 2000.

37. Diamond, H, Goldberg, E, and Janosky, JE: The effect of full-time faculty hospitalist on the efficiency of care at a community teaching hospital. Ann Intern Med 129:3, 197–203,1998.
38. Berlin, L, Stennett, J, and Bednash, G: 2003–2004 Enrollment and graduations in baccalaureate and graduate programs in nursing. American Association of Colleges of Nursing, Washington, DC, 2004.
39. American Association of Colleges of Nursing. Research Institutional Data System 2003. Unpublished data.

CHAPTER 7

Formulation and Approval of Credentialing and Clinical Privileges

Geraldine "Polly" Bednash, PhD, RN, FAAN
Judy Honig, EdD, CPNP
Linda Gibbs, BSN, RN, MBA

Geraldine "Polly" Bednash, PhD, RN, FAAN, was appointed Executive Director of the American Association of Colleges of Nursing in December 1989. Dr. Bednash oversees the educational, research, governmental affairs, data bank, publications, and other programs of the only national organization dedicated exclusively to furthering nursing education in America's universities and 4-year colleges. From 1986 to 1989, Dr. Bednash headed the association's legislative and regulatory advocacy programs as director of government affairs. Dr. Bednash currently serves as Vice President for Nursing of the Health Professions Education Council of the Association of Academic Health Centers and is a member of the editorial boards of several leading nursing publications. Her publications and research presentations cover a range of critical issues in nursing education, nursing research, clinical practice, and legislative policy. Before joining the American Association of Colleges of Nursing, Dr. Bednash was Assistant Professor at the School of Nursing at George Mason University and a Robert Wood Johnson Nurse Faculty Fellow in Primary Care at the University of Maryland. Her experience includes developing resource policy for the Geriatric Research, Evaluation, and Clinical Centers of the Veterans Administration and serving as nurse practitioner and consultant to the family practice residency program at DeWitt Army Hospital at Fort Belvoir, Virginia, and as an Army Nurse Corps staff nurse in Vung Tau, Vietnam. Dr. Bednash received her bachelor's of science in nursing from Texas Woman's University, her master's of science in nursing from Catholic University of America, and her doctorate from the University of Maryland.

Judy Honig, EdD, CPNP, is Associate Professor of Clinical Nursing and Associate Dean, Student Services at Columbia University School of Nursing. She has been faculty member at Columbia School of Nursing since 1988. In addition to her administrative responsibilities, she participates in funded research, curriculum development, classroom and clinical teaching, and faculty/practice. Dr. Honig has practiced as a pediatric nurse practitioner for 20 years in active, academic, and faculty practices in urban community-based pediatric practices. She has had admitting privileges at Children's Hospital of New York since 1994. Currently, she is a primary care provider in a predominantly Latino practice and maintains a subspecialty in behavioral pediatrics.

Linda Gibbs, BSN, RN, MBA, from 2001 to 2003 served as Assistant Professor of Clinical Nursing and Associate Dean for Practice Development at Columbia University. In this capacity, she served as administrator of the Columbia Advanced Practice Nurse Association and was involved in developing the hospital credentialing process for Columbia University School of Nursing faculty. Prior to joining the Columbia faculty, Linda was with Price Waterhouse Coopers, LLP, as a health care consultant in strategic planning. Her other work experience includes financial planning at the Medicaid Assistance Program in New York City, utilization review at the Health Insurance Plan of New York, and clinical practice at Mount Sinai Hospital. Ms. Gibbs received a BS in Nursing in 1993 from the University of Michigan and an MBA from Columbia Business School in 1999.

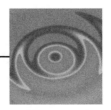

Formulation and Approval of Credentialing and Clinical Privileges

CHAPTER OBJECTIVES

After completing this chapter, the reader will be able to:

1 Analyze the differences between certification and licensure and the manner in which each is used in the regulation of advanced practice.

2 Engage in a dialogue regarding the issues surrounding multistate licensure and the importance of this to advanced practice nurses (APNs).

3 Compare and contrast the scopes of practice for each of the four traditional APN roles authorized by the nurse practice act in the state in which an APN intends to practice, including barriers to practice.

4 Discuss the differences between clinical and full staff privileges.

5 Contact a local hospital and obtain information and materials necessary for applying for clinical privileges.

Licensure, certification, and clinical privileges are interwoven components of advanced nursing practice. The first two are the gates through which the clinician must successfully pass to be granted the authority and the recognition for practice. The third can be an obstacle or a pathway for extending practice and functioning as a comprehensive clinical provider. Unfortunately, gaining either of the first two does not always automatically provide APNs with the authority to acquire clinical privileges to practice in nursing homes, hospitals, clinics, and a variety of other settings. However, APNs must be well versed in how to acquire these professional standings or to challenge barriers placed in their way.

REGULATION: PROFESSIONAL AND PUBLIC

The regulation of professional practice is accomplished in a variety of ways. Licensure, certification, and professional standards of practice represent variations on the regulation of practice. Each is structured on the basis of different value sets to control safety and quality in practice. Standards of practice are internally directed and professionally controlled entities. Professions such as nursing, medicine, and law engage in thoughtful deliberation regarding the standards that represent their efforts to self-regulate.[1] Professional self-regulation provides accountability to the society served by the profession and acknowledges that the profession will engage in efforts to protect the public from unscrupulous and unsafe practice. Professional nursing organizations such as the American Nurses Association, the American College of Nurse-Midwives (ACNM), and the American Association of Nurse Anesthetists (AANA) establish professional standards of practice through their collective members. These professional standards may be used as a mechanism for judging the practice of individual APNs and may also serve as a measure of quality of practice in legal assessments of a clinician's capabilities.

External regulation can occur through licensure or certification of the individual practitioner. Licensure is a publicly controlled operation in which the state or governing authority sets minimum standards for safe practice. The individual must meet these standards in order to be granted the privilege of practicing in a particular jurisdiction.[1] Licensure is a public function that has been delegated to the states and territories by the Constitution. Unlike licensure, certification is voluntarily sought by the professional. The professional agrees that certification has value and engages in a process of testing to establish that the standards developed by the certifying body, usually a nongovernmental and professionally monitored organization, have been met. In contrast to licensure, which validates the clinician's minimum level of competence, certification is a mechanism to document that the clinician has achieved a higher level of competence and perhaps specialization.[2]

For APNs, public regulation and professional certification have become intertwined as employers and regulators increasingly seek APNs to deliver safe, appropriate, and cost-effective care. Professional certification and licensure are receiving a great deal of scrutiny as policymakers, regulators, professional associations, and employers attempt to bring some order to the confusing array of regulations affecting advanced practice nursing. This chapter will capture the system in this period of rapid change.

Current Issues in Regulation

The regulation of advanced practice nursing has undergone significant upheaval in recent years. A number of factors have led policymakers to question the appropriateness or adequacy of the current systems of regulation for APNs. These include regulatory barriers to practice, difficulties with interstate mobility, lack of uniformity in public regulation of APNs, and increased use of telecommunications to deliver care. In addition, the dramatic changes in the health care delivery system have caused policymakers to carefully scrutinize the regulation of all health professionals. A number of commissions and advisory bodies have engaged in review of the spectrum of licensure and certification activities for health professionals.[3-5] The Pew Health Professions Commission report, *Reforming Health Care Workforce Regulation: Policy Considerations for the 21st Century,*[6] represents one of the most comprehensive overviews of regulation in all the health professions. This report raised a number of regulatory issues that have affected, and will continue to affect, advanced practice in nursing.

The Pew Report was the result of a year-long review by a commission task force of current public regulation systems and their usefulness in protecting the public. The commission task force made 10 recommendations for reform of regulatory systems (Table 7–1) and strongly urged the implementation of these to produce standardized, accountable, flexible, effective, and efficient regulatory structures. The Pew commissioners and others reviewed the complex array of issues affecting access to health care and identified a growing concern that the regulation of professional practice often decreases access to health care rather than protects it. Regulations very often serve professional interests and are used to draw regulatory lines around practice domains and to limit the care activities in which professionals can "legally" engage.

The Pew report provides an important backdrop to policy discussions regarding the current evolution of health care delivery. The report makes clear that the regulation of practice should be based on demonstrated competencies, not on the ability of one clinical group to draw territorial lines around a domain and proclaim dominance. This recommendation has been most widely supported by APNs, who have had limits placed on their practice that were either politically or professionally motivated rather than factually based.

The Pew commissioners appropriately cited current changes in the health care system as they raised questions regarding the appropriateness or utility of regulatory structures that limit access to or the use of a variety of health care providers, including APNs. The growing costs of delivering health care services has enhanced the willingness of both employers and the public to seek care from APNs and fostered an interest in reconceptualizing how care is delivered or who is capable of delivering it.

"Bottom-line" concerns drive much of the decision-making for health care,

TABLE 7–1. Reforming Health Care Work Force Regulation: Policy Considerations for the 21st Century
Statement of Recommendations
1. States should use standardized and understandable language for health professions' regulation and its functions in order to describe them clearly for consumers, provider organizations, businesses, and the professions.
2. States should standardize entry-to-practice requirements and limit them to competence assessments for health professions to facilitate the physical and professional mobility of the health professions.
3. States should base practice acts on demonstrated initial and continuing competence. This process must allow and expect different professions to share overlapping scopes of practice. States should explore pathways to allow all professionals to provide services to the full extent of their current knowledge, training, experience, and skills.
4. States should redesign health professional boards and their functions to reflect the interdisciplinary and public accountability demands of the changing health care delivery system.
5. Boards should educate consumers to assist them in obtaining the information necessary to make decisions about practitioners and to improve the board's public accountability.
6. Boards should cooperate with other public and private organizations in collecting data on regulated health professions to support effective work force planning.
7. States should require each board to develop, implement, and evaluate continuing competency requirements to ensure the continuing competence of regulated health care professionals.
8. States should maintain a fair, cost-effective, and uniform disciplinary process to exclude incompetent practitioners in order to protect and promote the public's health.
9. States should develop evaluation tools that assess the objectives, successes, and shortcomings of their regulatory systems and bodies to best protect and promote the public's health.
10. States should understand the links, overlaps, and conflicts between their health care work force regulatory systems and other systems that affect the education, regulation, and practice of health care practitioners and work to develop partnerships to streamline regulatory structures and processes.

Report of the Taskforce on Health Care Workforce Regulation. (1995). Reforming Health Care Workforce Regulation: Policy Considerations for the 21st Century. San Francisco, CA: Pew Health Professions Commission.

today, and shape the utilization of health care professionals. These new dynamics have created a marked and growing demand for APNs. Much of the interest in using APNs has been based on the APN's ability to substitute for more costly providers such as physicians. More importantly, there is also a growing awareness that APNs are safe, competent, and cost-effective providers of health care services who have been able to operate within an appropriate independent practice domain. Finally, a growing body of research has documented the different, and enhanced, outcomes achieved by APNs: more cost-effective interventions, higher patient satisfaction, increased compliance with therapeutic regimens, to name a few. Increasingly, these enhanced outcomes have caused policymakers and employers to question the logic or appropriateness of regulatory policies that limit the practice of APNs.[8–10]

Regulation of Advanced Practice Nursing: Variety and Confusion

Large, multifaceted health care organizations have created practice domains that stretch beyond state boundaries, which usually defined practice regulation. This expansion, in turn, has created interest in greater mobility among APNs and in greater consistency in the requirements for public regulatory oversight. Against this backdrop, however, the APN practices in a regulatory environment that varies widely, is sometimes conflicting, and often is very limiting.

Unlike the uniform standard for licensing of entry-level nurse clinicians, APNs face a panoply of state requirements for licensure. Each state or territory of the United States maintains some form of regulatory oversight over APNs. In 18 states, APNs are granted a second license for practice.[12] In the remaining states, APNs are granted some form of state authority to practice in the advanced role entitled "recognition" or "certification."[12] Unfortunately, state regulatory initiatives for APNs lack any evidence of consistency in the form of titling, practice privileges, or prescriptive authority.[13] APNs are licensed, certified, or recognized by state boards of nursing. In addition, the types of APNs who are authorized for advanced practice or recognized by the state regulatory boards also vary across the states.

In all states, nurse practitioners (NPs) have achieved statutory recognition and some form of state authority to write prescriptions.[15] Certified registered nurse anesthetists (CRNAs), clinical nurse specialists (CNSs), and certified nurse mid-wives (CNMs) receive recognition as APNs in almost all states. although frequently state laws or regulations limit their prescriptive authority. In addition, in many states, the CNS is recognized only in particular areas of specialization (e.g., psychiatric–mental health nursing or pediatrics) or is not recognized as an APN. In an analysis of state regulatory environments, *The Scope of Practice and Reimbursement for Advanced Practice Registered Nurses: A State-by-State Analysis,*[14] conducted by the George Washington University Intergovernmental Health Policy Institute, concluded:

> The lack of standardization among states' scopes of practice provisions for [advanced practice registered nurses] APRNs causes confusions for APRNs, other health care providers, insurance companies and consumers, and inhibits national unity among APRNs. (p. 3)

A major criticism of APN regulation has been the great array of titles that are recognized by states. Pearson[15] provides an annual update of the recognized state authorities, prescriptive limitations, and titles. The array of titles and acronyms reported as recognized by state regulations has created tremendous confusion for employers, other health professionals, policymakers, and APNs. Safriet[16] was harshly critical of this inconsistent titling as a source of confusion and loss of potential support by regulators seeking to limit practice by a clinician group.

Safriet's work on the confusing array of regulatory authorities and their some-times illogical word choices has provided many groups, both nursing and non-nursing, with a clearer picture of the failure of public regulation. Safriet noted that these often illogical regulatory structures most often are based on a concept of advanced practice nursing as a purely substitutive professional role that is secondary to the presence of physician practice. This limitation is not based on fact or experience and fails to take into account the large body of research documenting the efficacy of advanced practice nursing.

Safriet's work has been instrumental in effecting a great deal of change in public regulatory structures, as evidenced by the increasing number of states that have expanded APNs' authority to practice and prescribe. Moreover, the work of Sekscenski, et al,[17] reviewing the effect of state regulation on the availability of advanced practice clinicians, has documented that restrictive regulatory environments are negatively correlated with the presence of APNs. These researchers noted that those states with the most restrictive regulatory structures have the lowest per capita densities of APNs.

Sekscenski et al[17] noted that mobility of APNs is severely hindered by the lack of consistency in practice regulation. This inconsistency inhibits intrasystem mobility in the emerging large corporate health care structures. Integrated networks can span state lines in their scope-of-care responsibilities. However, neighboring states can have markedly different regulating policies for the practice of APNs. In addition, in many instances, APNs living along the borders of states often may have practice sites in several states. Finally, with the growing use of telehealth and distance-mediated health care, it is often not clear to regulators if the care provider is covered under laws of the state in which the provider is located or in which the patient is receiving care. The "brave new world" of cyberspace has created new modes of care delivery, such as computer- and video-transmitted patient-care experiences that can create uncertainty about where care is being delivered and who has authority for oversight of the professional's authority to practice.

Some employers argue that if oversight of practice were organizationally based, the issue of practice location would not be limited by state boundaries. Proponents of corporate-controlled regulation of APNs and other health professionals note that such a licensure procedure would provide organizations with more flexibility in the use of APNs, thus overcoming the artificial or inappropriate barriers to their full utilization. The nursing profession historically has been opposed to the notion of institutional licensure for professional nurses. Opponents of this approach to the regulation of APNs contend that quality of care could be hindered by the use of inadequately prepared clinicians who are educated by the corporation and are authorized to practice in a system that is more concerned with cost than quality. Questions also arise as to the ability of these corporate structures to engage in the expensive process of testing and evaluation necessary to ensure competence for advanced practice.[18]

Emerging Issues in the Advanced Practice Licensure Process

The growing concerns regarding interstate or across-state-boundary practice by registered nurses (RNs) and APNs has led the National Council of State Boards of Nursing (NCSBN) to create a model for licensure of individuals who practice across state boundaries. Termed the Multistate Licensure Compact, the NCSBN model allows individuals to practice in a state without a license for that specific state, provided the state of residence and the state of practice have joined a multistate compact. The compact is modeled after compacts that control driving privileges. Individual drivers are not required to hold a driver's license in each state in which they drive but are granted this privilege through agreements across states. The first step in creating a multistate licensure compact focused on basic RN practice.

Currently, 20 states have signed or are in the process of approving the implementation of a multistate compact for RN practice.[19] The common practice by APNs to engage in either telehealth or multistate practice and the confusing array of advanced practice licensure mechanisms, titles, and authorities have also created the need for a multistate compact guiding APNs. In March 2004, Utah became the first state to enter the APRN compact.[19]

As part of the development of a multistate compact for advanced practice, multiple nursing organizations have worked with and given consultative advice to the NCSBN on the uniform standards for advanced practice education and regulation that will frame the APN compact. The organizations represent the full spectrum of practice, credentialing, and education for advanced practice as a nurse practitioner, nurse anesthetist, nurse midwife, or clinical nurse specialist. In development of the compact, consensus has been sought on multiple logistical and standard issues, such as the basic level of education necessary to be covered under the compact or the types of certification that would be mandated for coverage. This process resulted in the development of a NCSBN statement on *Uniform Advanced Practice Registered Nurse Licensure/Authority to Practice Requirements.*[20] Several issues remain to be resolved among the national certification bodies for APNs, educational associations, and the NCSBN regarding their statement on uniform requirements. A major concern of the groups is the decision by the NCSBN to require the presence of a nationally recognized certification examination as a prerequisite to authority to practice. In the view of many who oppose this requirement, certification examinations are developed as practice evolves and cannot be developed absent some critical mass of clinicians who will test and expand conceptualizations of practice. Examinations cannot be developed absent clinicians already practicing in the role. Some organizations have asked the NCSBN to consider a phase-in process for clinicians practicing in new specialties to allow development of certification examinations. Early drafts of the Uniform Advanced Practice Standards did provide this option with a time limit for this "alternative mechanism" for certification. This remains as an unresolved issue.

To be granted initial licensure to practice, all nurses must successfully pass the NCLEX examination, which is developed and administered by the NCSBN. The NCSBN, a national membership organization that represents individual state or territorial boards of nursing, has engaged in a variety of efforts that have brought more urgency to the issue of advanced practice regulation. In 1993, the NCSBN House of Delegates approved a position statement mandating that all APNs be granted a second license for practice and that APNs be required to hold a master's degree to be eligible for this license. The position statement noted that second licensure already existed in a number of states, that APN practice was markedly different from that authorized through the RN licensure process, and thus that advanced practice required a new regulatory mechanism.

The second-licensure issue was opposed by a number of nursing organizations, including a variety of specialty certifying organizations and the American Association of Colleges of Nursing. These groups argued that the use of two levels of licensure was both confusing and unnecessary and that the existing use of professional certification was adequate to ensure the skills and competence of APNs. The

NCSBN cited inconsistent requirements and the limitations to mobility that resulted from these inconsistencies as significant factors in the development of the second-licensure proposal. Most nursing organizations, however, did not oppose the proposed graduate degree requirement also included in the 1993 NCSBN position statement and experienced some conflict that second licensure and graduate degree requirements were tied to the same proposal.

As previously noted, all states and territories engage in some formal recognition of advanced nursing practice. The second-licensure proposal was an attempt to bring uniformity to titling and educational requirements. The NCSBN House of Delegates adopted this position at its 1993 meeting.[21] However, because all states grant some type of practice recognition equivalent to the pure definition of licensure, the requirement that this additional recognition be termed a "license" to practice would not expand states' authority to regulate, a right already granted to the states by the Tenth Amendment of the Constitution.

The NCSBN's proposal to require a master's degree as eligibility to practice as an APN has received mixed support. In states where the state regulatory bodies have set target dates for meeting this requirement, extensions of these deadlines have been granted in the face of opposition to this higher standard. However, the master's degree requirement has become largely irrelevant, as increasing numbers of certifying examinations require the master's degree as a prerequisite to sitting for the examinations.

Despite the NCSBN's passage of the second-licensure proposal, this initiative was never enacted. Through a collaboration of nursing certification bodies and nursing regulators, agreement was reached to recognize the standardized and approved certification examinations as a proxy for a licensure process for APNs. As part of the process to reach agreement, the national certifying organizations agreed to undergo a review process that would "accredit" their examinations and provide assurance of the psychometric quality of them. Two national organizations that review and validate (accredit) the certifying organizations' capabilities are the American Board of Nursing Specialties (ABNS) and the National Commission for Certifying Agencies of the National Organization for Competency Assurance (NOCA_NCCA). See Tables 7–2 and 7–3 for information on the ABNS. Nursing regulators who had previously questioned their ability to ensure the competence of recently graduated APNs agreed that the certifying bodies, after undergoing this extensive review and validation process through these agencies, could validate APN safety for practice. The NCSBN Delegate Assembly agreed that the nursing certification bodies had made significant changes in the standardization of the examinations and uniformity of expectations across the NP certification organizations, thus creating what the NCSBN termed "legally defensible, psychometrically sound, nurse practitioner examinations that are sufficient for regulatory purposes."[20] States also recognize education and training as an additional mechanism for documenting qualifications for practice. If the education or training requirements for certification closely match the state's requirements for practice, then these documented qualifications can be accepted by the state. In many states, the regulatory agencies governing advanced nursing practice have agreed to accept proof of successful completion of professional APN certification as validation of eligibility to

---

TABLE 7–2. American Board of Nursing Specialties

The American Board of Nursing Specialties (ABNS) is the peer review body in nursing that oversees development of national professional certification processes. The ABNS, established in 1991, was the result of a 3-year project funded by the Macy Foundation to bring uniformity to professional certification in nursing and to ensure that certification was a mechanism for enhancing the quality of care delivered. The purposes of the ABNS are:

1. Provide a forum for nursing certification collaboration
2. Promote the value of nursing certification to various publics
3. Provide a mechanism for accreditation and recognition of quality nursing specialty certification accreditation

The ABNS has established 19 standards that must be met in order for a certification program to be recognized by the ABNS. Individuals who successfully complete professional certification examinations from an organization that is ABNS-recognized are considered "board certified." The following organizations have been recognized by the ABNS:

1. American Board for Occupational Health Nurses, Inc.
2. American Board of Neuroscience Nursing
3. American Legal Nurse Consultant Certification Board
4. American Nurses Credentialing Center
5. Board of Certification for Emergency Nursing
6. Certification Board of Perioperative Nursing
7. Council on Certification of Nurse Anesthetists
8. National Board of Certification for Hospice and Palliative Nurses
9. Nephrology Nursing Certification Board
10. Oncology Nursing Certification Corporation
11. Rehabilitation Nursing Certification Board

For information on ABNS standards, contact:

Executive Director
610 Thornhill Lane, Aurora, OH 44202
EDatABNS@aol.com
(330) 995–9172
www.nursingcertification.org

---

practice in the advanced practice role. As a result of the agreement reached by the certification bodies and the NCSBN, NP certification through one of these accredited organizations is now accepted as a valid mechanism for granting authority to practice to NPs in many states.

Professional certification, as defined by the American Nurses Credentialing Center (ANCC; http://nursingworld.org/ancc/), is the process by which an organization, based on predetermined standards, validates an RN's qualifications, knowledge, and practice in a defined functional or clinical area of nursing. Professional certification is reserved for those nurses who have met the requirements for clinical or functional practice in a specialized field, have pursued education beyond basic nursing preparation, and have received the endorsement of their peers. On satisfying these criteria, nurses are eligible to take certification examinations based on nationally recognized standards of nursing practice that demonstrate special knowledge and skills surpassing those required for state licensure.[22]

The use of professional certification as evidence for validation of public authority to practice intermingles the domains of professional certification and public regulation. The credentialing organization, separate and distinct from the

---

TABLE 7–3. National Commission for Certifying Agencies

National Commission for Certifying Agencies (NCCA) is the accreditation body of the National Organization on Competency Assurance (NOCA). The mission of the NCCA is:

1. Establish accreditation standards
2. Evaluate compliance with the standards
3. Recognize organizations/programs that demonstrate compliance
4. Serve as a resource on quality certification

NCCA has established 21 standards with which an organization must demonstrate compliance in order to be recognized. The following organizations have been recognized by NCCA:

1. American Academy of Nurse Practitioners
2. American Association of Critical-Care Nurses Certification Corporation
3. American Nurses Credentialing Center Commission on Certification
4. ACNM Certification Council
5. Council on Certification of Nurse Anesthetists
6. Pediatric Nursing Certification Board
7. National Certification Corporation for the Obstetric, Gynecologic, and Neonatal Nursing Specialties
8. Oncology Nursing Certification Corporation

For information on NOCA–NCCA standards, contact:

NOCA
2025 M Street, NW, Suite 800
Washington, DC 20036
(202) 367–1165
www.noca.org

---

professional membership or specialty organization, bases its credentialing examination on the standards and scope-of-practice definition set by the membership of the professional practice organization. After an in-depth job analysis, a test development committee, composed of individuals who by their education and experience are recognized as experts in the specific area of practice, identifies relevant content, areas of focus, and professional competencies to be measured. Next, examination questions are solicited from nurses certified in the specialty area and other experts throughout the country. The submitted questions undergo rigorous review, critique, and rating for accuracy and relevancy by a psychometrician. The panel of experts or test development committee then selects a representative sample of the questions for inclusion in the certifying examination.

Many professions also require practical tests and oral reviews to supplement written examinations in determining a candidate's qualifications for certification. Although written examinations are the most frequently used form of evaluation, 47 percent of certification organizations use only written examinations, and an additional 28 percent use written examinations in combination with practical tests and/or oral reviews. While the means of testing depends on the occupation or profession, written examinations can effectively evaluate knowledge. Manual or verbal skills for a particular profession often must be demonstrated through a practical test or oral presentation. Approximately 25 percent of certification programs use a practical test, and 11 percent use an oral review.[23]

Prior to the agreement by the NCSBN to recognize certification examinations as a proxy for licensure, there was great variety among the states in the use of national certifying examinations as a precursor to state recognition. In addition to NCSBN member boards' concerns regarding the psychometric properties of the testing mechanisms used by certifying bodies and questions regarding the tests' abilities to ensure the competence of an individual to serve in the expanded APN role, other critics of state reliance on professional certification processes pointed to the inconsistencies in the criteria for allowing an APN to sit for certification as a weakness. Educational requirements, graduate degree requirements, and precertification practice requirements varied among certifying organizations. In many instances, some organizations reportedly applied varying degrees of scrutiny to the educational credentials of certification applicants and allowed some applicants to waive such requirements. The collaborative efforts of NCSBN and the four organizations that certify NPs created a laudable model for ensuring both professional accountability in setting standards of practice and public oversight of practice authority.

NCSBN delegates began their work by focusing on NP practice, but there is widespread understanding that the concerns for regulation of advanced practice extend to concerns about the preparation of CNSs for advanced practice. In fact, current requirements in NCSBN's *Uniform Advanced Practice Registered Nurse Licensure/Authority to Practice Requirements*[20] apply to all APNs, including CNSs. As this issue has evolved, the relationship between public regulation and private credentialing has become more widely understood and debated. A variety of other concerns has been expressed regarding the regulation of APNs. Remaining current in skills and knowledge and the method by which such continuing competence is evidenced are at issue. Moreover, as noted previously, the development of new specialties in advanced practice for which certification examinations do not yet exist has created unintended barriers to practice in states that require national certification for practice authority. Continuing discussions of these issues are driven by concerns for protecting the public and for allowing APNs to function to their fullest capacity. These issues bear watching in each state. In any event, it appears certain that the regulation process will continue to evolve as issues related to multistate practice and specialty practice definitition are addressed by regulators.

PROFESSIONAL CERTIFICATION FOR APNs

Eight professional organizations offer certification for APNs: four for NPs, two for CNSs, one for nurse midwives, and one for nurse anesthetists. (A list of the professional organizations and specialties certified is shown in Table 7–4.) Some variation in philosophy, criteria, and requirements exists among the certifying organizations, particularly those that certify NPs. The most obvious difference is the requirement for a master's or higher degree in nursing.

Three of the organizations that certify NPs—ANCC, the American Academy of Nurse Practitioners (AANP) (http://www.aanp.org/), and the Pediatric Nursing

TABLE 7–4. Professional Organizations that Certify Advanced Practice Nurses

Certifying Body	Areas of Certification
American Academy of Nurse Practitioners Certification Program	Adult NP Family NP
American Association of Critical-Care Nurses Certification Corporation	Acute and Critical Care-Adult CNS Acute and Critical Care-Pediatric CNS Acute and Critical Care-Neonatal CNS
American College of Nurse-Midwives Certification Council	Certified Midwife Certified Nurse Midwife
American Nurses Credentialing Center (ANA)	Acute care NP Adult NP Family NP Gerontological NP Pediatric NP Adult Psychiatric Mental Health NP Family Psychiatric Mental Health NP Advanced Practice Palliative Care Nurse Community health CNS Gerontological CNS Home health CNS Medical-surgical CNS Adult psychiatric and mental health CNS Child and adolescent psychiatric and mental health CNS Pediatric CNS
Council on Certification of Nurse Anesthetists (American Association of Nurse Anesthetists)	Certified Registered Nurse Anesthetists
National Certification Corporation	Neonatal NP Women's health NP
Pediatric Nursing Certification Board	Pediatric NP Acute Care PNP (beginning 2005) Advanced Oncology Certified NP (beginning 2005) Advanced Oncology Certified Clinical NP (beginning 2005)
Oncology Nursing Certification Corporation	Advanced Oncology Certified Nurse (until 2005)

Certification Board (PNCB) (http://www.pncb.org/)—require a master's or higher degree for certification examination eligibility. The National Certification Corporation on Women's Health and Neonatal Nursing (NCC), the only organization that does not have a master's degree requirement for NP certification, convened representatives of all women's health NP and education organizations to examine this issue and to develop and implement a plan that would provide the foundation for a move to requiring a master's degree. These groups produced a consensus statement issued in September 1995 recognizing the existence of a national movement from certificate to graduate education for NPs and the need to identify and support mechanisms to provide an orderly transition of women's health care NP education from certificate to graduate education.[24] Effective January 1, 2007, the NCC will require individuals seeking certification as a women's health care or neonatal NP to hold either a master's degree in nursing or a post-master's certificate.

In its certification materials, the AANP[25] states that "certification is offered to graduates of approved Master's level adult and family NP programs" (p. 1). The AANP goes on to state that NPs who have not graduated from approved master's-level adult and family NP programs that meet the same criteria as master's degree programs may petition the Certification Board for permission to sit for the examinations. The Oncology Nursing Certification Corporation (ONCC),[26] which offers certification for both NPs and CNSs in advanced nursing oncology, also requires NPs and CNSs to hold a master's degree in nursing to apply for certification. The ONCC examination does not test for specific NP or CNS competencies; rather, it focuses on the clinical science base of oncology nursing practice.

The ACNM Certification Council (ACC) (http://www.acnm.org/), the only body that certifies nurse midwives, requires graduation from an accredited program but does not require an advanced degree in nursing. ACNM Division on Accreditation (ACNM-DOA) currently accredits certificate, graduate, and precertificate nurse midwifery education programs. In addition, ACNM also accredits non-nurse midwifery programs. To date, two midwifery programs for individuals without a nursing degree have been accredited by the ACNM-DOA. These programs are a combination of physician assistant and midwifery programs. Graduates of these programs are required to acquire the same competencies and to sit for the same certification examination as nurse midwives. Midwifery certification examinations are administered by the ACC.

The AANA (http://www. aana.com/crna/) offers certification for nurse anesthetists. To be eligible for the certification examination, the individual must be a graduate of a nurse anesthesia program accredited by the Council on Accreditation of Nurse Anesthesia Educational Programs of AANA. Under AANA standards adopted in November 1994, a master's or higher degree was required by January 1998. Not all nurse anesthesia programs are located in schools of nursing, and therefore a number of programs may offer a non-nursing master's degree.[27]

The following four sections provide overviews and comparisons of the certification requirements for each of the advanced practice nursing specialties. Requirements for certification are revised regularly. For more detailed and current information regarding eligibility requirements for certification or recertification in each of the specialty practice areas, the APN should contact the respective professional organization.

NP Certification

Four professional organizations offer NP certification programs specific to NP practice: the AANP, the ANCC, the NCC, and the PNCB (see Table 7–4). Certification is offered in a number of specialties: acute care NP, adult NP, family NP, gerontological NP, neonatal NP, pediatric NP, psychiatric/mental health NP, school NP, women's health care NP, advanced oncology nursing, and others. The newest NP certification under development by the PNCB is designed to test for practice as a pediatric acute care NP. The ONCC offers certification in advanced nursing oncology for NPs and CNSs: the same examination is used for both. As noted above, the process does not test for separate role capabilities. For this reason, many state boards of nursing do not recognize this examination as evidence of an individual's capabilities to practice in the NP role. However, results of the most recent role delineation study on NP and CNS practice in oncology did show differences in functions and tasks; therefore, separate examinations are being developed.[54]

The various NP certification bodies have differing requirements for the educational experience of individuals seeking certification. Individuals seeking entry into an APN program are encouraged to assess and document whether the program they are considering has met the requirements of the certifying body. In addition, individuals should determine state and national certification requirements and document that the program and certification will allow them to follow their chosen career path. In some instances, two or more organizations offer examinations for the same specialty practice area but hold different expectations of the educational program.

Before the collaborative development of the Acute Care Nurse Practitioner Certification Examination by the American Association of Critical Care Nurses Certification Corporation and ANCC in 1995, NPs prepared in acute care did not have a mechanism for obtaining national certification, creating a barrier to practice in those states that had enacted legislation requiring national certification by a professional organization for NP practice. Similarly, prior to development of the psychiatric NP certification examination, individuals prepared for this role frequently experienced difficulty with state recognition for their authority to practice. The continued evolution of advanced practice and the lag period necessary for the evolution of new certification examinations will continue to create challenges for individuals prepared in specialties for which no tests exist. Currently, discussions regarding the Multistate Licensure Compact are focused heavily on these concerns as individuals with different perspectives on the definition of specialty practice struggle to create a uniform policy on practice authority requirements.

Recertification requirements also vary among the five professional certifying organizations, with lengths of certification terms ranging from 5 to 6 years. The most common requirements for recertification include either reexamination or documentation of a specified number of hours in direct patient care in one's area of specialization and a specified number of hours of continuing education. A number of states now require the individual to have a specified number of continuing education hours annually in pharmacology to maintain one's prescriptive privileges. The adequacy of continuing education requirements in ensuring practitioner competence has been seriously questioned, however, by the 1995 Pew report titled *Reforming Health Care Workforce Regulation*.[6]

The PNCB provides two options for maintaining one's certification as a pediatric NP. An individual can take a scored self-assessment learning exercise, an independent study educational tool each year, or earn a specified number of continuing education credits. The self-assessment activity must be completed, however, in at least two of the years in the 6-year recertification cycle.[28]

CNS Certification

CNS certification is offered by the ANCC, the American Association of Critical Care Nurses Certification Corporation (AACN-CC), and the ONCC. The ANCC areas of CNS certification include medical-surgical nursing, gerontological nursing, community health nursing, home health nursing, adult psychiatric and mental health nursing, child and adolescent psychiatric and mental health nursing, and others. As noted previoiusly, the ONCC offers an advanced oncology nursing certification that is not specific to CNS practice but which CNSs can take. To become certified in any of these specialty areas, the candidate must have a master's degree or higher in nursing.

Each of these certification programs requires that candidates have a minimum number of hours in direct patient care in their areas of specialization. ANCC certification as an adult or child and adolescent psychiatric and mental health CNS requires both documentation of a specified number of hours in direct patient care and a minimum number of hours of consultation and supervision by a nurse who is ANCC-certified or eligible for certification as a CNS in psychiatric and mental health nursing.[22]

The AACN-CC offers certification programs in adult, neonatal, and pediatric critical-care nursing. To qualify for any of these examinations, an individual must hold a current RN license, have a master's degree in nursing with specific preparation as a CNS, and document a specified number of clinical practice hours in direct care of the critically ill patient.[29]

Nurse Midwife Certification

The ACNM Certification Council is the only professional organization that offers certification for midwifery. To be eligible for the national certification examination, the individual must hold a current RN license to practice in the United States and must document satisfactory completion of a nurse midwifery program or a midwifery program for non-nurses that is either accredited or preaccredited by the ACNM Division of Accreditation[30] (see http://www.acnm.org). Core competencies for basic nurse midwifery are clearly delineated by ACNM for each of the components of nurse midwifery care: preconception, antepartum, intrapartum, postpartum, neonatal, and family planning and gynecological care.[31]

Nurse Anesthetist Certification

Professional certification for nurse anesthetists is offered solely by the Council on Certification of Nurse Anesthetists, an arm of the AANA. To be eligible to take the certification examination for registered nurse anesthetists, candidates must hold a current and unrestricted RN license in the state in which they practice and must have completed a nurse anesthesia educational program accredited by the

Council on Accreditation of Nurse Anesthesia Educational Programs[32] (see http://www.aana.com). In its requirements for program accreditation, the Council on Accreditation of Nurse Anesthesia Educational Programs delineates the number and type of patient experiences required for graduation. In addition, the number of required experiences and specific types and methods of anesthesia are also defined.[33]

CLINICAL PRACTICE AND INSTITUTIONAL PRIVILEGES

APNs must have access to a variety of health care settings to provide the full range of comprehensive health care services within the scope of their practice and to allow the consumer a full choice of high-quality, cost-effective health care services. Traditionally, privileges to practice in a given health care institution have been reserved for members of the institution's medical staff, and admission to this group has been closely guarded. All health providers must be privileged to practice in a given health care setting. Clinical privileges permit APNs and hospitalists to provide inpatient services to their patients. APNs with admitting privileges care for patients in the hospital and, in addition, admit and discharge. Past battles waged by APNs and other health professionals to obtain admitting privileges have laid the groundwork for today's APN practice. As the number and diversity of APN specialties increase and as the move toward an integrated health care delivery system gains momentum, more APNs will seek privileges, including admitting privileges, to practice in all types of health care settings, from acute care to community-based settings.

Clinical Practice Settings for APNs

The number of APNs who currently hold clinical privileges at a health care institution is not known. However, general information on practice settings and arrangements in which APNs in the various specialties are located is available.

According to the ACNM, in 2002 more than 50% of CNMs worked primarily in an office or clinic. Most CNMs also listed a hospital or physician as their place of employment.[43] Also in 2002, 99 percent of all births attended by CNMs occurred in a hospital, 0.26 percent occurred in a free-standing birth center, and 0.59 percent occurred in the home.[34]

According to 1995 demographic data published by the AANA, 10,358 (40.4 percent) of all CRNAs were institutionally employed. More than 11 percent were self-employed or part of a CRNA group practice, and another 25 percent were practicing in a joint nurse anesthetist/anesthesiologist (CRNA/MDA) group practice. Of those in a joint CRNA/MDA practice, only 0.8 percent were partners or joint partners.[35]

As a group, CNSs and NPs are more diverse in their practice settings and scopes of practice. Data regarding the practice arrangements of CNSs and NPs are minimal; however, some inferences can be drawn based on known data. In 1992, the estimated number of NPs not working with a physician or a psychologist was 398 (1.8 percent), implying that this small percentage of NPs were in independent practice. An additional estimated 466 NPs (2.1 percent) were in a practice arrangement in which the NP paid a consultant's fee to a physician or psychologist. Only an estimated 3.4 percent of NPs were not on a salary and received only fee-for-service practice receipts. The estimated percentage of CNSs who did not work with a physician or a psychologist was 18.4 percent. An estimated 8.6 percent of CNSs paid a consultation fee to a physician or psychologist. An estimated 27.8 percent of all CNSs received fee-for-service practice receipts only. However, this number decreased to only 2.3 percent when psychiatric–mental health CNSs were removed from the sample.[36]

In general, APNs who specialize in the management of hospitalized patients are becoming more numerous. Like the physician hospitalist, the model of inpatient care being transferred to a hospital employee has developed rapidly and has improved in-patient efficiency without compromising quality.[50] More than 94 percent of all neonatal NPs were employed in inpatient hospital-based settings. The second highest percentage of specialty NPs employed in inpatient hospital-based practices were adult NPs (11.5 percent). More than one-third of gerontology NPs were employed in a nursing home or an extended-care facility (34.3 percent). Medical-surgical CNSs constituted the largest group of CNSs employed in an inpatient hospital-based setting (62.9 percent). However, only 22 percent of adult psychiatric CNSs were employed in inpatient hospital-based settings.[36]

The number of APNs in all specialty areas involved in independent practice is increasing slowly. All APNs, whether they are practicing in an independent practice setting or not, are responsible for the comprehensive health care of clients. The ability of APNs to deliver comprehensive care is compromised by their inability to coordinate and provide services to these clients when their conditions warrant admission to a health care institution. The financial and quality-of-care benefits associated with the possession of admitting privileges are becoming increasingly evident.

Factors Governing Institutional Privileges

An APN's ability to obtain privileges at an institution is governed by three entities:

1. State law and regulations
2. Joint Commission on Accreditation of Healthcare Organizations (JCAHO)
3. Institutional bylaws

State Law and Regulations

State law and regulations define the scope of advanced practice nursing within the particular state. The state nurse practice acts under which APNs practice determine the scope of practice and the amount of dependence or independence with which they may practice. Clinical privileges granted to an APN must be in accordance with these state laws and regulations. The number of states that have enacted laws allowing independent practice of APNs has increased dramatically, and additional state boards of nursing and advanced practice nursing groups are considering similar legislation.

Joint Commission on Accreditation of Healthcare Organizations

The APN's ability to obtain privileges is also influenced by the standards for institutional accreditation established by JCAHO. JCAHO first revised its medical-staff standards in 1983 to allow hospitals to extend clinical privileges to nonmedical practitioners. This change in policy was spurred by antitrust case law, changes in reimbursement laws, an increased emphasis on cost control, expanded numbers and types of providers, and an increased spirit of competition.[37] The 1984 JCAHO standards stipulated that medical staff must include physicians but also allowed hospitals to grant medical-staff membership to other licensed practitioners permitted by law and the hospital to independently provide patient care services.[39] The 2001 JCAHO standards describe the medical staff as:

> MS.1.1.1 It includes fully licensed physicians and may include other licensed individuals permitted by law and by the hospital to provide patient care services independently in the hospital (both physicians and these other individuals are referred to as "licensed independent practitioners").[51]

JCAHO goes on to define a licensed independent practitioner as "any individual permitted by law and by the organization to provide care and services without direction or supervision, within the scope of the individual's license and consistent with individually granted clinical privileges."

JCAHO provides the APN with a framework by which to obtain privileges:

> MS.6.5 The management of each patient's care is the responsibility of a qualified licensed independent practitioner with appropriate clinical privileges.[51]

It is also clear which provider can direct patient care:

> MS.6.5.1 Management of a patient's general medical condition is the responsibility of a qualified physician member of the medical staff.[51]

Institutional Bylaws or Policy

The governing board of a hospital grants membership to the medical staff of the institution. The board must also delineate the specific functions that may be performed by individual practitioners if allowed to provide patient care services independently in the institution, whether or not they are members of the medical staff. Even when federal case law, state law, and accreditation standards stipulate that APNs may obtain privileges at a health care institution, the individual institution may determine the specific credentials deemed acceptable and the specific clinical privileges allowed. The privileges delineated by the institution may be more restrictive than those allowed under state nurse practice acts.

Since the revision of the JCAHO accreditation standards to allow hospitals to grant privileges to "other independently licensed" providers, many institutions have created a separate category to encompass nonphysician providers. Such terms as "affiliate," "associate," or "allied health staff" are some of the more commonly used terms to denote nonphysician staff membership and privileges.

The granting of affiliate staff privileges generally does not grant the APN full standing on the institution's medical staff. The most common difference between full medical and affiliate/associate-staff privileges is that APNs are not allowed to admit and discharge patients under their own name. Affiliate or allied staff membership also does not include medical staff voting privileges. Another difference that may exist is that an affiliate staff member might not be allowed to serve on any of the medical staff committees that make recommendations to the institution's governing board regarding rules and regulations by which the medical staff operates.

Many hospitals that have created an affiliate staff category have also delineated specific circumstances under which the practitioner who is granted affiliate staff status may practice and specific functions that may be performed. These criteria and functions often are more restrictive than the scope of practice allowed by state law. Although it may be seen as self-serving and protective of the medical staff, an institution's board of governors is permitted to establish rules and procedures that maintain and protect the quality of care delivered to patients at that institution. In addition:

> MS.1.1.3 All medical staff members and all others with delineated clinical privileges are subject to medical staff and departmental bylaws, rules and regulations, and policies and are subject to review as part of the organization's performance-improvement activities.[51]

Privileges at an Institution

APNs as well as physicians and other nonmedical staff must be credentialed for privileges at an institution. In this chapter privileges are separated into two categories: clinical and admitting. Clinical privileges grant the practitioner the ability to treat patients within the institution. All health care practitioners within the institution must have clinical privileges before caring for patients. Admitting privileges allow the APN to admit his/her patient to a certain institution. When applying for clinical privileges to an institution, the APN can also request to be granted admitting privileges. Credentialing is a part of the privileging process due to the mere fact that practitioners' privileges are predicated on their credentials. The credentialing process usually involves the collection and review of data to qualify the practitioner for patient care within the institution.

During the credentialing process, JCAHO requires that four core elements be examined:

> MS.5.4.3.1 For an applicant for initial appointment to the medical staff and for initial granting of clinical privileges, the hospital verifies information about the applicant's licensure, specific training, experience, and current competence provided by the applicant with information from the primary source(s) whenever feasible. [51]

An institution credentialing a practitioner would request the following from a practitioner[52]:

- Proof of education
- Evidence of state licensure as an RN and second licensure/certification as an NP
- Drug Enforcement Agency (DEA) number

- Proof of national certification as an NP in specialty field
- Current life support certification
- Summary of employment history and history of other locations at which privileges have been held
- Membership in professional associations
- References
- Malpractice insurance
- Written collaborative practice agreement
- Practice protocols
- Privileges request form
- Curriculum vitae
- Health assessment

In addition to the review of a practitioner's credentials, hospitals and institutions will also utilize the National Practitioner Data Bank (NPDB) and criminal background checks. The NPDB will list a practitioner if he/she has been involved in the settlement of a malpractice case, regardless of the practitioner's innocence or guilt. Failure of an applicant to disclose his/her involvement in a suit to the institution may lead to a termination or denial of privileges.

Clinical Privileges

All APNs who are employed by a hospital-based institution must have clinical privileges. These APNs are most often credentialed by the department of nursing, a special committee for the privileging of allied health professionals, or the hospital human resources office in the form of a job description.[52] APNs and midwives who practice as licensed independent practitioners and not as employees of the institution, according to JCAHO, need to be privileged through the medical staff office. Clinical privileges identify the specific patient care services that can be delivered by an individually qualified practitioner within the institution. Delineation of privileges is defined as an "accurate, detailed, and specific description of the clinical privileges granted."[37]

Admitting Privileges

Those APNs in practice outside of the institution, applying for clinical privileges, can request to be granted admitting privileges. Admitting privileges allow the APN to have access to his/her patient for continuity of care. In 1983, the District of Columbia enacted legislation that prohibited hospitals or any other health care facility from denying clinical privileges or medical staff membership for qualified CRNAs, CNMs, certified NPs, podiatrists, or psychologists. This legislation was expanded in 1985 to include CNSs. Five states—Alaska, Arizona, Arkansas, Oregon, and Wisconsin—allow APNs to admit patients to an institution.[53] In most states, hospital admitting privileges for APNs are not regulated and are granted at the discretion of the hospitals. Many hospitals will grant privileges to APNs only if their collaborating physicians have staff privileges at the hospital.

A number of benefits to possessing admitting privileges have been cited in the literature.[38,39,41] These include:

- The ability to continue to provide and direct the care received by a patient if admission to a health care institution is necessary
- The ability to ensure that the patient is discharged back to one's care
- The ability to observe or assist in a patient's surgery
- The ability to review and write in the patient's chart without permission
- The ability to obtain reimbursement from third-party payers for visits made to patients
- The ability to oversee the care received by a patient, including the referral to specialists for consultation
- A means of demonstrating one's credentials and competencies or a way of obtaining a "stamp of approval" from the health care profession at large
- Preferred provider organizations (PPO) or managed care companies may use hospital privileges as a means of measuring a provider's competence or as a method of quality assurance for the PPO
- A means of gaining recognition as a legitimate health care professional in a competitive health care market
- A way to maintain an ongoing relationship with a patient, including serving as a patient advocate
- A way to increase one's knowledge of, and ability to discuss, a patient's potential hospital experiences
- A means of keeping one's skills and knowledge of technology and procedures current
- The ability to become involved in setting the rules and regulations governing practices at the health care institution
- The ability to more fully market one's services to the consumer
- The ability to maintain one's self-esteem
- The ability to meet physicians' and consumers' demands for services provided by APNs

Along with the benefits of obtaining admitting privileges, APNs must be willing to assume the increased accountability and responsibility for the services they provide to patients. APNs must participate fully in the decision-making processes involved in providing care to patients and in ensuring that appropriate coverage is provided 24 hours a day. APNs are liable for their own actions, just as physicians or institutions are liable for negligent actions involving the care of patients. In addition, APNs may be held liable for not referring a patient with a problem beyond their level of competence. With full medical-staff membership and privileges comes the ability and responsibility to serve on one or more medical staff committees. Not only does this provide the practitioner with the ability to participate more fully in the decision-making and policy-making processes of the institution; it also requires a significant amount of time away from one's other professional and personal commitments.

The hospitalist role is being utilized more frequently by health care institutions to increase the efficiency and decrease the cost for inpatient stays.[50] Many of these institutions have realized cost savings by having an individual familiar with the hospital's policies and capabilities oversee an admitted patient. In addition, many primary care physicians (PCPs) have chosen not to direct their patients' care while hospitalized based on the same cost-benefit analysis. PCPs are finding that taking time out of their schedule to see hospitalized patients interferes with seeing patients in the office and requires more time of them. As a result, their potential reimbursement is affected by the reduction of patients seen along with the notion that not all visits to patients within the hospital are reimbursable.

Both APNs and physicians who are designated primary care providers are continuing to fulfill their duties as PCPs alongside the hospitalist. The responsibility and accountability for that patient has decreased while the patient is hospitalized, but not the continuity of care. PCPs do work with hospitalists to provide a team approach to the hospitalized patient so that follow-up care, once the patient is discharged, can be seamless. This arrangement also allows the PCP some flexibility in terms of visiting the hospitalized patient.

Appeal for Denial of Privileges

Denial of medical staff membership and privileges to an individual APN may be due to inadequate credentials or because the institution does not want that type of provider practicing in the institution despite adequate credentials. An institution has the responsibility and right to deny medical staff membership and privileges to any practitioner if there is inadequate documentation of competence, if there is evidence of prior incident of disciplinary action, and/or if references do not support the granting of clinical privileges. If an application is disapproved, the appeals process documented in the bylaws must be followed. If privileges have been awarded previously to APNs in a given specialty, it is very difficult to prove that privileges were denied due to discrimination.

In attempting to reverse an adverse decision by an institution's board, the appeals process must be followed carefully and exhausted before turning to alternative actions. An alternative mechanism that may be tried is to wait a reasonable amount of time and reapply. Changes in the health care arena are occurring, and political pressure may be brought to bear on an institution. Alliances with medical and other health professional colleagues and consumers must be sought. Opponents of granting medical staff membership to APNs may retire or leave the institution. As consumers become more attuned to, and involved in, health care issues, state legislatures are becoming more willing to enact laws that broaden the scope of advanced nursing practice. This movement will pave the way for increasingly independent practice and the increased use of APNs to provide comprehensive health care services across all health care delivery sites.

Legal action, particularly if taken as an individual practitioner, is a lengthy and extremely costly process in terms of both financial and emotional resources. In many instances, the entire appeals process has extended over 13 years. In some instances, decisions have been made in a more timely fashion but generally involve an out-of-court settlement. If legal action is deemed necessary, several courses of action are available; these are most appropriately determined and explained by legal counsel.

Federal Trade Commission

The Federal Trade Commission (FTC) has the ability to investigate a complaint made by an APN or group of nurses regarding anticompetitive practices of an institution. Although the FTC has refused to hear numerous cases regarding discrimination against APNs, there is some evidence of its willingness to mediate well-documented instances of discrimination. On January 28, 1988, the FTC issued a consent agreement involving a group of nurse midwives and the medical staff of the Memorial Medical Center in Savannah, Georgia. The complaint brought by the nurse midwives alleged that in 1983 the hospital medical staff's credentials committee voted to allow a nurse midwife to perform deliveries at the medical center in the presence of a physician, as authorized under Georgia law. Shortly thereafter, members of the medical staff protested and threatened to shift their patient admissions to another hospital. One month later, the committee reversed itself and denied the nurse midwife hospital privileges, without stating any reasonable basis for the decision. Under the consent agreement, the medical staff agreed not to deny or restrict hospital privileges for any nurse midwife, unless the staff was able to provide a reasonable basis for believing that such restriction would serve the interest of the hospital in providing health care services.[42]

Antitrust Rulings

Legal action in response to the denial of medical-staff membership and clinical privileges may also be sought in federal court, alleging violation of the Sherman Antitrust Act. Although extremely expensive and lengthy, such legal recourse has been successful in several cases involving APNs.

As early as 1976, health care providers were subject to federal antitrust laws. In *Hospital Building Company v Trustees of Rex Hospital,* 428 US 738 (1976), the U.S. Supreme Court held that health care is a commercial business operated for economic benefit and thus subject to the Sherman Antitrust Act.[44] The act [45] prohibits conspiracies "in restraint of trade or commerce among the several states" (Section 1) and prohibits monopolizing "any part of the trade or commerce among the several states" (Section 2). Many health care practitioners have asserted that a hospital's refusal to permit them to practice at a hospital was illegal under one or both of these provisions of the Sherman Antitrust Act. Health care practitioners who have been denied privileges because of exclusivity contracts or because they were members of certain professions, including nursing, have also brought suit against hospitals under the Sherman Antitrust Act.[46] Most states also have enacted similar antitrust legislation that may be a viable alternative to action at the federal level.

For a case to be brought under the Sherman Antitrust Act, two preliminary criteria must be satisfied. First, it must be shown that the case or controversy involves interstate trade or commerce. In some cases, the required nexus between the identified conduct and interstate commerce has been implied from facts showing that some patients have come from out of state, that equipment used is purchased from out of state, that the hospital or institution has out-of-state shareholders, and/or that insurance payments have come from out-of-state companies. In other, more restrictive cases, the court has ruled that to qualify under the Sherman Antitrust Act, the practitioner's business or the denial of access to the practitioner must directly affect or involve interstate commerce.[47]

The second criterion that must be proved is that there has been a conspiracy in restraint of trade. The conspiratorial action must have the effect of restraining competition in a relevant or defined market. The conspiracy may involve little more than a joint understanding or action. For example. in the case of *Bhan v NME Hospitals,* the court noted that the five hospitals operated within the area indicated that the defendant hospital's policy of not allowing nurse anesthetists to practice was not a restraint of trade.[47] However, in *Oltz v St. Peter's Community Hospital,* a decision was obtained in favor of the nurse anesthetist where the defendant hospital was the only hospital equipped to do general surgery in the area.[47]

In *Bhan v NME Hospitals,* several precedents relevant to advanced nursing practice and antitrust case law were established. Mr. Bhan, a CRNA, had worked for one of the NME hospitals on a fee-for-service basis for several years. Under a contract with the hospital, he and an anesthesiologist had provided all of the hospital's anesthesia services until the time that the hospital hired a second anesthesiologist. At that time, Bhan's anesthesiologist associate urged the hospital to drop Bhan from the staff and to rely on himself and the other anesthesiologist, and the hospital followed this recommendation. Mr. Bhan claimed that the all-anesthesiologist policy was adopted as part of a conspiracy to eliminate competition. The federal trial court dismissed the lawsuit on the grounds that nurses and doctors do not compete because, in California, CRNAs were not authorized to write orders and were required to work under a supervising physician. The U.S. district court of appeals reversed this decision, stating that although the legal restrictions on CRNAs create a functional distinction between them and anesthesiologists, such restrictions did not preclude their reasonable interchangeability. In effect, the court held that nurses have standing to sue under the antitrust laws when they are excluded from practicing as the result of anticompetitive arrangements between hospitals and physicians.[48]

In *Oltz v St. Peter's Community Hospital,* a federal trial court and the federal court of appeals agreed that the hospital had conspired with anesthesiologists to restrain the nurse anesthetist's practice. Mr. Oltz was an independent contractor providing anesthesia services, primarily for obstetric cases. The facts demonstrated that Mr. Oltz was popular with the obstetricians, who preferred his services over those of the anesthesiologists. When the hospital decided to organize an anesthesia department, Mr. Oltz's contract was terminated. The contract was reinstated when the hospital received correspondence from Oltz's attorney and the state attorney general's office. Subsequently, three of the hospital's four anesthesiologists threatened to quit if Oltz's services were retained, and so his contract was once again terminated. After Oltz's departure, each anesthesiologist received a 40 to 50 percent salary increase. A monetary pretrial settlement was negotiated with the anesthesiologists, and Oltz proceeded successfully in obtaining a jury verdict against the hospital. This is one of the only cases in which a health care provider has been able to prove that the installation of an exclusive contract violated the Sherman Act and caused economic damages.[44]

In a case involving a nurse midwife, *Nurse Midwifery Associates v Hibbett*,[49] the nurse midwives attempted to invoke the Sherman Antitrust Act and the Tennessee state antitrust laws to prohibit the defendants (three hospitals, one pediatrician, three obstetricians, and an insurance carrier) from denying staff privileges to nurse midwives. The nurse midwives alleged that the defendants' denial of privileges had put them out of business. One of the obstetricians, Hibbett, was also a member of the board of trustees of the insurance company. The court denied the claim against one hospital and the insurance company for various reasons, the most important being that the nurses failed to prove a conspiracy by these defendants. The court did decide that the claims against two of the hospitals and Hibbett warranted a trial. After 13 years, an out-of-court settlement was reached.

The description of antitrust rulings presented here should be considered illustrative cases rather than a comprehensive discussion of case law. The reader should be familiar with the concepts referred to in antitrust rulings as they relate to APNs. Any decision to enter into an antitrust legal case should be made only after lengthy discussion with qualified legal counsel.

SUMMARY

Regulation of advanced practice nursing is in a state of flux. Several factors, such as the increased numbers of APNs in the various practice specialties, the number of practice specialties, changes in the health care delivery system, increased consumer involvement in health care, and public demand for accountability by health care providers for high-quality, cost-effective care, have and will continue to have a significant impact on the regulation of advanced practice nursing. APNs must assume a leadership role both in the delivery of health care services and in the professional and public regulation of nursing practice. To assume such a role, APNs must be able to understand and articulate the authorized scope of their practice. The ability to understand the interrelationships among the processes used by the public and the profession to regulate advanced practice nursing and to respond appropriately to these processes is crucial.

SUGGESTED EXERCISES

1 Review the statutory and regulatory standards for advanced practice nursing in the state in which you expect to practice after graduation. Determine the correct state regulatory agency, and then make a request for the state authority-to-practice guidelines.

2 Identify the advanced practice nursing certifying organization that administers the examination most relevant to your expected area of practice, and request information regarding the standards for practice, the process of application for certification, and the process for renewal of certification.

3 Acquire a copy of the Pew Health Professions report on licensure and regulation, and compare that report's recommendations to the standards for regulation in the state in which you will practice.

4 Obtain a copy of the bylaws of a hospital to determine the process used to delineate and grant clinical and admitting privileges. Based on the hospital's bylaws, determine whether an APN is eligible for membership on the medical staff.

5 Review the annual update of *The Nurse Practitioner* on licensure and prescriptive privileges, and identify changes that have occurred from the previous year. How does the state in which you practice compare with other states in the area of independent practice, scope of practice, prescriptive authority, and reimbursement for all APNs?

REFERENCES

1. American Nurses Association: Nursing's Social Policy Statement. American Nurses' Association, Washington, DC, 1995.
2. Malson, LP: Credentialing in Nursing: Contemporary Developments and Trends. American Nurses Association, Kansas City, MO, 1989, p. 1.
3. Cox, C, and Foster, S: The Costs and Benefits of Occupational Regulation. Bureau of the Federal Trade Commission, Washington, DC, 1990.
4. Friedland, B, and Valachovic, R: The regulation of dental licensing: The dark ages? Am J Law Med 17:249, 1991.
5. Maine Health Professions Regulation Taskforce: Toward a More Rational State Licensure System for Maine's Health Professionals: A Report to the Governor and Maine Legislature. Medical Care Development, Maine Health Professions Regulation Task Force, Augusta, Maine, 1995.
6. Pew Health Professions Commission: Reforming Health Care Workforce Regulation: Policy Considerations for the 21st Century. Pew Health Professions Commission, San Francisco, 1995.
7. Starr, P: The Social Transformation of American Medicine. Basic Books, New York, 1982.
8. Burl, JB, and Bonner, A: Demonstration of the cost-effectiveness of an NP/physician team in long-term care facilities. HMO Pract 8:157, 1994.
9. Frampton, J, and Wall, S: Exploring the use of NPs and PAs in primary care. HMO Pract 8:164, 1994.
10. Schultz, JM, Liptak, GS, and Fioravanti, J: Nurse practitioners' effectiveness in NICU. Nurs Manage 25:50, 1994.
11. National Council of State Boards of Nursing: What regulation of advanced nursing practice can offer health care reform. Issues 14:4, 1993.
12: NCSBN: Using Nurse Practitioner Certification for State Nursing Regulation: A Historical Perspective. Author, 2003, Chicago. At ncsbn.org/public/regulation/licensure_aprn_practitioner.html.
13. King, CS: Second licensure. Adv Pract Nurs Q 1:7, 1995.
14. Henderson, T, Fox-Grage, W, and Lewis, S: The Scope of Practice and Reimbursement for Advanced Practice Registered Nurses: A State-by-State Analysis. Intergovernmental Health Policy Institute, Washington, DC, 1995.
15. Pearson, L: Fifteenth annual legislative update: How each state stands on legislative issues affecting advanced nursing practice. Nurse Pract 1:26–58, 2003.

16. Safriet, BJ: Health care dollars and regulatory sense: The role of advanced practice nursing. Yale J Regul 9(2), 1992.
17. Sekscenski, E, et al: State practice environments and the supply of physician assistants, NPs, and certified nurse-midwives. N Engl J Med 331:1266, 1994.
18. American Nurses Association: Institutional Licensure: An Historical Perspective. House of Directors Action Report. American Nurses Association, Washington, DC, 1995.
19. National Council of State Boards of Nursing. http://www.ncsbn.org/nlc/rnlpvncompact_mutual_recognition_state.asp Accessed March 2004.
20. National Council of State Boards of Nursing (2000) Uniform Advanced Practice Registered Nurse Licensure/Authority to Practice Requirements. Author, Chicago.
21. National Council of State Boards of Nursing: What regulation of advanced practice can offer health care reform. Issues 14:4, 1993.
22. American Nurses Certification Corporation: 1996 Certification Catalog. American Nurses Certification Corporation, Washington, DC, 1995.
23. National Certification Corporation: Certification Committee Newsletter. National Certification Corporation, Chevy Chase, MD, 1995.
24. Association of Women's Health Organizations and Neonatal Nurses, National Association of Nurses in Reproductive Health, and Planned Parenthood Federation of America: Consensus Statement on Women's Health Care Nurse Practitioner Education (September 15, 1995). Washington, DC, pp. 19–35.
25. American Academy of Nurse Practitioners. National Competency-Based Certification Examinations for Adult and Family Nurse Practitioners. American Academy of Nurse Practitioners, Austin, TX, 1996.
26. Oncology Nursing Certification Corporation: Oncology Nursing Certification Corporation Test Bulletin. Oncology Nursing Certification Corporation, Pittsburgh, PA, 1996.
27. American Association of Nurse Anesthetists.
28. National Certification Board of Pediatric Nurse Practitioners and Nurses: Pediatric Nurse Practitioner Certification and Certification Maintenance Programs. National Certification Board of Pediatric Nurse Practitioners, Cherry Hill, NJ, 1995.
29. American Association of Critical Care Nursing Certification Corporation: Certification Renewal Handbook. American Association of Critical Care Nursing Certification Corporation, Aliso Viejo, CA, 1996.
30. American College of Nurse-Midwives Certification Council: Statement on Eligibility Requirements for Application to Take the National Certification Examination. American College of Nurse-Midwives Education Committee, Washington, DC, February 1994.
31. American College of Nurse-Midwives Education Committee: ACNM Core Competencies for Basic Nurse-Midwifery Practice. American College of Nurse-Midwives Education Committee, Washington, DC, 1992.
32. Council on Certification of Nurse Anesthetists: 1996 Candidate Handbook. Council on Certification of Nurse Anesthetists, Park Ridge, IL, 1996.
33. Council on Accreditation of Nurse Anesthesia Education Programs: Standards for Accreditation of Nurse Anesthesia Educational Programs. Council on Accreditation of Nurse Anesthesia Education Programs, Park Ridge, IL, 1994.
34. National Vital Statistics Report, vol. 50, no. 5, February 12, 2002. Accessed June 2003 from www.aacn.org/prof/display
35. American Association of Nurse Anesthetists: Demographic Information for All CRNA Members, Excluding Students. Chicago, IL, 1995.
36. Department of Health and Human Services: Survey of Certified Nurse Practitioners and Clinical Nurse Specialists: December 1992. Department of Health and Human Services, Public Health Service, Health Resources and Services Administration, Bureau of Health Professions, Division of Nursing, Rockville, MD, 1994.
37. Joint Commission on Accreditation of Healthcare Organizations: 1995 Accreditation Manual for Hospitals, vols 1 and 2, 1992. Joint Commission on Accreditation of Healthcare Organizations, Oakbrook Terrace, IL, 1994.
38. Rose, M: Laying siege to hospital privileges. Am J Nurs 84:613, 1984.
39. Stevens, JE: The question of hospital privileges for allied health professionals. Quality Rev Bull 10:17, 1984.
40. Miles, J: Antitrust implications of allied health practitioner privilege decisions and hospital-physician exclusive contracts. Med Staff Counselor 2:19, 1988.
41. Smithing, RT, and Wiley, M: Hospital privileges: Who needs them? J Am Acad Nurse Pract 1:150, 1989.

42. American College of Nurse-Midwives: Hospital staff settling charges they illegally denied hospital privileges to nurse-midwife. J Nurse-Midwifery 33:152, 1988.
43. Readership and Practice Profile of the ACNM: Findings of a Direct Mail Survey. J Nurse Midwifery, vol. 39, no. 1. Accessed from www.midwife.org/prof/display June 2003.
44. Cushing, M: Safeguarding the spirit of competition. Am J Nurs 89:1035, 1989.
45. Sherman Act, 15 USC 1 & 2.
46. Blumenreich, GA: Anesthesia Advantage, Inc. vs. Metz. J Am Assoc Nurse Anesthetists 58:335, 1990.
47. Blumenreich, GA: Antitrust protection against a hospital's denial of access. J Am Assoc Nurse Anesthetists 56:383, 1988.
48. American Association of Nurse Anesthetists: News Release: U.S. Ninth Circuit Court of Appeals Backs Nurse Anesthetists. American Association of Nurse Anesthetists, Chicago, IL, 1985.
49. Nurse Midwifery Associates v Hibbett, 918 F2d 605 (6th Cir 1990).
50. Wachter, RM, and Goldman, L: The hospitalist movement 5 years later. JAMA 287: 487, 2002.
51. Joint Commission on Accreditation of Healthcare Organizations: Comprehensive Accreditation Manual for Hospitals. Joint Commission on Accreditation of Healthcare Organizations, Oakbrook Terrace, IL, 2000.
52. Kamajian, MF, Mitchell, SA, and Fruth, RA: Credentialing and privileging of advanced practice nurses. AACN Clin Issues 10: 316, 1999.
53. Pearson, L: Fourteenth annual legislative update. Nurse Pract 27:10, 2002.
54. Oncology Nursing Certification Corporation, http://www.oncc.org/Accessed May 2004.

CHAPTER 8

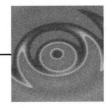

Reimbursement for Expanded Professional Nursing Practice Services

CHAPTER 8

Michael J. Kremer, DNSc, CRNA, FAAN
Margaret Faut-Callahan, DNSc, CRNA, FAAN

Michael J. Kremer, DNSc, CRNA, FAAN, received his doctorate from the Rush University College of Nursing. His master's of science in nursing is from Seattle Pacific University, Seattle, Washington. He received his nurse-anesthesia education at the University of Illinois in Springfield, Illinois, and undergraduate psychology and nursing degrees from Northern Illinois University in DeKalb, Illinois. He is Associate Professor of Adult Health Nursing and Assistant Director of the Rush University College of Nursing Nurse Anesthesia Program. Dr. Kremer chairs the American Association of Nurse Anesthetists (AANA) Foundation, is a Chair Reviewer for the Council on Accreditation of Nurse Anesthesia Educational Programs, and is an Associate Editor of the *Journal of the American Association of Nurse Anesthetists.*

Margaret Faut-Callahan, DNSc, CRNA, FAAN, received her master's and doctoral degrees at the Rush University College of Nursing and attended Loyola University in Chicago, Illinois, for her undergraduate education. She is a Professor and Chair of Adult Health Nursing and Director of the Nurse Anesthesia Program at the Rush University College of Nursing. Dr. Faut-Callahan is a recognized leader in nurse anesthesia education, having been an early proponent of the master's degree in nursing as the exit degree for nurse anesthesia programs. She developed the first doctoral program in nursing with a focus on nurse anesthesia. She has served in many elected and appointed positions at the local, state, and national levels. She currently chairs the Council on Accreditation of Nurse Anesthesia Educational Programs.

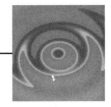

Reimbursement for Expanded Professional Nursing Practice Services

CHAPTER OBJECTIVES

After completing this chapter, the reader will be able to:

1 Discuss the components of a traditional economic system.

2 Describe the criteria for an economic system in relation to health care.

3 Note the effect of changes in price, supply, and demand for health care.

4 Become familiar with cost considerations in the provision of health care by and reimbursement for physicians and advanced practice nurses.

5 Demonstrate familiarity with key terms in finance and reimbursement.

An important policy shift in health care that emerged during the 1980s was the adoption of traditional market forces in an attempt to achieve greater efficiency in the production of health care services. A reliance on regulatory control of health care financing, such as the certificate of need system implemented in the 1970s, failed to contain health care costs. Regulatory control was advocated ostensibly from a quality standpoint, but providers, professionals, and insurers favored only the weakest mechanisms to ensure quality while supporting regulations that advanced their economic self-interests and enabled them to create monopolistic positions in their respective health care markets.[1] The monopolies created determined the type and amount of health care provided and obtained regulatory barriers to protect professionals from others seeking to enter markets over which they had control. Buerhaus[2] posited that if health care had been governed less by regulations and more by traditional market forces, the genesis of monopolistic forces would have been stifled. In that case, market forces would have predominated, and professionals would have been forced to compete on the basis of price, quality, and the extent to which they provided services that were responsive to the preferences of consumers. This chapter discusses these economic trends as well as the components of the economic system.

Rising costs of health care require advanced practice nurses (APNs) to be cost-effective and knowledgeable regarding reimbursement of their services within rapidly expanding managed care organizations. However, the rapid pace of change in reimbursement legislation, policies, and procedures makes this a daunting task. The current American health care system hardly resembles the one in place a decade ago. Managed care organizations (MCOs) and preferred provider organizations (PPOs) dominate health care, and large provider networks have emerged as a result of consolidations and mergers. As patient care has moved out of the inpatient arena into outpatient delivery services, MCOs have increasingly stressed the importance of health maintenance, preventive services, management of chronic illness, and patient education. The rationale for this focus is that improved client health ultimately translates into improved health of the MCO's financial ledger. The managed care industry has grown and changed at a rapid pace and has recently had to respond to negative public perceptions about care quality and access. As a result of public and legislative pressure, more than 100 laws that restrict managed care administrative or clinical practices were enacted by state legislatures between 1996 and 1999. At the federal level, Congress continues to grapple with legislation that calls for improved access, quality assurance, and patient's provider choice.[3]

APNs can no longer rely on administrators, office managers, and physician employers to protect and promote their interests. If barriers to reimbursement currently experienced by APNs are to be addressed, it will take a concerted effort of nurse educators, professional nursing organizations, and savvy practicing nurses to lobby elected bodies and the managed care industry for full and unobstructed participation within MCOs.[3]

THE ECONOMIC SYSTEM

The economic system consists of the network of institutions, laws, and rules created by society to answer the following universal economic questions:

- What goods and services shall be produced?
- How shall they be produced?
- For whom shall they be produced?

Every society needs an economic system because human, natural, and manmade resources are scarce relative to human wants, because the resources have alternative uses, and because there is a multiplicity of competing wants. Thus, decisions must be made regarding the use of these resources in production and the distribution of the resulting output among the members of society.[4] The U.S. spent $1.4 trillion on health care in 2001, and the amount continues to increase.[39] Difficult decisions must be made regarding allocation of health care resources. Some relevant questions include:

- Who will receive health care services?
- By whom will these services be provided?
- At what cost will these services be provided?

CRITERIA FOR AN ECONOMIC SYSTEM IN RELATION TO HEALTH CARE

Given the scarcity of resources and the existence of competing goals, the economic system with respect to health care should result in:

1. An optimum amount of resources devoted to health care
2. The combination of these resources in an optimal way
3. An optimal allocation of resources between current provision of health care and investment in future health care through research, education, and similar efforts

The general rule for reaching such optima is "equality at the margin"[4] (p. 13). For instance, the first criterion would be met if the last dollar's worth of resources devoted to health care increased human satisfaction by exactly the same amount as the last dollar's worth devoted to other goods.[4] The contrast between this view of a social optimum and the notion of optimal care as used in health care needs to be discussed. The relation between health and health care inputs can usually be described by a curve that may rise at an increasing rate at first but then decreases and eventually levels off or declines (Fig. 8–1). Optimal care could be defined as Point A, where no further increment in health is possible. The social optimum, however,

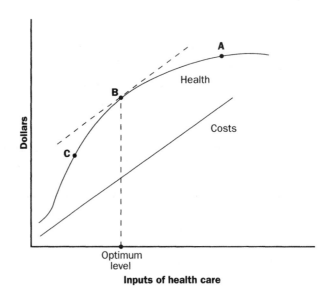

FIGURE 8–1   Determination of optimum level of health care utilization.

requires that inputs of resources not exceed the point at which the value of an additional increment to health is exactly equal to the cost of inputs required to obtain that increment, or Point B. At Point C, where the ratio of benefits to costs is at a maximum, additional inputs still add more to benefits than to costs.

TYPES OF ECONOMIC SYSTEMS

Economists have identified three "pure types" of economic systems:

1. Traditional
2. Centrally directed
3. Market price

Every actual economy is a blend of types, but their relative importance varies. Primitive and feudal societies relied on basic economic decisions that were made by one person or a small group of people; the former Soviet Union is an example of such a system. The United States, Canada, and most countries of Western Europe have relied on a market system for the past century or two.[4]

A market system consists of a collection of decision-making units called households and another collection called firms. The households own all the productive resources in the society. They make these resources available to firms, who transform them into goods and services that are then distributed back to the households. The flow of resources and of goods and services is facilitated by a counterflow of money.[4]

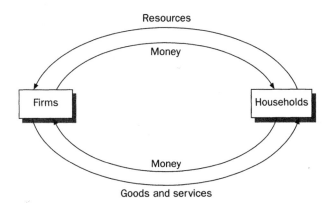

FIGURE 8–2   Elementary model of a market system.

In a market system, as shown in Figure 8–2, the exchanges of resources and of goods and services for money take place in markets where prices and quantities are determined. These prices are the signals or controls that trigger changes in behavior as required by changes in technology or preferences. The market system is sometimes referred to as the price system.[4]

In the markets for resources, the households are the suppliers, and the firms provide the demand. In the markets for goods and services, the firms are the suppliers, and the households are the sources of demand. In each market, the interaction between demand and supply determines the quantities and prices of the various resources and the goods and services. Figure 8–3 demonstrates a typical market. The income of each household depends on the quantity and quality of resources available to it and the prices of those resources; the amount of household income determines its share of the total flow of goods and services. The household is assumed to spend its income in such a way as to maximize its utility, or satisfaction. It does this by following the principle of equality at the margin; that is, it adjusts its purchases so that marginal utility, or the satisfaction added by the last unit purchased of each commodity, is proportional to its price.[4]

It is assumed that firms attempt to maximize profits, or the difference between what they must pay the households for the use of resources and what they get from them for the goods and services they produce. To maximize profits, they too must follow the rule of equality at the margin, adjusting their use of different types of resources so that the marginal products (the addition to output obtained from one additional unit of input) are proportional to price.[4]

The essence of a competitive market is that:

- There are many well-informed buyers and sellers, no one of whom is large enough to influence price.
- The buyers and sellers act independently (that is, without collusion).
- There is free entry for other buyers and sellers not currently in the market.

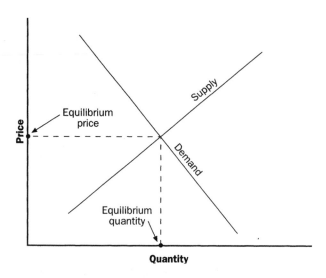

FIGURE 8–3   A typical market.

The U.S. economy departs in many respects from the competitive market model; this departure is particularly noticeable in the health care sector. Most health care markets depart substantially from competitive conditions, sometimes inevitably and sometimes as a result of deliberate public or private policy.[4]

MARKET COMPETITION

In a competitive industry, firms have strong economic incentives to minimize the costs of producing their products and services so they can be priced competitively and sold in the marketplace. To minimize production costs, firms must be innovative in their use of capital and labor, endeavoring to find the least costly number and combination of resources to produce their goods. Because consumers consider both price and quality of goods and services when making purchases, firms attempt to improve the quality of their products without causing significant price increases. Firms conduct market research to determine consumer preferences and initiate promotional activities to inform the public on the price and quality of their products as well as to differentiate their products from those of competitors.[2]

In a competitive marketplace, consumers are given a variety of choices in the goods and services they may purchase. Influenced by their level of income, their tastes and preferences, and the amount of information available on the product, consumers consider the trade-off between price and quality and purchase those items that are most satisfying. Those in control of supply and demand in competitive markets are in touch with each other; however, satisfying the consumer is the only way that firms can sell their products and earn profits.[2]

Much of the health care system has been built on what Enthoven[5] called "cost-unconscious" demand. The lack of sensitivity to the price of health care has occurred for several reasons. Current tax law permits the exclusion of employer-paid health insurance premiums from the taxable income of employees. This has led to the purchase of more health insurance coverage than would be the case if employees bought the insurance directly using after-tax income. This tax policy has resulted in an overconsumption of health care because employees are not conscious of the price of services they consume, and providers, who know that an insurance company will pay for the services, have no economic incentive to restrain the cost of providing a treatment or the amount of care provided.[6] As long as the patient and provider are insensitive to price and are spared from fiscal accountability for their actions, patients will continue to demand more health care than they may require, and providers will supply that care. In this system, neither party has economic incentives to consider the costs or benefits of consuming additional amounts of health care; each behaves as if more is better.

Employers, in most instances, have also fostered cost-unconsciousness by constructing their health insurance offerings so that the employee who chooses the lowest-priced health plan is not permitted to keep any of the savings.[4] The prevalence of employers subsidizing the more costly fee-for-service third-party payer system against cost-minimizing health maintenance organizations (HMOs) and competitive health care plans removed incentives for employees to shop around and select the least costly health insurance plan. This practice stymied price competition among health care plans because lower-cost plans cannot take business away from the next-lowest-priced plan by cutting the price paid to the people actually making the choice[4] (p. 369).

It was thought that employers persisted with this irrational strategy because, in addition to the perverse incentives to purchase fee-for-service plans inherent in the tax treatment of employer-paid health insurance premiums, unions have historically insisted that their members have 100 percent comprehensive health coverage. Employers were reluctant to use their considerable purchasing power to stimulate price competition among health care plans.[2]

A major economic force having an impact on health care delivery and its cost was the increasing cost of health care to employers in the late 1980s and after. The cost of health care to employers undermined the ability of the industry to be price-competitive in a global marketplace. Employers have since become motivated to adopt reforms demanding health services that stimulate greater price competition among health care plans and other supply-side providers. It is in the best interest of the nursing profession to become involved in research and management efforts seeking to find solutions to some of these supply, demand, and cost problems in health care and to prepare for a far more competitive health care system.[2]

One recent example of public economic policy having an impact on reimbursement in health care is the Medicare payment policies affecting physicians. In 1996, the federal government completed the 4-year phase-in of the resource-based relative value scale (RBRVS), its payment system for physicians under part B of the Medicare program. Although the program seemed to be accomplishing one of its primary objectives—to transfer payments away from tests and procedures and apply them toward evaluation and management services—physicians experienced a number of dissatisfactions with the program. The Physician Payment Review Commission (PPRC), which monitors the implementation of the fee schedule, expressed concern that low Medicare RBRVS payments may negatively affect the access of beneficiaries to physicians. Other investigators[7,8] have shown that low Medicaid fees hamper access to office-based physicians and encourage the use of hospital outpatient departments and emergency services, both of which only reinforce PPRC concerns about the link between physician payments and decreased access to care. Should federal budget deficit pressures result in prolonging inadequate RBRVS payments (approximately 75 percent of Medicare physician payments are financed using general tax dollars) and should physicians respond by reducing the medical care provided to an increasing number of Medicare beneficiaries, then additional demand for APNs could develop.[9]

Groups such as the American Medical Association (AMA) and their component societies lobby state legislatures, Congress, and the Center for Medicare and Medicaid Services (CMS) to restrict the definition of primary care provider to physicians and to limit reimbursement laws and regulations to an equally narrow providership. Their success has been mixed. In response to increasing acceptability of APNs in the workforce, numerous state legislatures have legitimized APN practice autonomy in laws and regulations. To date, 26 states have statutes granting APNs the right to practice without physician supervision or collaboration. Eighteen states mandate their direct reimbursement by private insurers, HMOs, MCOs, and Medicaid.[38] The 1997 Balanced Budget Act guarantees Medicare reimbursement for nonphysician providers (NPs, CNSs, and PAs) regardless of setting and is expected to be a model for reimbursement practices that will be adopted by states and other health plans. Although this act authorizes direct APN reimbursement, it also requires collaboration with physicians.[40] This requirement is a problem in states where collaboration is not required because APNs in those states who have established independent practices are not able to bill Medicare without changing their practices and obtaining physician collaboration.[3]

The potential economic consequences of the pricing decisions of an advanced nursing practice, including the anticipated effects on physicians and consumers, are discussed later in this chapter. To describe these consequences adequately, it is necessary to first discuss key economic terms and concepts that underpin the relationship between price and the firm's demand, amount of total revenues, profitability, and economic responses by physicians and consumers.[9]

DISEQUILIBRIUM

One disturbing characteristic of some health care markets is the failure of price to reach a level of equilibrium, or the level at which the quantity demanded and the quantity supplied are equal.[4] Most recently, payers have provided greater incentives for primary versus specialty care services, leading to an economic disincentive for the use of specialty services. The persistence of a price disequilibrium is a clear indication that the market departs substantially from the competitive norm. In the case of excess demand, rationing ensues. Services such as hemodialysis or major organ transplantation may not be available to all members of society.

SUPPLIER-INDUCED DEMAND

Figures 8–4 and 8–5 illustrate excess demand and supply, assuming constant initial supply, demand, price, and quantity conditions. An increase in the number of physicians in this market shifts the supply curve, resulting in a reduction in price and an increase in the quantity of care. Assuming that demand is inelastic with respect to price, physicians' incomes will decline, which will induce physicians to recommend additional units of service. This results in a shift in the demand curve. In this case, both price and quantity increase in response to the physician-induced demand. In contrast to the theoretical expectation that an increase in supply raises quantity and reduces price in a competitive market, findings suggest that an increase in the supply of physicians is accompanied by an increase in quantity and a constant or rising price.[10]

Such results are consistent with the demand-shift hypothesis. The health care provider is hypothesized to shift demand to attain a target income. The target income is the amount of money earned through comparison with other physicians of the same specialty training and geographic location. Empirical studies of the impact of increases in the physician-population ratio on utilization indicated no decline in utilization associated with increases in physician supply. A modest positive

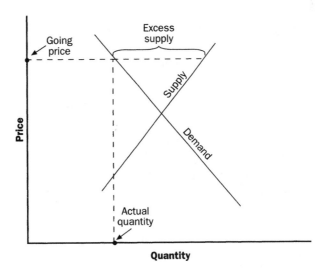

FIGURE 8–4   Excess supply.

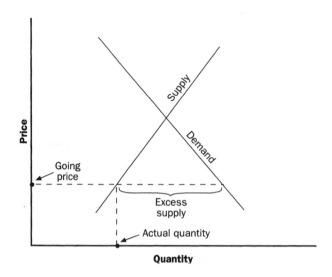

FIGURE 8–5   Excess demand.

relationship was found between utilization and the physician-population ratio. Estimated elasticities varied widely, ranging from 0.03 to 0.80.[10]

The inducement hypothesis questions the appropriateness of increased cost sharing by consumers as an approach to controlling utilization and moderating growth in health care expenditures. Additional cost sharing and the concomitant decrease in consumer-initiated demand not only reduce the earnings of physicians but also induce providers to increase demand, thereby reducing the impact of higher net prices on total health care spending. Moreover, the inducement hypothesis suggests that controls placed on fees charged by physicians are unlikely to successfully constrain total spending on health services. Rather, price controls are likely to expand utilization and induce the substitution of more expensive services for less costly ones.[10]

Several important problems must be considered when undertaking empirical studies of the demand for health care. The first is the adequacy of using health insurance information to obtain estimates of the price of health services. The second is the effect of provider influence on demand; for example, the extent to which supply creates its own demand. The third problem is the effect of health status on the demand for health care. Exclusion of a health status variable will bias the results in terms of the importance of the other independent variables. Empirical studies indicate that the demand for health services is inelastic with respect to price and income. The demand-for-health model recognizes that health services are purchased to obtain better health. Moreover, other items purchased, such as tobacco products, fatty foods, or alcoholic beverages, also have an impact on health status. One example of this model is that older persons, to retard the depreciation in health status caused by advancing age, increase their purchase of health services.[9,10]

THE EFFECTS OF CHANGES IN PRICE, SUPPLY, AND DEMAND FOR HEALTH CARE

The hospital sector is the most inflationary component of the health services industry. As is the case with other aspects of the health services industry, general inflation is responsible for the bulk of the increase in hospital expenditures. However, the increase in intensity, or acuity, per visit accounts for more of the increase in hospital expenditures than for physicians' or nursing home services.[10]

After almost 10 years of low growth rates in hospital costs, since 1998 the United States has again experienced increased hospital inpatient expenditure growth. Whereas the recent rate of expenditure growth has not been as high as those of pharmaceuticals and outpatient services, because hospital inpatient care represents the largest single component of health care expenditure, even small rates of growth can have a large effect on health care expenditure. From 1998 to 2001, hospital inpatient expenditures constituted about 34 percent of the growth of total health care expenditures. During this period, inpatient expenditures increased by an average of 5.9 percent annually, twice the overall annual rate of inflation during this same period. The mean U.S. expenditure for a hospital stay in 2000 was $10,915, based on an average cost per day of $1,850 and an average length of stay of 5.9 days.[41]

The key drivers of inpatient expenditures, based on state-level health care and inpatient expenditure data, are:

- The overall level of economic activity, e.g., disposable income, local prices and wages
- Level of hospital technology, including cost of technology, consumer demand, and backlash against managed care
- Hospital market and financial structure, e.g., competitive markets, hospital closures, and profit versus nonprofit status
- Health care labor force, particularly nursing supply shortages
- Prescription drugs and medication errors

It is estimated that more than 800 financially distressed hospitals will close or merge between 2000 and 2005.[49] The combination of a highly competitive marketplace, hospital specialization, and heavy regulatory and legislative burden will result in continued widespread hospital closures.[50] Despite projections that the recent increase in growth of hospital costs will be short-lived and that technological change will ultimately support a trend away from hospitalization toward outpatient care,[51] emerging evidence indicates that inpatient costs will continue to escalate if the current pace of medical technology adoption is allowed to continue unchecked.[52]

Given the strong relationship between economic activity and hospital inpatient expenditure, it is likely that the current economic slowdown will relieve some of the cost increase pressure.[53] The last economic slowdown, in 1991 to 1992, triggered a number of aggressive health care and hospital cost containment strategies that held the rate of health care expenditure growth in check for several years. On the other hand, the primary mechanism that was employed at the time involved moving more consumers into managed care health insurance plans and aggressively discounting provider reimbursement levels. Experts in the insurance industry speculate that these options have been pushed about as far as they can go and will not substantially alter future inpatient and health care cost trends.[41]

The issue of the magnitude of economies of scale in the production of hospital services has been studied for many years. Past evidence indicates only a slight tendency for average costs to decline as output increases. However, there is stronger evidence of scale economies for particular types of medical services. Case mix (for example, patient acuity and type of payer) is an important factor that must be taken into account when considering the effect of hospital size on average costs.[10]

State regulation of hospital costs has become increasingly widespread in the past 20 years. Rate regulation has been found to have a moderate impact on cost per admission, cost per patient day, and per capita expenditures. In addition, the growth in labor cost has slowed with prospective payment.[10] During the 1980s, the federal government began to run up annual budget deficits in excess of $200 billion. As the amount of the national debt grew, a greater portion of the federal government budget each year was required to pay interest on the debt, which reduced the amount of dollars available for other discretionary spending. Since the beginning of the Medicare and Medicaid programs in 1966, total public spending on health care has increased tremendously; it reached approximately $507 billion in 1997.[11]

In 2000, data from the Organization for Economic Cooperation and Development (OECD) were used to compare the health systems of the 30 member countries. Total health spending, which is the distribution of public and private health spending in the OECD countries, was analyzed. U.S. public spending as a percentage of gross domestic product (GDP) was 5.8 percent, very similar to public spending in the United Kingdom, Italy, and Japan (5.9 percent each), and slightly lower than in Canada (6.9 percent). While the United States spends more overall on health care than any other country, the difference in spending is caused by its higher prices for health care goods and services.[54]

At the beginning of the 1980s, several private and public sector initiatives appeared and acted both independently and interdependently to stimulate the beginning of economic competition among hospitals and physicians. The first of these initiatives occurred as a result of several events. American businesses were struck by double-digit inflation during the Carter administration, followed by a sharp economic recession during the Reagan administration. The volume of lower-priced imported goods rose substantially, as did competition from Japan and other countries. Many American businesses became aware of, and concerned about, the effects of steadily rising health care premiums, which were increasing the costs of labor. Employers started to fear that, if left unchecked, rising health care costs could thwart the ability to price their products competitively in a global market. Businesses sought to reduce costly inpatient hospital stays by beginning programs that mandated prehospital testing and screening and utilization review, required second opinions for surgery, and pressured insurance companies to cover the cost of less costly outpatient settings. Even before Medicare implemented diagnoses-related groups (DRGs), these private-sector actions were causing a decline in hospital occupancy rates and the number of admissions.[6]

While prospective payment has succeeded in moderating the growth in current expenditures, there is little evidence that regulations designed to limit capital formation have succeeded. Even in situations where regulation of capital expenditures were successful in limiting growth in the number of beds, hospitals substituted investment in new services for beds. Declining government support for capital regulation and industry are advanced as possible reasons for the ineffectiveness of controls on hospital capital formation.[10]

COST CONSIDERATIONS IN PROVISION OF CARE AND REIMBURSEMENT FOR PHYSICIANS AND APNs

Price of Services

Greater availability of primary and preventive care has been tied to cost savings and improved quality. Nonphysician practitioners are cost-effective with regard to the costs of their educational preparation and perhaps also with regard to their practice patterns and fees. How these professionals are paid and which of their services are covered have been contentious issues for more than two decades. This is evidenced by the patchwork of policies governing payment for their services, even within a single-payer system such as Medicare, and by substantial variation in payment rates among state Medicaid services.[12]

The extraordinary rise in health care costs and the inability of nursing to show cost savings have been a barrier to obtaining direct payment. Despite the breakdown of public and private spending on health care outlined above, the portion of the gross national product constituted by health care grew from 5.3 percent in 1960 to 12.5 percent in 1990, increasing from $42 billion to almost $647 billion. In 2000, health spending in the United States. reached 13 percent of the GDP, compared with only a little over 7 percent in the United Kingdom.[42] Congress has shown its concern about the rise in the health care budget by enacting new cost-containing Medicare payment systems for hospitals and physicians' services. Congress has exhibited restraint in the annual funding of other health programs, frequently increasing funding only to cover inflation. Reimbursement legislation for the services of APNs is almost always evaluated as a cost item. APNs are defined as nurse practitioners (NPs), clinical nurse specialists (CNSs), certified nurse midwives (CNMs), and certified registered nurse anesthetists (CRNAs). A summary of federal reimbursement for APNs is shown in Table 8–1. The Congressional Budget Office has long held that if the number of providers is increased, the costs for health care will increase because of the greater number of services provided.[13]

TABLE 8–1.	Current Status of Federal Reimbursement for Nurses in Advanced Practice[38]			
Federal programs	**NP**	**CNM**	**CRNA**	**CNS**
Medicare, Part B	Yes	Yes	Yes	Yes
Medicaid	Yes[a]	Yes	State discretion	State
CHAMPUS[b]	Yes	Yes	Yes	Yes[c]
FEHBP[d]	Yes	Yes	Yes	Yes

[a] Limited to pediatric NPs and family NPs
[b] Civilian Health and Medical Program of the Uniformed Services
[c] Limited to certified psychiatric nurse specialists
[d] Federal Employee Health Benefit Program[12]

Access Issues

Paying APNs directly allows them to provide care and improve needed access to care. Changes in federal health programs enacted by Congress were made to improve health care access to underserved populations, such as nursing home residents, low-income women and children, and people in rural areas. Direct reimbursement gives APNs recognition and visibility as primary care providers. More than 41 million U.S. citizens lack health insurance, and most of these people lack access to primary care.[39] To meet the needs of this uninsured population, additional primary care practitioners will be needed. Direct reimbursement of APNs eliminates one of the most significant barriers to greater utilization of these nurses.[13]

The Omnibus Budget Reconciliation Act (OBRA), enacted by Congress in 1990, allowed NP and CNS services to be reimbursed when provided in a rural area. This law was enacted because Congress wanted to improve access to care for rural Medicare beneficiaries. Although the NP and CNS had to work in collaboration with a physician, they did not have to submit claims through their employer; they were allowed to submit claims directly. The payment level was at 85 percent of the fee schedule for outpatient services and at 75 percent for inpatient services.[14]

The Balanced Budget Act (BBA) of 1997 removed economic disincentives for the utilization of APNs by authorizing direct Medicare reimbursement for NP and CNS services in all settings. NPs who wish to submit claims for services must apply for a UPIN number under their own name. Under the terms of the BBA, both urban and rural NPs can practice in all valid places of service. NPs are required to work in collaboration with a physician. However, because NPs do not need the immediate availability of a supervising physician, they have more latitude in where and how they practice. Before the BBA, urban-based NPs were reimbursed at 85 percent of physician fee schedules for all services. Rural NPs were reimbursed at 75 percent of physician fee schedules for hospital services and 85 percent of physician fee schedules for other services. Now, urban and rural NPs are compensated at 85 percent of physician fee schedules across the board and can be employed or self-employed. In addition, before the BBA, rural-based NPs were reimbursed at 65 percent of physician assist-at-surgery fees. Now, urban- and rural-based NPs are reimbursed at 85 percent of physician assist-at-surgery fees.[15] However, the U.S. General Accounting Office (GAO) has recommended that advanced practice clinicians not receive reimbursement as surgical first assistants under the physician fee schedule (PFS). Instead, reimbursement for these services would be included in the inpatient prospective payment system (PPS) that pays hospitals.[55]

In January 2004, CMS announced the adoption of the National Provider Identifier (NPI) as the standard unique identifier number for all health care providers to use when filing and processing health care claims and other transactions. The final rule will go into effect May 2005. The standard NPI was mandated by the Health Insurance Portability and Accountability Act of 1996 (HIPAA). The NPI will replace all identifiers previously issued. A health care provider will be assigned only one NPI, and that identifier will not change over time. All health care providers, whether or not they are covered entities under HIPAA, are eligible to be assigned an NPI. All covered health care providers must obtain an NPI and must use the NPI in standard transactions no later than May 2007 or May 2008, depending on the size of the health plan.[34]

Health Care Plans and Health Insurance Policies

The forces that evolved in the 1980s and early 1990s culminated in the development of health care price competition because cost-conscious purchasers of health care sought to obtain greater value for each dollar spent. The evolution of managed health care delivery has become a significant force with which APNs must be familiar.

Managed care involves the application of standard business practices to health care delivery. Managed care purports to represent the best of the American free enterprise system. New methods of providing finance and reimbursement for health care services require hospitals and health care providers to make tremendous transitions to entirely new business models.[16] Today, health care providers are confronted with price competition and the need to control costs rigorously while facing increasing demands for data documenting the quality of clinical outcomes.[17]

For the first time, in 1993, 51 percent of employees with employer-sponsored health insurance were enrolled in managed care plans. In addition, many traditional insurance plans had managed care features, insofar as they subjected provider services to external utilization reviews, second opinions, and so forth. In 2001, 93 percent of Americans with health coverage were in some form of managed care plan.[43] Preferred provider plans were the primary form of managed care, covering 48 percent of workers with health coverage.[44] The only reversal in this managed care trend was in Medicare beneficiaries, which went from 16 percent in 2000 to only 12 percent in 2002.[45] As payers, providers, and consumers of health care seek solutions to ever-increasing costs, managed care in the United States has experienced explosive growth. The purchasers of health care, including private and public payers as well as patients, have become particularly interested in managed care as a flexible means for reducing health care expenditures while preserving high-quality patient care. Insurers are under intense pressure from employers to reduce premiums. Accomplishing this without reducing profits means decreasing costs, which in turn requires insurers to limit expenditures, generally by controlling provider services.

Recent developments in health care coverage reported by the U.S. Bureau of the Census[56] include:

- Percentage of people covered by employment-based health insurance was 63 percent in 2002
- 25 percent of individuals were covered by government health insurance programs
- Medicaid provided coverage for 11 percent of the population
- 12 percent of all children did not have health care coverage
- Although Medicaid insured 13.3 million people, an additional 10.1 million "poor" people still had no health insurance in 2001
- Racial and ethnic disparities in health care coverage persist
- Full-time and part-time workers were more likely to have health insurance (83 percent); however, among the poor, workers were less likely to be covered (51 percent) than nonworkers (63 percent).

The growth of prepaid capitated health care networks will be aided by continuing regulatory and market-based adjustments designed to ensure that providers compete fairly on the basis of price and quality. APNs can expect that more of the clinical and economic forces that shape their practices and determine their incomes will be driven by impersonal and unambiguous incentives that govern price-competitive industries. Providers and health professionals will be rewarded only to the extent that they keep their prices low and quality high.[9]

The evolution of prepaid capitated firms, or the managed care industry, has been a significant and positive development for APNs, whether they are employed by managed care firms or decide to compete independently as solo providers or in group practice arrangements. From the economic perspective, the major difference between practicing as an employee of an HMO or practicing independently is that as an employee, the APN functions as an economic complement, whereas APNs in independent practice function largely as economic substitutes to an HMO or medical group practice.[9]

APNs are an economic complement so long as providing their services increases the productivity of the managed care firm and the profits of the owners. The complementary role is not unlike that of hospital-employed RNs, whose nursing practice functions to increase the productivity of physicians by allowing them both to treat inpatients and to maintain an office-based practice. Because an HMO operates according to a prepaid capitated budget, it has an economic incentive to keep the total costs of providing health care as low as possible. In this way, any amount of unspent dollars can be retained as profit. Thus, HMOs have an economic interest to provide enrollees with more preventive care and health education so they can reduce future consumption of HMO resources by treating fewer enrollees for preventable acute and chronic illnesses. HMOs try to reduce admissions to costly hospitals, negotiate discounts on the purchase of pharmaceutical products and medical devices, and pursue other methods to reduce costs.[9] The only barrier to incentivizing the provision of preventive health care services is the tendency for participants of one managed care plan to jump to another plan when premiums rise or employer options change. Therefore, many MCOs have been hesitant to spend these health care dollars up front.

Fagin[18] suggested that adequately educated APNs have proven competence and are capable of working without physicians' supervision. Many of the clinical services that APNs provide can closely substitute for those provided by physicians. Because APNs are less costly to an HMO in terms of salary and benefit requirements, it makes sense that they represent an economically attractive opportunity for an HMO to fill gatekeeping and other provider roles. As purchasers increasingly demand that HMOs lower the premiums charged per enrollee lest they induce their employees to enroll in a different and lower-cost HMO, price competition among HMOs is expected to intensify significantly. HMOs will continue to face greater pressures to keep their costs low, which, one could argue, would further increase demand for APNs. Because managed care firms will increasingly be motivated to keep their premiums priced competitively, it has been proposed that they will develop new roles for APNs and experiment with delivery models that will be tailored extensively around APNs. The purpose would be to find new ways to lower costs while increasing enrollee satisfaction and attainment of desired clinical outcomes.[9]

For at least two economic reasons, APNs must anticipate that physicians will resist the increasing employment of APNs. As more APNs become available, the total supply of health professionals will increase relative to the available number of managed care positions. Consequently, this will place downward pressure on the salaries that managed care firms are able to offer and still hire all the providers they want. If the supply of primary care physicians increases, additional physicians will seek employment with managed care firms and compete for available positions with APNs who have a comparative cost advantage.[9] In contrast, however, if the number of primary care positions decreases and more primary care providers are available, physicians will be forced to accept lower levels of compensation, thus coming into direct competition with APNs who have continued to seek higher salaries.

A second possible reason to expect physicians to resist the expansion of APNs in managed care is that many firms might adopt policies directing that APNs' caseloads comprise the "less difficult cases." But by having to care for "difficult cases," primary care physicians may be unable to obtain appropriate outcomes or levels of patient satisfaction to qualify for a year-end bonus. Hooker[19] reported that the Kaiser Permanente HMO system determined as far back as 1980 that 83 percent of the care provided by HMO physicians could be provided by an APN or PA. In primary care, that percentage is said to jump to 93 percent. In any health care system, the highest cost is labor. If a health care provider is able to provide the same services as physicians, with similar quality and outcomes, the only true barrier to this type of APN-PA utilization is physician attitudes.[19]

In the Hooker study, research findings demonstrated that PAs and APNs could see as many or more patients per day as physicians at 50 percent less than physicians' cost. From a workload standpoint, adult medicine physicians, PAs, and APNs at Kaiser Permanente Northwest appeared to see similar numbers of patients on hourly, daily, and annual bases. In addition, the types of patients seen by PAs and APNs in adult ambulatory settings were generally similar to those seen by physicians. From this standpoint, Hooker[19] concluded that "APNs and PAs were substitutes, rather than complements for, physician services" (p. 134).

Therefore, APNs must understand that, although they present economic benefits to owners of prepaid health plans, they represent an increasingly visible economic threat to primary care and specialist physicians. For these reasons, it should be no surprise that organized medicine has taken action aimed at monitoring and limiting any expansion in APN scope of practice.[46] The position that organized medicine has adopted is that APNs must practice under the supervision of a physician.[12] Mirr[20] noted that the lack of direct reimbursement for APN services decreases the overall effectiveness of these nursing professionals. Further, Timmons and Ridenour[21] reported that NPs have been billing patients for years under the title of physicians. In group practices, services provided by APNs are often billed under physician provider numbers. This practice has promoted economic dependence of the APN on the physician and has made the APN a "ghost" provider in the health care system.

The legality, or even the ethics, of billing for APN services under physician provider numbers must be questioned, particularly in states that have had APN reimbursement laws on the books for some time. APNs must be proactive to ensure their employers use billing practices that entail direct reimbursement for APN services. Direct billing enables tracking of revenue generated by APNs. APN fiscal data, patient outcomes, and performance indicators are necessary to negotiate contracts and assess cost-effectiveness. Failure to link APN provider numbers to their patient encounters makes accurate compilation of data and evaluation of APN cost-effectiveness impossible.[3]

Competition

APNs need to understand who their competitors are, how many of them exist, where they are located, what services they offer, how much they charge, and how they are paid. This information will tell APNs a great deal about what other providers have found effective or ineffective, sparing practicing APNs from making time-consuming and costly mistakes. Knowing as much as possible about the competition will also make it possible for APNs to determine how they can fill gaps in service, how they can take advantage of market niches, and how they might provide care creatively and at a lower cost.[9] This type of knowledge can be obtained by contracting with health marketing research firms, by developing a strategic plan with consultation as necessary, and by formulating an appropriate business plan based on the information gathered in this process.

Marketers take a large heterogeneous group of prospective buyers and divide them into smaller, more homogeneous groups who want approximately the same thing. This process is called market segmentation; each subgroup is called a market segment. Markets are segmented by variables such as age, sex, and income. Each segment is evaluated using a set of predetermined criteria. If two or more target markets are chosen, the organization is practicing a multisegment strategy. The process of gathering the information necessary to operate any business is called market research. Formal research techniques rely on systematic gathering of information from sources inside and outside the firm. Surveys, experimental designs, expert panels, and subscriptions to proprietary or syndicated research reports are typical of the formal research effort. Information that is routinely gathered, codified, analyzed, and stored is part of a marketing information system, which becomes a ready information source for decision makers.[22]

A marketing mix includes the following components:

- Product
- Branding
- Packaging
- Price
- Place
- Promotion
- Product positioning

Branding is important from the standpoint of professional identification. Clients must realize that health care services are available from appropriately prepared and credentialed APNs. Packaging is a function of the image projected by the product, in this case, the APN. Clinical competence, affability, availability, and a professional demeanor help to prepare an appealing package when APNs market their services. Price is another important consideration with multiple objectives; nearly all objectives will have to be related to long-term profitability. The marketer must estimate demand at the price level and forecast the response of competitors. Marketers typically create channels of distribution to move the product from producer to user. Channel members must focus on the needs of the final consumer as well as their own needs. Promotion informs, persuades, or reminds customers about a product, such as APN services. Promotion management begins with an understanding of the target markets the firm has chosen to serve. This means one must know which media, such as newspapers, television, and so on, the market uses to get information and understand how the market processes information and makes decisions. The organization or individual marketing services must develop a promotion strategy consisting of specific goals, plans to achieve them, an adequate budget to support this effort, and a method for evaluating results.[22]

A promotion plan includes some combination of promotion tools, referred to as the promotion mix. Like the marketing mix, it is a synergistic blend of elements. The four groupings of promotion tools are:

- Advertising
- Sales promotion
- Public relations and publicity
- Personal selling

Advertising is the use of impersonal messages sent through paid media, such as television, radio, newspapers, magazines, transit and highway billboards, telephone and business directories, and direct advertisements. Public relations activities are designed to foster goodwill, understanding, forgiveness, or acceptance. Publicity is not always favorable.[22] As the marketplace for health care providers contracts, a mixture of conciliatory and defensive posturing is seen in published interviews such as the following: A newspaper interview with two APNs and a physician was titled "Nurse Practitioner Supervision at Issue: RNs Push for Collegial Practice."[23] The physician commented that nurses had the ability to "treat a sore throat" but lacked the medical education and judgment and hours and hours of supervised experience that allow them to look at the entire differential of what a sore throat may be.[23]

The physician's perception was that nurses and physicians should "be a team" and that patients should know whether they are seeing "a board-certified physician or a board-certified advanced practice nurse." Despite some positive comments from the NPs interviewed for this story, the physician was able to cast some doubt as to the capabilities of APNs, thereby leaving the impression in the consumer's mind that the NP may not be able to provide quality care without physician supervision.

Antitrust Issues

The economic threat that APNs represent to physicians leads to occasional difficulties with antitrust issues. The American Nurses Association (ANA) and other APN organizations watch the development of antitrust protection very carefully. ANA points out that regulations are necessary to prevent any of the following possible events:

- Use of practice arrangements that prohibit nurses from performing patient care activities within the scope of a state's nurse practice act
- Use of practice arrangements that limit the activities of nurses recognized as advanced practitioners
- Imposition of insurer limits on the availability and accessibility of liability coverage for nurses or the requirement for physician supervision as a prerequisite for coverage
- Use of insurance surcharges to increase malpractice premium coverage and other insurance-related impediments to physician-nurse collaboration
- Subjective or arbitrary insurance reimbursement policies, such as denial of reimbursement for services performed within the scope of any licensed provider's practice if there is coverage for that service provided by the physician
- Denial of staff privileges at health care facilities, including prescriptive authority for those authorized by state law to prescribe.[53]

Without federal protection and clearer guidelines, every time APNs are denied basic rights to practice, they would have to enter into lengthy litigation and demonstrate their legal right to compete. Case law exists that states that some specialty nurses and physicians do compete. See *Oltz v St. Peter's Community Hospital,* 861 F2d 1440, 1443 (9th Cir 1988), and *Bahn v NME Hospital,* 772 F2d 1467, 1471 (9th Cir 1975). Not only is this an issue of paramount importance to nurses, it is a priority issue of the Coalition for Quality Care and Competition, which represents more than 400,000 nonphysician providers. Issues important to this coalition include:

- Prohibition of any entity or plan from discriminating against a class of health care professional
- Elimination of restrictions in current law that pose barriers for nonphysician providers to practicing in accord with state licensing acts
- Federal provisions guaranteeing nondiscriminatory access to qualified health providers being uniformly applied to all states, entities, and plans
- Replacement of the term "physician" with the term "qualified professional" in health care regulatory language

These positions go a long way in qualifying the needs of nonphysician providers in regulatory arenas. However, without federal protection and a mandate that states must adopt these provisions, the nonphysician provider will be in a situation of fighting for practice privileges and the right to provide care.[16]

If APNs in solo or group practice arrangements are to survive in a competitive market, they will need to be alert, seek ways to innovate and keep their costs as low as possible, and be willing to make frequent adjustments in the quality, pricing, and marketing of their services. It is recommended that APNs set their prices below the prevailing market price of services provided by physicians or their nearest competitors.[9] In addition, identifying services not provided or inadequately provided in a given market, e.g., ongoing management of clients with chronic conditions or health education services, will make the APN viable in an extremely competitive environment.

Many policy makers and researchers argue that there are problems with physician oversupply and imbalance in the specialty mix. Some have argued that these would be resolved as a more competitive health care market developed, predicting that cost-conscious integrated systems would change the demand for physicians' services. As a result, physicians would experience lower incomes or potential unemployment, sending a signal to students and educators to change behavior. A systematic analysis has not been done assessing the impact of changes in the organizing and financing of health care on the physician labor market. However, two types of changes were predicted for medical education:

1. The effect of increasing demand for generalists on changing specialty mix
2. The question of whether the market would create incentives to train fewer physicians overall[24]

Although there have been changes in the marketplace, it is difficult to know whether these changes signal a departure from previous trends. Positions in generalist fields have become somewhat more attractive, but changes in incomes have been modest, and the number of specialists continues to increase. Reported trends in graduate medical education include a growing number of subspecialty programs, which increased in 2001 by 65 to over 3,800. A smaller number of specialty programs exists, with a reported decrease of 25 to 4,203, accompanied by a corresponding shift in the number of residents training in them.[29]

Cooper,[47,48] however, in contrast to other health resource analysts, projects that by 2020 there will be a deficit of over 200,000 physicians, more than 20 percent of the projected demand. Based on demographic changes in the population and an increasing number of nonphysician clinicians providing primary care, he also stresses that this deficit will be primarily a growing shortage of specialists.

KEY TERMS IN FINANCE AND REIMBURSEMENT

Fee-for-Service Versus Capitation

The traditional health care billing system in which a health care provider charges a patient separately for each service is the fee-for-service system. This type of system allows patients to have free choice in health care providers and does not require providers to assume risk for the provision of care. For example, providers are more likely to be reimbursed proportionally for providing care in a fee-for-service system than in a managed care system.

Using nurse anesthesia as an example, fee-for-service and traditional indemnity insurance plans will be described in the context of reimbursement for services provided by these APNs. In the early years of the 20th century and through the 1950s, CRNAs were usually paid employees of either a surgeon or a hospital. In rural areas, CRNAs often contracted with hospitals to provide services based on fee-for-service structures, that is, a set amount of compensation per case as opposed to straight salary for hours worked.[25]

Blue Cross and Blue Shield were among the first private payers to emerge, which was during the 1930s. Early insurance plans paid only for physician or hospital charges and would not directly reimburse other health care providers, such as CRNAs, psychologists, and physical therapists. To obtain payment for their services, these providers would submit charges to the hospital or physician. The hospital or physician would then obtain reimbursement for services as "incident to" their own and pass the money on to the nonreimbursed provider.[27]

Health care costs escalated under the private payer systems of reimbursement. Reasons cited for this trend were often attributed to the failure of payers to reimburse lower-cost providers such as nonphysicians; preferential reimbursement of higher-cost care systems, such as hospitals, rather than ambulatory or outpatient services; and the insistence of physicians that harm would come to the physician-patient relationship if the fee-for-service structure were not maintained and strengthened.[25]

In an effort to control escalating medical costs, Medicare instituted a prospective payment system (PPS) in 1983. Initially, this legislation affected only Medicare, Part A (hospital costs); however, it would soon have an effect on Medicare, Part B (physician and nonphysician costs). Before 1983, Medicare reimbursed hospitals for CRNAs on a cost-based system in which the hospital passed along the actual costs of providing the Medicare portion of CRNAs' services directly to Medicare.[25]

As a result of the OBRA of 1986, all CRNAs, regardless of their practice setting, were able to receive reimbursement from Medicare directly or to assign their billing rights to their employer. All CRNA services are subject to Medicare assignment (no balance billing). A subsequent law allowed rural hospitals with 500 or fewer surgical cases per year requiring anesthesia and one full-time CRNA to "pass through" the costs of anesthesia services. In 1992, final regulations were published that detailed procedural definitions of the 1986 legislation.[25]

Most health insurance plans have undergone rapid change, attempting to control spiraling health care costs. APNs can expect reimbursement rates to decrease or remain flat in the near future, affecting all types of APNs in various practice settings, whether self-employed or not. In many markets, fee-for-service reimbursement structures are a thing of the past, giving way to the more cost-efficient "managed care" plans, in which all providers, including physicians, are salaried.

In contrast, capitation is prepayment for services on a per-member per-month basis. Providers are paid the same amount of money every month for a member regardless of whether that member receives services and regardless of how expensive these services are. To determine an appropriate capitation, it is important first to determine what will be covered in the scope of services, including all services that the provider will be expected to deliver. Certain services are difficult to define, such as diagnostic testing, prescriptions, surgical procedures (what if the same procedure is performed by the primary care provider and by a referral physician?), and so forth. Other services such as immunizations, office care, and so forth, are easier to define. Most performance-based compensation systems also hold the primary care provider accountable for nonprimary care services, either through risk programs or through positive incentive programs. Providers need to be able to estimate costs for each capitated service.[26] Some other relevant concepts in managed care related to reimbursement are described in the next section of this chapter.

Copayment, Coinsurance, and Deductibles

A copayment is that portion of a claim or medical expense that a member must pay out of pocket. This is usually a fixed amount, such as $15 in many HMOs and PPOs. Coinsurance describes a provision in a member's coverage that limits the amount of coverage by the plan to a certain percentage, commonly 80 percent. Any additional costs are paid by the member out of pocket. It is a significant challenge for clinicians to provide services to clients with varying amounts of insurance coverage. A deductible is that portion of a subscriber's (or member's) health care expenses that must be paid out of pocket before any insurance coverage applies, commonly $100 to $300. Deductibles are common in indemnity insurance plans and PPOs but are uncommon in HMOs. Deductibles may apply to only the out-of-network portion of a point-of-service plan. Point-of-service plans provide a difference in benefits (for example, 100 percent coverage rather than 70 percent) depending on whether the member chooses to use the plan, including its providers, and is in compliance with the authorization system to go outside the plan for services.[26] Increasing copayments and deductibles are two mechanisms health plans and purchasers of health plans use to control rising costs of health insurance premiums.

Adverse Selection

Adverse selection is a situation in which an insurance carrier or benefit plan has a disproportionate enrollment of adverse risks, such as an impaired or older population, with a potential for higher health care utilization than budgeted for an average population. Adverse selection occurs when premiums do not cover the cost of providing services.[27] Therefore, insurers may indicate that it is fiscally essential for them to avoid providing health insurance coverage to higher-risk individuals.

Community Rating

Community rating involves setting health insurance premiums based on the average cost of paying for services for all covered people in a geographic area, regardless of their history or potential for using health services. Community rating is a method of calculating health insurance premiums that sets the same price for the same health benefit coverage for all individuals in a pool of insured and does not take into account such variables as the claims experience of the group, age, sex, or health status. Community rating helps to spread the cost of illness evenly over all health plan enrollees (the whole community) rather than charging the sick more for health insurance.[27]

Experience Rating

With experience rating, health insurance premiums are based on the average cost of actual or anticipated health care used by various groups and takes into account such variables as previous claims experience, age, sex, and health status. It is the most common method of establishing premiums for health insurance in private programs.[27] However, with increasing managed care penetration in many markets and the move toward fully capitated systems, competition between insurance plans will likely intensify. Underbidding for contracts between competing managed care plans may be part of that process, regardless of the methods used to derive premium costs.

Even when APNs are employed by large HMOs, it is important to be aware of issues such as fluctuations in the numbers of enrollees, because the current health care marketplace is dynamic, and competing provider groups vigorously bid for contracts. APNs seeking to affiliate themselves with HMOs and PPOs need to consider what type of plan structure is employed. The plan may be a corporation, partnership, for-profit, or not-for-profit. The sponsorship of HMOs and PPOs provides a key to the underlying philosophy and initial purpose of the plan. The sponsorship could also reflect the receptivity of the plan to discussion regarding APN services. Typical sponsors include insurance companies, providers, investor ownership, consumer ownership, third-party administrators (PPOs), and entrepreneurial arrangements.[28]

APNs must ascertain the current arrangement between the MCO and providers. To some extent, this is determined by the model of the HMO or PPO. The current arrangements will affect the approach that should be taken by the APN in the negotiating process. The following information should be gathered:

- Who are the existing providers for the plan, and what hospitals are they associated with? What is the size of the network? How long have the providers been participating? How many new providers are added each year? How many providers have left the plan?

- Are the providers contracted with as a physician association, a joint venture, or as individual physicians or physician groups? If the plan contracts with one large association of physicians, providers may have to "subcontract" with this organization before contracting with the plan. Even if contracting is possible directly with the plan, the physician association usually has more influence than in less centralized organizations and may have to be included in discussions between APNs and the plan. If the plan contracts with groups or with individual physicians, the ability for new provider groups to contract directly with the plan is improved.

- Does the plan contract with other health care providers, such as nurse anesthetists, podiatrists, optometrists, chiropractors, and mental health professionals? To the extent that a plan has already broadened its panel of providers beyond that of medical doctors, some of the groundwork has already been achieved. Such plans already appreciate the quality of service and cost containment ability of contracting with nonphysician providers. The doorway is probably open for nonphysician providers who can demonstrate the efficacy and cost-effectiveness of their services.

- What are the reimbursement arrangements with providers? As much information as possible should be gathered on the current reimbursement and risk arrangement with existing providers. Such information will help determine the feasibility of various (discounted, capitation, fee schedule) arrangements that a group of APNs might consider, as well as the extent to which the plan typically shifts the risk to providers.[28]

Entrepreneurial APNs need to be prepared to accept risk when contracting with managed care entities. If clinical services performed by the APN cost less to provide than the contracted amount per member per month, profit is achieved. However, if the APN provides more services than the contracted amount, loss is incurred by the APN or APN group, not by the MCO.

Global Budgeting

Global budgeting is an overall budget limit on health care services, regardless of where the funds originate. Global budgeting can take the form of a state or federal maximum limit on total health care expenditures, but it usually implies federal limits. In some contexts, global budgeting has come to mean setting a limit on spending within sectors—for example, specific allocations for physicians, APNs, or hospitals.[28]

Canada has used global budgeting for health care with varying results. One of the authors provided cardiac anesthesia services for British Columbia residents who were unable to undergo timely cardiac surgery in Canada. The Canadian government in that situation had to contract with the state of Washington to provide open heart surgery services. The National Health Service in Great Britain coexists with private indemnity insurance carriers. Certainly, physicians and other health care providers working for salaries under global budgets or in capitated systems have less financial incentive to provide services than under traditional fee-for-service care delivery.

REIMBURSEMENT FOR SPECIFIC APN GROUPS

Failure of many MCOs to recognize APNs as reimbursable care providers is an issue of concern. Lack of provider status may result in denial of payment for services rendered by APNs even if the services are delivered within the legal scope of APN practice. As documented annually by Pearson,[38] laws in each state vary in their definitions of and processes for APN reimbursement practice. Laws in several states require Medicaid agencies to recognize APNs as primary care providers, but these laws do not apply to all third-party payers. Some states leave the decision about APN recognition up to individual MCOs, and other states have no nursing reimbursement laws.[3] For an up-to-date resource on state reimbursement laws and regulations, see the annual *Legislative Update* published in the January issue of *The Nurse Practitioner.*

Many APNs who deliver services within physician or group practices are frustrated that their patient encounters are billed under physician provider numbers or "incident to" the physician's services. Practices may choose to bill for APN services in this manner to ensure that the practice receives 100 percent of a typical physician fee reimbursement rate for services. Unless the APN service was truly delivered under the criteria for "incident to" service, reimbursement for the service should be billed under the APN's own provider number. Medicare and Medicaid reimbursement rates for services provided by APNs vary from state to state and differ among nongovernmental third-party payers, ranging from 70 percent to 100 percent of a typical physician's fee. Physicians and office managers may be unfamiliar with state laws pertaining to APN reimbursement, causing APN employers to bill inadequately and not receive proper payments from third-party payers.[3] In the following sections, reimbursement issues for specific APN groups will be discussed.

CNMs

In a study of CNMs practicing in the United States, Ament[30] reported that more than 77 percent of respondents were reimbursed by salary; 14 percent were reimbursed on an hourly wage basis; 17 percent of respondents reported having profit sharing; and another 17 percent were reimbursed by percent of production. See Table 8–2.

Personal reimbursement data were also reported, both salary and hourly wages, for four categories of CNMs: new CNM employee, 2 to 5 years of experience, 6 to 10 years of experience, and 11 or more years of experience. The majority of respondents worked as physician employees (21 percent) or as hospital employees (17.6 percent), and 18.3 percent of respondents were in solo/private practice.

TABLE 8–2. Reimbursement Data by Years of Experience[30]		
Experience	Salary, Mean	Salary, Range
New CNM	$51,000	$15,000–70,000
2–5 years	55,000	19,200–80,000
6–10 years	58,600	25,000–90,000
≥11 years	61,500	20,000–100,000

Respondents were also asked what percentage of their population was covered by various reimbursement types, what percentage of the usual and customary physician fee they received for each reimbursement type, the average time to negotiate a provider contract for each reimbursement type, and whether the reimbursement type was a capitated or global fee.[30] See Table 8–3.

Respondents were asked to identify data needed to apply for a provider contract (Table 8–4). More than three-quarters of respondents indicated they needed evidence of their CNM/RN license, certification, and professional liability coverage to apply for a provider contract.[30]

When asked who had primary responsibility for obtaining and/or maintaining provider contracts in their practice, 51 percent said their business manager, 22 percent said the CNM director, 14 percent said the physician director, and 7 percent said someone else. Other groups with primary responsibility included hospital administration, marketing department, an outside agency, office staff, and the university department. Five percent of the responding CNMs said this question did not apply to them.

TABLE 8–3. CNM Reimbursement Data by Reimbursement Type[30]			
Reimbursement Type	% Physician Fee	Average Contract Negotiation Time (months)	Capitated or Global Fee
Medicare	100	2	Global
Managed care Medicare	80	2	Global
Medicaid	100	2	Global
Managed Care Medicaid	100	6	Global
CHAMPUS	100	1.5	Global
Managed Care CHAMPUS	75	9	Capitated
FEHBP	100	3	Global
Managed Care FEHBP	100	3	Global
Primary Care FEHBP	80	9	Global
Commercial carriers	100	2	Global

TABLE 8–4. Evidence Needed for CNMs to Apply for a Provider Contract[30]	
Document	Frequency %
CNM/RN license	86
Evidence of certification	82
Evidence of professional liability coverage	77
Physician name and number	62
Curriculum vitae	57
Evidence of hospital privileges	55
Evidence of independent hospital privileges	17
Evidence of dependent hospital privileges	23
Evidence of courtesy hospital privileges	5
Evidence of prescriptive authority/DEA number	48
Physician practice agreement	47

Slomski[31] described CNM practice arrangements. In one practice, the obstetrician/gynecologist had 65 percent of the practice patients; however, the CNM performed 60 percent of the deliveries, delivering all her own patients and splitting calls with the physician. This CNM stated that she assisted with C-sections, performed circumcisions, comanaged diabetic patients, and gave public lectures on a variety of topics, e.g., perimenopause, which had significantly increased the size of the practice. In another practice, the CNM described a 4 percent to 5 percent lower C-section rate in her practice, compared with the national rate of 21 percent. Slomski pointed out that the lower professional fees collected for vaginal deliveries versus cesarean sections may present a real economic consideration for some practices.[31] However, this may be desirable from a payer perspective.

Medical malpractice premiums are rising rapidly for obstetricians and other specialty physicians. The economic impact has been profound, as some hospitals have discontinued offering obstetrical services. Implications for CNMs are twofold: collaborating physicians may become scarce while demand for their services may increase; and the entire specialty of obstetrics and gynecology may be profoundly affected by the increased costs associated with malpractice premiums.

CRNAs

Anesthesia care, in the past decade, has become one of the more highly contested terrains in advanced practice. Cromwell[32] noted that the supply of anesthesiologists has grown rapidly despite evidence that nurse anesthetists provide equally good care at a fraction of the cost. In addition, attempts by the federal government to make Medicare payments more efficient and equitable by lowering economic return to physicians specializing in anesthesia have created a hostile work environment.

Anesthesia is an example of the choices and challenges facing society regarding the future workforce mix. Two providers currently administer anesthesia in the United States—physician anesthesiologists (MDAs) and CRNAs. Over the past 26 years, the supply of anesthesiologists has tripled while the number of CRNAs has grown 75 percent. Consequently, the growth in anesthesia providers has out-paced the growth in demand for services (operations). The rapid influx of MDAs into what had been predominantly a nursing domain runs counter to the growth in managed care plans that has placed a heavy priority on the use of allied health personnel.[32]

Given the increased emphasis on health care cost containment, the willingness of hospitals to adopt a more costly anesthesia workforce is puzzling. Competitive market theory would have predicted that rapidly rising anesthesia costs, in the face of heightened public and private efforts to control outlays, would have resulted in the hiring of more CRNAs and curtailing of anesthesiologist employment. An anesthesiologist's base salary ranges from $199,872 to $285,770 nationally, while CRNA base salaries range from $99,675 to $117,771.[33] Moreover, CRNAs and anesthesiologists are highly substitutable, as evidenced by the distribution of the two types of providers across hospitals and regions.

Because of their more extensive medical training and higher hourly cost, the anesthesiologist's role, at least in the operating suite, is logically one of medical di-rection or consultation. It does not make economic sense for anesthesiologists to displace CRNAs and take over the myriad tasks already ably performed by CRNAs at half the cost. Nor does it make sense given the lack of evidence on differences in outcomes between the two provider groups. Finally, the Joint Commission on Accreditation of Healthcare Organizations (JCAHO) does not require the presence of an anesthesiologist on the staff in order to accredit hospitals. Despite the evi-dence of substitutability and lower costs, over the past 30 years, CRNAs have seen their role in the workplace diminish to a point at which they are the minority provider. With efficient payment policies, unhampered by hospital organizational and state licensing rigidities, these trends in the anesthesia workforce mix would be far different than the current one in which anesthesiologists (35,000) outnumber CRNAs (28,000) in the United States.[32]

Historically, insurers have paid either on a discounted-charges basis or on ac-tual costs, both highly inflationary. Payers almost always divide their payments into two components, one for the hospital and another for the physicians. Consequently, many private payers, even today, cannot report what average total outlays are for a particular operation across different hospitals. Bifurcated payments for anesthesia have been more problematic due to the great amount of substitution between CRNAs and anesthesiologists and the opportunities for "double billing." Hospitals bill only for the anesthesia costs they incur. Until recently, CRNAs, like other nurses, were employed by the hospital, in which case the institution billed for their services, sometimes directly, but more often indirectly as an overhead support cost to surgery. Anesthesiologists nearly always bill directly for their professional ser-vices. With CRNA costs "hidden" in hospital bills, it has been difficult for payers to isolate the true full costs of anesthesia and make comparisons of costs and work-force mix across institutions.[32]

Finally, and in some respects the most inflationary, there are the opportunities for anesthesiologists to supervise. These opportunities exist precisely because of the close substitution of CRNAs for physicians. Private insurers have allowed anesthesiologists to double-, triple-, or quadruple-bill their time in overseeing the activities of CRNAs without significant prorating to account for the modest time they personally spend with each patient.[32]

Under Medicare, anesthesiologists have always been paid differently than other physicians on the basis of a dollar "conversion factor" multiplied by corresponding base and time units involved in a given case. In the early years of the program, anesthesiologists directly employing and supervising CRNAs were paid their full allowable charge under Part B with no separate CRNA charge. There were no limits to the number of concurrent cases the physicians could bill for. The program made a distinction when the CRNA was hospital-employed, in which case the MDA's time units, but not the base units, were halved. The rationale was that the program was also paying the nurse anesthetist's salary to the hospital under Part A. When Congress passed the OBRA of 1987, it sought to correct the problem by reducing base units by 10 percent, 25 percent, and 40 percent when MDAs were supervising from one to four cases at once.[32]

Medicare changes implemented in 1998 removed economic incentives for anesthesiologists to medically direct two CRNAs on two simultaneous operations. As if the Medicare program sees no value in anesthesiologist involvement on two cases over and above the services performed by the CRNA, their time is considered a pure substitution. For CRNAs employed by physicians, the situation is potentially quite different. The MDA practice must still bill 50–50 for the two providers on concurrent cases. But when the practice receives the full Medicare allowable payment in two components, the practice can reimburse its (usually) salaried CRNAs the going market hourly wage, which is usually less than half the Medicare allowable fee. Hence, while the program implicitly recognizes the two providers as equal in terms of payment on a per-case basis, the potential impact on existing CRNA employment arrangements is far from neutral.[32]

The Medicare program has established a set of conflicting incentives antithetical to the most efficient anesthesia team arrangement through a set of well-meaning but short-sighted policy changes. First, it mandated that the anesthesiologist be personally involved in seven key tasks throughout the anesthetic procedure. Secondly, its split-billing rule established an effective pay rate for CRNAs essentially equal to that of physician anesthesiologists who have acquired several more very expensive years of education. Medicare has struggled with anesthesiologist payment almost from the program's inception for two reasons. First, because CRNAs dominated the profession in the mid-1960s, the program stipulated that an anesthesiologist need not be present for CRNAs to deliver anesthesia under a surgeon's direction. Yet, at the same time, it recognized the value added from anesthesiologist supervision through additional direct payment to this one specialty instead of treating the whole service as hospital-based and falling under Part A. By allowing direct billing by anesthesiologists under Part B, the program failed to grasp the fact that delivery of anesthesia is fundamentally a Part A, hospital-based service.[32]

Given the rapid growth in the supply of anesthesiologists, coupled with the changes in Medicare reimbursement policies antithetical to team anesthesia, occupational licensure has become a major battleground. In the growing competition for hospital-based anesthesia positions, the American Society of Anesthesiologists (ASA) has come to regard nurse anesthetists as "not quite professionals" who are encroaching on their domain. As mentioned earlier, anesthesia historically has been a nursing function. In 1949, for example, there were 3,678 active U.S. CRNAs in practice versus only 1,837 anesthesiologists. Anesthesiologists have justified their own "encroachment" by making a fine distinction between "practicing medicine," which is what physicians do, and "practicing nursing," which is what nurses do. It does not seem reasonable to conclude that nurses are encroaching on physician activities just because anesthesiologists (or any other specialty) enter a field and begin performing the same tasks as nurse anesthetists (or other nurses). According to ASA's own review of state regulations, no state requires CRNAs to be supervised by anesthesiologists. Undeterred, ASA continues actively to promote and support bills requiring anesthesiologist involvement in every surgical case.[32]

Cromwell[32] believes that until payers change the way they pay for anesthesia, unproductive incentives will continue to drive the system in the wrong direction. Payers, particularly Medicare, must stop paying anesthesiologists directly for their services if they want them to move into more supervisory and collaborative roles. While split billing by Medicare caps the program's outlays at what a solo anesthesiologist would cost, the payment is still far greater than what the program would pay under an optimal workforce mix at competitive salaries for the two providers. What is much worse, split billing is often antithetical to team anesthesia.[32]

Payers can achieve lower costs and a better workforce mix by negotiating a global payment for inpatient surgery that includes both the hospital and all physician services. For example, a small number of insurers, including Medicare, now carve out global bundles for specialized inpatient services, e.g., cardiac and orthopedic surgery, which puts the medical staff at risk for all, or most, physician services. Simply defining anesthesia as a Part A hospital service would accomplish even more. Were anesthesiologists unable to direct-bill Medicare (and private payers as well), they would either have to take salaried positions in the hospital or negotiate less favorable contract relationships. In either case, the hospital would be responsible for how much they were being paid. If anesthesiologists refused to take lower salaries or discounted fees, institutions would use fewer of them in more supervisory roles. This is beginning to happen in a few hospitals that are starting to compete their previously exclusive anesthesia contracts due to high charges to managed care payers. The staff model HMO, where all anesthesia costs are internalized, also results in higher CRNA-anesthesiologist ratios than in competing institutions where anesthesiologists are "free inputs" to the facility.[32] If Medicare persists with its split-billing arrangement and pays both providers equally, CRNAs will continue to be displaced. The resulting anesthesia workforce would be primarily physicians, earning less because the increased supply would attenuate demand for MDA services.

Many novel capitation arrangements already exist. In fully capitated, staff-model HMOs that own their own hospitals, incentives for using the optimal anesthesia workforce are strongest, again because all provider costs are internalized. A 1995 Kaiser Permanente internal study[35] concluded that a one-to-four MDA-CRNA ratio was more cost-effective than the more typical one-to-two ratio found in many West coast facilities. Because anesthesia costs tend to be a small part of the overall cost, private insurers building a hospital network pay scant attention to the cost or the workforce mix in anesthesia.[32]

It has been estimated that 80 percent of nurse anesthetists practice in the team mode, e.g., collaboratively with anesthesiologists. Anesthesiology lacks definitive outcomes data derived from prospective multicenter studies that demonstrate an optimal provider mix in terms of cost and quality. Cromwell's admonitions regarding the advisability of dismantling bifurcated payments for anesthesia, optimal use of nurse anesthetists, and the desirability of defining anesthesia as a Medicare Part A hospital-based service bear close study by the involved professional organizations, government agencies, and payers.

Clinical Nurse Specialists and Nurse Practitioners

Lindeke and Chesney[3], in a study of psychiatric-mental health CNSs and NPs, described perceived barriers to practice. Three themes emerged:

- Lack of APN recognition by MCOs and payers. Patient access to high-quality care provided by APNs is limited when health care systems fail to specifically designate them as providers of care. APNs are often not identified in advertising and promotional materials published by MCOs. APNs may not receive information regarding reimbursement regulations even when they are credentialed by the payers and have their own provider numbers. Credentialing of APNs is frequently a slow process. MCOs may be unfamiliar with APN scope of practice and national certification. As a result, some APNs practice without their own provider numbers and are employed by practices that do not attempt to obtain APN provider numbers.

- A lack of APN knowledge and education about reimbursement. APNs recognize their limited knowledge of reimbursement rules, regulations, and policies. APNs lacked knowledge regarding coding, billing, and insurance coverage, all of which affected their ability to effectively work within the system and wasted valuable time; were uncertain how their patient visits were being billed; and were unclear regarding the reimbursement they were actually receiving.

- Difficulty in coping with rapid change in reimbursement policies and procedures. The rapid pace of change within the health care system necessitates that APNs continually update their knowledge and understanding of reimbursement issues and policies. APNs may react to the rapid pace of change by claiming disinterest or a lack of understanding. Lack of understanding is not an excuse for inappropriate billing and is not an option in today's health care system for APNs committed to a favorable professional future.

Following the implementation of the BBA of 1997, several strategies were attempted by organized medicine to restrict the ability of NPs and CNSs to bill for Medicare reimbursement. The AMA developed a citizen's petition to be filed with the CMS. The petition demanded the implementation of a system that would ensure that Medicare reimbursement to APNs be made only if the services were provided in collaboration with a physician and were within the APN's state scope of practice. The petition was circulated and endorsement sought from all national medical specialty organizations and state medical associations.[36]

Since the BBA's expansion of opportunities for direct reimbursement to APNs, the appropriate relationship between physicians and APNs and the meaning of collaboration have been hotly contested. The AMA submitted extensive comments to CMS supporting restrictive definitions of collaboration and relationships of APNs and physicians. The AMA and other medical organizations failed to achieve this aim previously during the comment period, leading to CMS's final rule on the definition of collaboration. States vary in their requirements for APN-physician relationships; some are in the midst of change. Some require a collaborative relationship, but others do not. The authority of states to determine the appropriate relationship between APNs and physicians is recognized by federal statute, which defers to state law. In states that do not require collaboration, federal regulations require APNs to document their scope of practice and indicate the relationships they have to deal with issues outside their scope of practice.[36] The AMA stated that the Health Care Financing Administration (now the CMS) had no system for the assessment and review of claims made by APNs and urged that a system be developed to determine whether each APN complied with state law. The AMA asked the CMS to limit distribution and renewal of Medicare billing numbers to APNs who complied with the collaboration and scope-of-practice requirements and to conduct audits to ensure that Medicare payments to APNs are limited to services provided in collaboration with a physician and within the scope of practice allowed by state law.[36]

The arguments used by the AMA are just one means to retain authority for patient care to "recognize ... APNs, under physician leadership, as effective physician extenders."[36] An active Medicare fraud and abuse program already exists to cover all providers. If the actions demanded in the petition or similar restrictions were to be implemented, fiscal and other barriers to the full scope of APN practice would be created, which would, according to the ANA, "have a chilling effect on Medicare reimbursement opportunities for nurses."[36]

Economic Comparison of APNs, PAs, and Physicians

Primary care PAs in multispecialty groups gross slightly more than $3 for every $1 in compensation, according to the Medical Group Management Association (MGMA). Internists, in contrast, gross slightly more than twice their compensation. If an NP or PA produces $30,000 in annual profit—an attainable figure according to the MGMA—the physician practice or group partners can divide the money among themselves.[37]

PAs and NPs increase practice incomes in other ways. In managed care markets, they allow physicians to handle larger patient panels and receive a larger capitation check. In the fee-for-service realm, they free doctors to concentrate on more complex, better paying cases.[37]

APNs and PAs are also commanding generous reimbursement from commercial insurers: generally 80 to 100 percent of what physicians receive. NPs and

TABLE 8–5. How NPs, PAs, and CNMs Compare with Physicians on Pay and Productivity			
	Median Compensation	Median Gross Charges	Median Ambulatory Encounters per Year
CNM	$68,588	$230,195	1,469
NP	55,433	151,504	2,620
PA (primary care)	61,411	205,254	3,496
Family physician, No Ob-Gyn	138,277	320,213	4,407
Internist	140,951	327,873	3,353

Source: 1999 Physician Compensation and Productivity Survey, Medical Group Management Association[37]

CNMs have even had some success in a bigger battle: persuading managed care plans to allow enrollees to choose them as PCPs (Table 8–5).

PAs and NPs, often considered a cost center by hospitals and other employers, now represent a source of professional fee income. Table 8–6 contains a breakdown of current average costs/revenues generated by PAs and NPs based on MGMA's annual compensation report.

Because of increased reimbursement levels mandated by the BBA, net revenue generated by NPs and PAs should increase significantly. Many hospitals and other employers of APNs and PAs are now looking at them in a new light as revenue generators. In addition, the BBA has expanded the market from rural areas to all practice arenas. APNs need to be aware of market segmentation and competition that can affect their practices, especially with the level playing field in reimbursement for NPs and PAs created by the BBA.

For physicians and medical groups, NPs and PAs offer a less expensive means of practice expansion. By hiring these providers, a physician group can increase its capacity for a higher volume of patients or expand into new markets without incurring the level of risk associated with employing a new physician or with practice mergers. The broad expansion of covered service sites the BBA mandated offers an affordable way to grow areas of a practice that may have been unprofitable or less attractive if a physician had to provide the services. In addition, medical groups that

TABLE 8–6. Revenues and Costs of PAs and NPs			
	Revenue per Day	Cost per Day	Net Revenue per Day
NP	$570	228	342
PA	719	248	471

Source: Physician Compensation and Production Survey: 1998 Report (Based on 1997 data). Medical Group Management Association, Englewood, CO.

take on managed care risk can provide services less expensively and remain within global per-member, per-month budgets.[37]

Physicians and APNs have clashed over turf in the past, and the BBA may make such conflicts more prevalent. In effect, Medicare now views "midlevel" providers as acceptable lower-cost practitioners, meaning that they are a potential source of direct competition for physicians. When hospitals hire increased numbers of PAs and NPs, physicians may view this as a threat. Many physicians are learning to incorporate APNs and PAs into their practices as a complement to the physicians' services. Other physicians see APNs as part of a rising tide of providers threatening their position as the main contact or entry point into the health care system. An additional factor that could fuel competition is the growing number of NPs and PAs entering the market.[37]

SUMMARY

Reimbursement for APNs has been discussed in the context of traditional economic theory. The economic system, particularly as it relates to health care, was described. Concepts such as market competition, disequilibrium, and supplier-induced demand were explicated. Cost considerations in the provision of services by, and reimbursement for, physicians and APNs were discussed in relation to the price of services, access issues, health care plans, competition, and antitrust issues. Key terms in finance and reimbursement were defined.

Reimbursement is a challenging component of APN practice. APNs should be aware of market economics, use appropriate marketing strategies, and strive to provide high-quality cost-effective services. As health care providers assume more financial risk, fiscal rewards may be less predictable than in the past. However, APNs equipped with the necessary knowledge and skills can fill needed service niches in health care, practicing independently or collaboratively with physicians.

A debate is currently taking place in the United States on whether a surplus of physicians exists or will exist in the future. Most of the projected surpluses revolve around comparisons of fee-for-service versus much lower managed care demands. However, the projected national surpluses are small in proportion to the very large growth that is projected for the number of nonphysician clinicians. Ultimately, it will depend on how the responsibility for patients is divided among licensed clinicians and what our society will want physicians to do. The boundaries of medicine and nursing have always been ill defined. Whether APNs, highly cost-effective practitioners, will flourish over the next 20 years depends not so much on their training as on financial, organizational, and legal obstacles to their scope of practice.

SUGGESTED EXERCISES

1. An NP who has been employed for 15 years is told that her position is being eliminated. She is told that her position is "too expensive" for the proposed hospital budget under a reengineering plan. Consultants have told hospital administration to decrease fixed costs

such as payroll. The panel of patients seen by this NP would be given the option of being seen by other health care providers in the community. How might the NP retain her practice while capturing the income stream generated by her services?

2 A nurse educator who is active in professional organization activities repeatedly cites the benefits of care provided by APNs. These benefits include safe and cost-effective care. At one forum, the educator is closely questioned regarding the availability of data substantiating these benefits. How might the educator respond to these questions, based on the evolving health care marketplace?

3 An NP employed by an HMO contemplates relocating from an urban setting to a rural one, where she contemplates entering a joint practice arrangement with a physician who is anxious to collaborate with the NP. However, both the physician and the NP are unfamiliar with reimbursement mechanisms for services provided by NPs. What resources should these professionals consult to maximize reimbursement from their joint practice arrangement?

REFERENCES

1. Felstein, P: The Politics of Health Legislation: An Economic Perspective. Health Administration Press Perspectives, Ann Arbor, MI, 1988.
2. Buerhaus, P: Nursing, competition, and quality. Nurs Econ 10:21, 1992.
3. Lindeke, LL, and Chesney, ML: Reimbursement realities of advanced nursing practice. Nurs Outlook 47:6, 1999.
4. Fuchs, V: The Health Economy. Harvard University Press, Cambridge, MA, 1986.
5. Enthoven, A: Managed competition: An agenda for action. Health Aff (Millwood) 7:25, 1988.
6. Feldstein, P: Health Care Economics, 4th ed. Delmar Publishers, Albany, NY, 1993.
7. Cohen, J: Medicaid physician fees and use of physician and hospital services. Inquiry 30:281, 1993.
8. Lee, D, and Gillis, K: Physician responses to Medicare physician payment reform: Preliminary results on access to care. Inquiry 30:417, 1993.
9. Buerhaus, P: Economics and healthcare financing. In Hickey, J, Ouimette, R, and Venegoni, S (eds): Advanced Practice Nursing. Lippincott, Philadelphia, 1996.
10. Sorkin, A: Health Economics, 3rd ed. Macmillan, New York, 1992.
11. EBRI Online Facts from EBRI, National Health Care Expenditures, 1997. http://www.ebri.org/facts/0199afact.htm Accessed July 6, 2003.
12. Hoffman, C: Medicaid payment for nonphysician practitioners: An access issue. Health Aff (Millwood) 13:140, 1994.
13. Mittelstadt, P: Federal reimbursement of advanced practice nurses' services empowers the profession. Nurse Pract 18:46, 1993.
14. Lewin, I: To the Rescue: Toward Solving America's Health Care Crisis. Families USA Foundation, Washington, DC, 1993.
15. Pryor, C: Balanced budget act enhances value of physician assistants, nurse practitioners. Health Care Strategic Manage 17:12, 1999.
16. Faut-Callahan, M: Economics of anesthesia. Unpublished manuscript, 1995.
17. Bradford, B: Personal communication, April, 1996.
18. Fagin, C: The cost-effectiveness of nursing care. In Aiken, L, and Fagin, C (eds): Charting Nursing's Future: Agenda for the 1990s. Lippincott, Philadelphia, 1992.
19. Hooker, R: The Role of Physician Assistants and Nurse Practitioners in a Managed Care Organization. Association of Academic Health Centers, Kaiser Permanente Center for Health Research, Sacramento, CA, 1993.
20. Mirr, M: Advanced clinical practice: A reconceptualized role. AACN 4:599, 1993.
21. Timmons, G, and Ridenour, N: Legal approaches to the restraint of trade of nurse practitioners: Disparate reimbursement patterns. J Am Acad Nurse Pract 6:55, 1994.
22. Fugate, D, and Freese, G: Nursing marketing. In Decker, P, and Sullivan, E (eds): Nursing Administration. Appleton & Lange, Norwalk, CT, 1992.
23. Petrakos, C: Nurse practitioner supervision at issue: RNs push for collegial practice. The Chicago Tribune, Nursing News, p 3, 1996.
24. Schwartz, A: Will competition change physician workforce? Early signals from the market. Acad Med 71:15, 1996.

25. Simonson, D, and Garde, J: Reimbursement for clinical services. In Foster, S, and Jordan, L (eds): Professional Aspects of Nurse Anesthesia Practice. FA Davis, Philadelphia, 1994.
26. Kongstvedt, P: Compensation of Primary Care Physicians in Open Panels. The Managed Health Care Handbook, 2nd ed. Aspen, Gaithersburg, MD, 1993.
27. Michels, K: Healthcare reform glossary of terms. J Am Assoc Nurse Anesth 62:19, 1994.
28. American Association of Nurse Anesthetists: Practice Management in Changing Environments, sections 4–1 and 4–2. The American Association of Nurse Anesthetists, Park Ridge, IL, 1994.
29. Brotherton, SE, Simon, FA, Tomany, SC: US graduate medical education, 1999–2000. JAMA 284:9, 2002.
30. Ament, L: Reimbursement, employment, and hospital privilege data of certified nurse-midwifery services. J Nurse Midwifery 43:305, 1998.
31. Slomski, A: "We Don't Just Catch Babies." Med Economics 77:186, 2000.
32. Cromwell, J: Barriers to achieving a cost-effective workforce mix: Lessons from anesthesiology. J Health Politics, Policy Law, 24:1331, 1999.
33. www.salary.com Accessed April 2004.
34. Federal Register: January 23, 2004, Volume 69, Number 15. Rules and Regulations pp 3433–3469. From the Federal Register Online via GPO Access (wais.access.gpo.gov.) http://a257.g.akamaitech.net/7/257/2422/14mar20010800/edocket.access.gpo.gov/2004/04 Accessed April 9, 2004.
35. Kaiser Permanente: An Inter-Regional Examination of Operating Room Best Practices. Unpublished report, 1995.
36. Minarik, P: Alert! Strategy initiated to restrict advanced practice nurses' ability to bill Medicare. Clin Nurse Specialist 14:250, 2000.
37. Guglielmo, W: In the trenches, it's cooperation that matters. Med Economics 77:194, 2000.
38. Pearson, L: Fifteenth annual legislative update. Nurse Pract 28:1, 2003.
39. Alliance for Health Care Reform Covers the Uninsured Week on Campus Resource Guide. Washington, DC: Robert Wood Johnson Foundation. March 10–16, 2003.
40. Department of Health and Human Services Office of the Inspector General: Medicare Coverage of Non-Physician Practitioner Services OEI-02-00-00290, June 2001.
41. http://bcbshealthissues.com Accessed June 28, 2003.
42. Alliance for Health Reform: Sourcebook for Journalists 2003: Chapter 8: Health Care Costs. http://www.allhealth.org/sourcebook2002/ch8_8.html Accessed June 28, 2003.
43. Kaiser Family Foundation: Trends and Indicators in the Changing Health Care Marketplace. 2002.
44. U.S. Health care Costs Expected to Double by 2007. Foresight 5:4 1998. http://www.kltprc.net/emergingissues/Chpt_60.htm Accessed June 26, 2003.
45. Alliance for Health Reform: Sourcebook for Journalists 2003: Chapter 11: Managed Care. http://www.allhealth.org/sourcebook2002/ch11_1.html Accessed June 28, 2003.
46. American Medical Association. AMA Young Physicians Section Interim 2003 Delegate's Report. http://www.ama-assn.org/ama/pub/category/9982.html Accessed June 28, 2003.
47. Cooper, R, Getzen, T, McKee, H, and Laud, P: Economic and demographic trends signal an impending physician shortage. Health Aff 21:1. 2002.
48. Cooper, R: There's a shortage of specialists: Is anyone listening? Acad Med 77:8, 2002.
49. Rapsilber, L, and Anderson, E: Understanding the reimbursement process. Nurse Pract 25:36, 2000.
50. McKeon, E: Medicaid reimbursement for APRNs. Am J Nurs 102:23, 2002.
51. Strunk, B, Ginsburg, P, and Gabel, J: Tracking Health Care Costs: Growth Accelerates Again in 2001. Health Tracking: Trends Web Exclusive September 25, 2002.
52. Edmunds, M: Why don't we receive equal reimbursement? Nurse Pract 27:47, 2002.
53. http://www.nursingworld.org. Accessed July 3, 2003.
54. Anderson, D, and Hampton, M: Physician assistants and nurse practitioners: Rural-urban settings and reimbursement for services. J Rural Health, 15:252, 1999.
55. Herrick, T: Surgical specialties threatened Clinician News 8:1, 2004.
56. http://www.census.gov Accessed July 2, 2003.

CHAPTER 9

Marketing the Role: Formulating, Articulating, and Negotiating Advanced Practice Nursing Positions

Christine E. Burke, PhD, CNM

Christine E. Burke, PhD, CNM, has had a clinical practice in nurse midwifery since 1976, when she earned her master's degree in nursing from Yale University. Dr. Burke is an educator whose teaching credentials include positions at the University of Colorado, Georgetown University, George Mason University, and Yale University. Pentimento Praxis, Dr. Burke's consultation practice, was established in 1992 after completion of her doctorate in nursing from the University of Colorado. The scope of her consultations includes creating caring communities, training teachers and community members in moral development and character education, caring for and preventing adolescent pregnancies, nurturing the perceptual palette, and providing parenting instruction. Dr. Burke lives in Denver, Colorado, where she currently works for The Denver Health Authority.

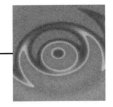

Marketing the Role: Formulating, Articulating, and Negotiating Advanced Practice Nursing Positions

CHAPTER OBJECTIVES

After completing this chapter, the reader will be able to:

1 Communicate the benefits that accrue to the target population or employer from utilization of the advanced practice nurse's (APN's) service offer through use of the 4 Ps.

2 Create a personal mission statement after reflection on personal values, beliefs, and quality-of-life issues that will influence your career pathways.

3 Interpret facts from major documents about cost, outcomes, and use of health services provided by APNs.

4 Create a marketing plan for an APN's service.

5 Create a succinct position statement for an APN's service that differentiates the service from alternatives and links it to target consumer needs and wants.

6 Demonstrate techniques and considerations in negotiating an advanced practice position from initial contact through the interview process to the contractual agreement.

7 Analyze existing network and use marketing techniques to further enhance and strengthen the resources.

Marketing, as a coordinated style of communicating information, is an essential skill for APNs. Success in the age of managed care and autonomous private practices and businesses demands an appreciation of market theories. APNs must understand a business plan as well as a nursing care plan to accomplish the goals of their independent practice. This chapter is bifocal in its presentation. The information shared is useful from either the employer's or employee's perspective. The skills necessary to gather and interpret marketing data, formulate marketing plans, and create essential written documents for the acquisition and development of APNs' services are presented through a marketing lens.

THE TRADITIONAL MARKETING APPROACH: THE 4 Ps

The marketing process is guided by the 4 Ps:

- Product
- Price
- Place
- Promotion

These concepts help to assess the needs and the available resources to be used in the promotion of the APN service.

The first P, the **product**, is interpreted in an APN's business plan, not as material goods, but rather as human services. Unlike material products, these services lack tangibility, efficient storage capability for later use, and cannot be exactly replicated with each client, factors that pose some of the challenges of creating a marketing plan that accurately projects the future of an APN's service. The difference of human service is important because it is at the core of patient satisfaction. The development of an APN's service as a product includes the consideration of the

market segmentation, or **target markets,** which describe who will be served; **product integrity,** or the balance of needs and resources; and the **competition,** or the other available health care services in the community.

Price, the second P, is the identification of the right cost for the services. This price must be neither too high nor too low and also must meet the existing financial mandates of insurance companies, managed care facilities, and federally funded Medicaid and Medicare plans. APNs' services can support their price for services from marketing research based on utilization and cost-effectiveness. Proof that the services meet the needs of the patients and are financially efficient has been determined in recent research, which is discussed later in this chapter.

The third P is for **place,** or where these services are delivered. The demands of the consumers direct this marketing concern. The geographic location and physical convenience of the APN service play heavily into the clients' decision-making among competitive health care services. The more accessible and the more easily usable a service is, the greater the acquisition of health care consumers. The simple matters of accessibility by public transportation, parking, and physically pleasant office spaces can ultimately sway potential clients from one service to another.

The final P is for **promotion,** or the ability to increase consumers' awareness of the APN's services offered and the communication of information that may attract consumers. The modes of promotion include advertisement, publicity, community presentations, and correspondence. In addition, promotion also includes the manner in which the APN reflects the quality of the service in speech, dress, and the conduct of business. The best method of promotion is word of mouth by satisfied consumers. By its nature, this method of promotion is grounded in familiarity and trust, and a good word from a previous employer or consumer can do more for successful marketing than many costly advertising promotions.[1]

In the early 1990s, the marketing firm of Burson-Marsteller introduced a fifth P, which relates to the **perception management** of your target audience. The customer perception of the APN as a capable, knowledgable health care provider is as important as the other 4 Ps of marketing services. The perception of the provider's skills becomes the reality for the consumer; the need to create a good perception is then obvious when an APN is marketing for employment. According to Burson-Marsteller, the perceptions motivate behaviors that create the business results. They further believe that the perceptions are built on the societal values that guide attitude formation and, ultimately, behavior. Woods and Cardin,[2] in their discussion of this aspect of perception, further discuss the need to consider the recognition of the emotional and the rational messages sent to consumers. These messages pass on the value of feeling safe with APN care, and this connects to the universal value we seek for peace of mind.

Marketing has changed some of its point of view. The 4 Ps are an old standard for creating marketing plans, but a new point of view has emerged that expands this to include the Four Cs: Customer value, Cost, Convenience, and Communication. Dr. Rick Crandall, a noted authority on marketing service rather than products, has stated that for service providers these four areas may prove to be more important than the traditional 4 Ps.[3]

Employment is one of the obvious goals of APN education. This goal is met through one of three pathways:

1. Employment in an established health care service that already employs APNs

2. Creation of new employment opportunities within a health care system that has the potential for expansion to include APNs.

3. Development of a private practice in the clinical or consultation arenas

In general terms, marketing is the activity that supports the buying and selling of products and services. The key to success in attaining employment involves matching the professional skills necessary for a job and the APN. By analyzing the health care needs of the target population and setting up a research-based plan to meet those needs, APNs are likely to create employment opportunities or, in marketing terms, to set up voluntary exchanges of goods and services.

A prerequisite to the successful marketing of an APN is knowledge. Each professional must spend time considering and developing self-knowledge and knowledge about the profession. Attention should be given to the following areas:

- Knowledge of personal values, professional skills, and practical necessities
- Knowledge of practice regulations
- Knowledge of existing services
- Knowledge of clients' health care needs and desires
- Knowledge of the target population's understanding of the role and scope of practice of the APN
- Knowledge of the utilization and cost-effectiveness of and satisfaction with APN services
- Knowledge of specific marketing elements

KNOWLEDGE OF PERSONAL VALUES, PROFESSIONAL SKILLS, AND PRACTICAL NECESSITIES

Developing a personal mission statement, or a statement of one's values, beliefs, and goals of practice, can assist in successfully communicating and selling one's view of health care. This statement will explain who you are. The personal mission statement typically includes one's values or guiding principles (e.g., trust, honesty, respect, responsibility, and caring) and one's professional skills and scope of services. Most important, it reveals the vision of the quality of life one needs (time for family, hobbies, political activity, and educational opportunities). This knowledge is usually acquired by introspection, by review of previous employment, and by consideration of personal needs, which are necessary for a reasonable life.

An example of guiding principles that have strongly affected the business community is Stephen Covey's *The Seven Habits of Highly Effective People.*[4] Covey developed a theory regarding the restoration of the character ethic. The habits are the intersection of knowledge, skill, and desire. Knowledge is the theoretical paradigm, or the "what to do"; skill is the "how to do"; and desire is the motivation. Covey divides these habits into three arenas:

1. The Private Victory
   - Be proactive, based on principles of personal vision.
   - Begin with the end in mind, guided by principles of leadership.
   - Put first things first, guided by principles of personal management.

2. The Public Victory
   - Think win-win, guided by principles of interpersonal leadership.
   - Seek first to understand, then to be understood, guided by principles of empathic communication.
   - Synergize, guided by principles of cooperation.

3. The Renewal
   - Sharpen the saw, guided by principles of balanced self-renewal.

The importance of this work is its universal message about human effectiveness. The translation of these theories into nursing practice will help create a stronger, more professional vision.

Questions helpful in the introspective process are:

- What about your work do you enjoy the most?
- What other interests do you have?
- What skills do you do well?
- Which need improvement?
- What support do you need to attain a proficient level of practice?
- What made you leave jobs in the past?
- How will this affect your future employment?
- Do you prefer to work alone or in a team?
- What about your team members is necessary for good working relationships?
- How do you see your role in relation to the health care system? What is your need for power or shared power?
- How do you handle stress?
- Will the job you are creating or applying for allow for some stress reduction management, such as exercise?
- What are your family needs (child care issues and emergency coverage, flexibility of hours to allow for family events)?
- How do you best communicate with others?

The time spent on a personal mission statement can save you from major career-related frustrations and problems. A considered mission statement can guide your job search with a clarity of purpose by defining both the professional and personal motivating factors. If salary and status hold greater value than free time and an active social life, focus the marketing efforts on demanding a financially fulfilling position. In all cases, be true to yourself.

Fisher and Brown,[5] of the Harvard Negotiation Project, in discussing the role of shared values with employers and employees, remind us that the fewer the differences in our shared values, the more likely we will have a basis for dealing with issues fairly. The opposite is not true, however; differences are not good for negotiations. It is often enriching for the work at hand to have some value differences that force the creation of new partnerships.

KNOWLEDGE OF PRACTICE REGULATIONS

The legal issues concerning advanced practice nursing are discussed in Chapter 13. Review this chapter and all related statutes and regulations. Place in a marketing portfolio the documents that will support an advanced nursing practice. Typically, these documents include:

- State nurse practice act
- State board of nursing regulations
- Prescriptive authority legislation
- Third-party reimbursement rules and regulations
- Practice protocols from similar APNs' services

An excellent resource for these regulatory issues is the annual legislative update compiled by *The Nurse Practitioner*.[6] *Nursing Economics* is another journal that keeps an eye on the legislative changes affecting nursing services. In the segment called "Capital Commentary," in-depth explanations and evaluations of health care policy issues are provided.[7]

KNOWLEDGE OF EXISTING SERVICES

Investigate the target market in which you wish to practice, with an eye toward answering the following questions:

- What services already exist in the community?
- Who uses the services?
- What are the needs for these services, based on the demographic data and the socioeconomic mix of the population (e.g., age, employment, unemployment, insured and uninsured)?
- Most important, what is not working with these services that an APN might be able to change (e.g., access to care, cost-effective care, patient education)?

Knowing the competition is the first step in creating a marketing strategy. Deciding how to position the service is the next. Positioning is a marketing strategy that works to separate the uniqueness of a product or service from the generic pack.

It begins with knowing your service and the competition's service and then finding a niche that allows your service to stand out.[8]

Ask what is needed by the consumer that an APN can meet. Knowing one's abilities and marketable skills is important, but it is more important to be in a position where someone will desire to use those services. This goal can be best accomplished by recommendations from people already highly respected by the target population or community. In a world full of well-qualified professionals, the APN or APN's service with strong recommendations will often rise above the competition and be hired.

Creating this **market niche,** the narrow market segment the APN can fulfill, can be accomplished by using a reverse marketing strategy. This consumer-driven process creates partners between the APN and the potential clients toward the common goal of health care satisfaction. The positioning process, therefore, demands a needs assessment of the actual or perceived consumer needs. This is accomplished by the use of interviews, surveys, and questionnaires.[3]

KNOWLEDGE OF CLIENTS' HEALTH CARE NEEDS AND DESIRES

Knowledge of the needs and desires of the clients involves watching and reaching people. Mark McCormack, in *What They Don't Teach You at Harvard Business School,* [9] described seven fundamental steps to reading people:

1. Listen aggressively to the what and how someone speaks.
2. Observe aggressively, and make note of all body language.
3. Talk less and you will learn more, see more, and hear more.
4. Take a second look at first impressions by reviewing what you first thought about a person or an idea.
5. Take time to use what you have learned by reviewing what you know about your job and the clients, and then consider how you will present your services.
6. Be discreet about what you have perceived about others and how they learn about your qualifications. Whenever possible, let others tell how great you are.
7. Be detached enough to step back from a heated business deal and watch what is happening so that your reaction is not overreaction. Always try to act rather than react as acting has more power.

Researching the health care needs of a target population includes McCormack's ideas of reading people on the interpersonal level and using the more global tools for reading a community, such as surveys. These surveys should offer a broader perspective of the health care needs from a mix of socioeconomic groups as well as from a variety of community members, consumers, health care administrators, insurance agents, and peer professionals.

KNOWLEDGE OF THE TARGET POPULATION'S UNDERSTANDING OF THE ROLE AND SCOPE OF PRACTICE OF THE APN

By survey, questionnaire, or personal contacts, determine the target market's level of understanding of an APN. Talk to prospective clients, employers, community leaders, insurance salespersons, hospital employees, and the medical community. Determine what, if any, previous experiences prospective employers have had with APNs.

Once the level of appreciation of the APN has been determined, formulate a plan for educating or increasing the awareness of your target population regarding the potential benefits of hiring an APN and their specific skills.

KNOWLEDGE OF THE UTILIZATION AND COST-EFFECTIVENESS OF AND SATISFACTION WITH APN SERVICES

Review and collect current literature that supports the role of the APN. Resource assessment and use are at the core of every economic strategy plan. A marketing plan should respect not only the fiscal and structural resources of the health care system but also the human resources necessary for health care provision. Encourage prospective employers or consumers to read the literature on utilization and suggest that they take the time to evaluate what costly physicians' services they might substitute with APNs' services. Research has shown that nonphysician health care professionals provide high-quality primary care and increased consumer access to care.

On the most basic level, APNs earn smaller salaries and, therefore, solely in terms of salary and benefits cost less than physicians. More important, APNs are more likely to prescribe improved nutrition, exercise, stress management techniques, and health promotion, modalities that are less likely to directly affect the clinic, hospital, or institutional budget. In addition, APNs are less likely to send each patient home with a prescription, potentially saving health care dollars.

Research in primary care has described the level of productivity and cost associated with patient delegation of nonphysician health providers (NHPs), NPs, physician assistants, and physician providers. These studies reveal that four NHPs can replace two to three physicians. The addition of an NHP to an office or clinic setting increased the total office visits by 40 to 50 percent. The substitution of one NHP for one physician resulted in an average savings of more than $34,000 per year.[10] Similarly, Greenfield et al[11] found that in an NHP system in a health care setting in which protocols were used, a 20 percent reduction on visit costs was realized. A meta-analysis of studies on NPs and certified nurse midwives (CNMs) provides our profession with excellent support for the use of professionals in these advanced practice nursing roles.[12] A 1986 study reported by the Office of Technology Assessment (OTA)[13] concluded that NPs and CNMs provided a quality of care equivalent to the care given by physicians. This study also concluded that in the areas of communication and preventive care, nurses were much more adept than physicians. A second study conducted in 1987 by Crosby, Ventura, and Feldman[14] reported findings similar to those of the OTA study. The 1987 study concluded that:

- Patients are satisfied with their care from NPs.
- The interpersonal skills of APNs are better than those of physicians.
- The technical quality of NPs is equivalent to physicians' care.
- NPs' patient outcomes are equivalent or superior to physicians' patient outcomes.
- NPs facilitate continuity of patient care and improved access to care in rural and other settings and provide care to underserved populations.

In November 1995, the Health Research Group of Ralph Nader's Public Citizen released a unique consumer guide[15] to certified nurse midwifery practices in the United States. The report concluded that CNMs will play an increasing role in American obstetric care because of the quality of care, cost-effectiveness, and overall patient satisfaction described by CNM clients. The Nader group found that 87 percent of CNMs serve low-risk clients, that 92 percent provide obstetric and gynecological care, that cesarean section rates for CNM clients were half that of the overall U.S. rate, and that CNMs use less technology and more patient education in prenatal visits. The endorsement of the use of CNMs by this prestigious research group can assist all CNMs to support their place in a health care system. These research findings can be incorporated in the marketing plan. Gathering research studies such as this for the marketing portfolio will act as a strong base of support, especially for systems that appreciate statistical proof of health care outcomes.

KNOWLEDGE OF SPECIFIC MARKETING ELEMENTS

Substitution and Complement Functions

In this changing health care climate, many physicians are concerned about their power, their income, and even their jobs. The rules are changing too quickly and too dramatically, causing discomfort for many providers, physician and non-physician alike. APNs have frequently found employment in areas less desirable for physicians. These areas are typically rural areas or underserved inner city clinics, which were not financially lucrative and were therefore less desirable to physicians.

In these areas, there is little argument about how APNs can be used both as substitution for and in complement with physician providers. For clarity, it helps to define these terms in the context of this chapter. Complement is defined as:

- Something that completes, makes up a whole, or brings to perfection; the quantity or number needed to make up a whole; either of two parts that complete the whole or mutually complete each other.
- Substitute is defined as one that takes the place of another, a replacement.[16] See Chapter 5 by Gilliss and Davis for additional discussion on complement versus substitute roles.

In an underserved area, any competent health care provider can reasonably argue for positions providing care that otherwise would be unavailable. This could mean working with a physician or physicians to "mutually complete" a health care partnership. It also could be as a substitute for a physician, "taking the place of" a physician in an area without one.

The arguments for positions in more competitive areas often are more difficult to make and may be less well received. In these areas, it is wise to focus on how APNs are different rather than how they are the same. If APNs are "the same as" physicians, it is often more difficult to break into the health care system where physicians are abundant. Practitioners may be more marketable if they "mutually complete" a health care partnership than attempt to replace one. In marketing roles in these settings, it is important to stress that APNs provide similar services but with an emphasis on health promotion and prevention.

In the ever-changing health care environment, APNs can no longer afford to be just clinicians. Marketing has become crucial to survival. Marketing is defined as the act or process of selling or purchasing in a market, an aggregate of functions involved in moving goods from producer to consumer.[16] Some factors to consider in the marketing process include:

- What is the product or service?
- How is the product or service different from others?
- How is the product or service better?
- Are APNs more consumer-oriented, more cost-effective, and so forth?

The Product or Service

The product or service generally is the APN, but the individualization depends on the particular area of practice. APNs are professionals with specialized knowledge or skills that are applied within a broad range of patient populations in a variety of practice settings.[17]

- CNMs are individuals educated in the two disciplines of nursing and midwifery, who possess evidence of certification according to the requirements of the American College of Nurse-Midwives (ACNM).[18] Nurse midwifery practice is the independent management of care of essentially normal newborns and women occurring within a health care system that provides for medical consultation, collaboration, or referral.
- Certified registered nurse anesthetists (CRNAs) are registered nurses who have completed a nurse anesthesia program accredited by the Council on the Accreditation of Nurse Anesthesia Education Programs[19] and have been

certified by the Council on Certification of Nurse Anesthetists. CRNAs provide the full range of anesthesia services in a wide variety of settings, including acute care, ambulatory surgical centers, and physician offices.

- Clinical nurse specialists (CNSs) serve as role models in delivery of high-quality nursing care to patients.[20] The CNS's client is the individual, nurse, or other health professional, and the focus is on nursing staff education, system analysis, and providing direct and indirect nursing care.[21]

- NPs provide a full range of primary and acute care health services, with a holistic patient and family focus. The NP's client is the patient, and the focus is on providing direct patient care.[22]

The Marketing Plan

After all the information has been collected from introspection, research data, personal communications, and target population surveys, the APN can create a marketing plan, or outline of strategies, for promotion of services. Marketing plans contain five major elements:

1. The statement of the purpose and the main objectives
2. The product description or what the APN's service has to offer
3. The big picture: where will the APN and APN's service be in 5 years
4. The immediate action plan or steps for getting to the big picture
5. The marketing tools and strategies to be used: including interviews, networking, and advertising

Figure 9–1 is an example of a marketing plan adapted for CNM practice.

A marketing plan should not be considered concrete, but rather ever-changing. It should be reviewed routinely and revised as needed to reflect changes in professional development or the needs of the target market. The possibility of health care and welfare reform in our country, for example, could change access to care. APNs must be ready to adapt to that change.

COMMUNICATION SKILLS

Networking

APNs are ideally positioned for the radical changes sweeping the health care field, but they will surely experience much struggle in the process. One way to cope with the inevitable struggle is through networking.

Networking is not new. It has been done on both an informal and a formal basis since the beginning of mankind. A network is simply a group of individuals with similar interests and/or problems who join together to provide support and to exchange information. With the advent of computer technology, contacts are no longer limited by geography or telephone bills. Networks easily span incredible distances, allowing even the most rural practitioners easy access to a peer group.

A. Describe your market: _____
   Age: _____
   Family size: _____
   Annual family income: _____
   Location: _____
   Health-care decision patterns: _____
   Reason to seek CNM care: _____
   Other: _____
   (Geographically describe your service area)
   (Describe your client base economically)
   How large is your market? _____
   Women of childbearing age or birth rate: _____
   Growing _____ Steady _____ Decreasing _____
   If growing, annual growth rate _____
B. Describe the service you will provide: _____
C. Describe your pricing/billing practices: _____
D. Describe the place you will provide services: _____
E. Describe referral sources: _____
F. Describe your competition: _____

G. Describe plans for practice promotion and continued marketing: _____

   _____

H. Describe any barriers to practice that might exist: _____

   _____

I. Describe any consumer or professional networking that will be done: _____

   _____

FIGURE 9–1   Developing a marketing plan. (Adapted from Collins-Fulea,[23] p. 25, with permission.)

Informal Network

An informal network has traditionally been part of the male-dominated business world, especially in the upper levels of certain disciplines. The network comprises acquaintances, colleagues, and friends from school, church, family, sports, and business. When a man needed a favor, he contacted someone in his network. Men grow up knowing how to network, partially because of the emphasis on team sports during boys' formative years. They learn quickly and well that they need one another in order to win the game, to get ahead.[24]

Formal Network

Professional organizations are a good example of a formal network. These organizations, through their membership, are able to disseminate information quickly and take action. When federal legislation is proposed that might have a negative impact on the public's health, the American Nurses Association is able to contact its network of state associations requesting that they enlist the support of their membership to oppose the bill. Networking can be an immeasurable benefit to success and happiness in an advanced practice role. Through networking, one can:

- Build support systems
- Share resources and avoid "reinventing the wheel"
- Identify similar practice issues, such as restraint of trade; credentialing difficulties; and physician opposition, direct or subtle[25]

The best place to learn about job opportunities is through one's network of friends and acquaintances. Networking, as related to job searches, is the process of enlisting other people to help one find employment. Most job openings are filled by word of mouth.[26] One never knows who can help!

- Build a base of contacts with alumni groups, professional organizations, PTA, and children's sports leagues.
- Expand this contact base.
- Get and use referrals.
- Follow up on all leads.

All leads are worth pursuing. When contacting someone from the network, let that person know that you are looking for a job and would welcome advice, suggestions, or ideas. It is probably better not to ask directly for a job. This can put people off and decrease the probability of assistance. The most important things that one can get from people are names of other people. Word of mouth is the most effective way to find a job. Other methods include:

- Newspaper advertisements: only 10 percent to 15 percent of job openings are advertised in newspapers
- Large-scale mailing of your résumé: the success rate for receiving a call for an interview is only 2 percent
- Temporary work: it can be a foot in the door and an opportunity for permanent work
- Executive recruiters (headhunters)
- Employment agencies
- Recruiting databases
- Going online with your résumé
- Browsing through job listings

The APN can get indirect knowledge of changes in job markets by reading the business pages and local business journals for hints to the "hidden job market." These include promotion announcements, transfers, retirements, company expansions, company relocations, awards, mergers, and takeovers.[27]

Rick Crandall has suggested that there are 17 ways to network better:

1. Keep track of who you know.
2. Regularly visit groups, and join the best.

3. Remember names better.

4. Make notes on business cards.

5. Pay attention.

6. Do research.

7. Project sincerity.

8. Do cold calling.

9. Improve your self-introduction.

10. Do online searches.

11. Listen more than you talk.

12. Follow up.

13. Ask for referrals.

14. Become a star.

15. Read the Monday business calendars.

16. Give a lot.

17. Volunteer.[28]

Dr. Crandall writes that another face of change in networking is online marketing. Web sites, your own and those of other people, as well as e-mail and searches on the Internet have broadened our capabilities for reaching possible employment opportunities and sharing our services with a broader audience.[29]

The Job Description

The purpose of the job description is to clarify the scope of practice and expectations of a professional position. See Figure 9–2 for an example of a job description. The job analysis mentioned previously helps create the framework of skills, educational requirements, licensure, reporting relationships, working conditions, and specific functions and responsibilities needed to fulfill a job description.

The job description is a guide for the prospective employee regarding these issues of practice. The components of the job description include:

- The job identification, which includes the official title, the salary, and the department of operations, if applicable.

- The job summary, which gives an overview of the scope of the job. The who, what, when, where, and why questions regarding the position should be succinctly answered in this summary.

- The functions and principal responsibilities, which should list the position functions and responsibilities precisely. These include such functions as physical assessment, laboratory result reviews, patient education, documentation, student teaching, clinic maintenance, community outreach, staff development, and research.

- The list of skills required, which should describe attributes such as good judgment, good interpersonal skills, and ethical practice.

POSITION TITLE: Certified Nurse-Midwife (CNM)

DEPARTMENT: OB/GYN   **GRADE:** 15a

JOB SUMMARY: Provides comprehensive, primary health care to a select population of essentially healthy women. Participates in the care of women with medical complications in collaboration with Obstetricians-Gynecologists.

Principal Functions and Responsibilities:
1. Performs accurate history and physical examinations on essentially healthy women.
2. Provides primary care in an ambulatory setting to women, including ordering and evaluating of diagnostic tests and management of minor complications.
3. Provides inpatient obstetrical care for essentially healthy women, including labor management, delivery of infant, repair of lacerations/episiotomies and management of minor complications. Initiates emergency care as needed.
4. Provides individualized client teaching and counselling utilizing the nurse-midwifery philosophy.
5. Identifies deviations from normal and consults, co-manages, or refers as appropriate.
6. Completes necessary documentation.
7. Participates in research and continuing-education activities.
8. Instructs and supervises nurse-midwifery students as assigned.
9. Performs other duties as assigned.

Skill and Ability Requirements:
1. Considerable degree of independent judgment, to monitor and respond to changes of a client's condition.
2. Interpersonal skills to work effectively with clients and other members of the health care team.

Work Conditions:
Normal client-care environment with some exposure to biological hazards and infectious diseases.

Education and Experience Requirements:
Graduation from an accredited school of Nurse-Midwifery
Certification by ACNM or ACC
State Licensure

Reporting Relationships:
1. Reports to the Director, Nurse-Midwifery Services
2. Indirectly supervises personnel involved with the care of assigned clients.

APPROVED BY: _____   **DATE:** _____

FIGURE 9–2   The job description. (From Collins–Fulea,[23] p. 114, with permission.)

- The working conditions, which should describe physical or time and space issues, including hours of patient care in clinic, on-call requirements, office space, clinic or hospital locations, and potential occupational hazards.
- The education and experience, which should state the minimum preparation necessary to practice and often includes a statement of preferred education and experience for the position.

- The reporting relationship, which is the key to the power structure in the job. This section should accurately describe who reports to whom and if anyone is reporting to the APN.

The job description will act as the template for the cover letters, résumés, and interviewing process.

The Cover Letter

The cover letter accompanies a résumé as a request for consideration for a job. It is the first impression one will make on a potential employer. The letter should be addressed to the appropriate person, clearly written, without spelling or grammatical errors. It needs to describe the specific job one is interested in, the period of one's availability, and contact information (a phone number, fax number, e-mail, and street address), and it should be written in a professional business style. The proper business format for the cover letter is as follows:

- The applicant's name and address
- The date
- The name and address of the person to whom one is sending the résumé
- The salutation ("Dear Dr. …")
- The opening statement, which gives the reason one is writing and indicates the job in which one is interested
- A brief paragraph stating why one is interested in the specific clinic or health care facility
- A closing paragraph, which includes a request for an interview and offers references if desired
- The complimentary closing ("Sincerely" or another acceptable closing), with a signature and a typed name beneath the signature.
- If the résumé is enclosed, be sure to write "enclosure" at the bottom left side of the letter. **Remember, keep copies of all correspondence.**

The cover letter is typically only one typewritten page (Fig. 9–3). This brevity requires the writer to consider what is most essential to entice the prospective employer to read the résumé and to communicate that information in a well-written and clearly presented manner. The cover letter should be written individually for each potential position. It should be printed on good quality bond paper and proofread carefully for any errors in grammar, spelling, and format.

The Résumé

Résumés vary in length and style, but all function to give a detailed outline of one's professional credentials, education, and experience. A résumé should be tailored to meet the needs and requirements of a specific job. Federal government positions generally require very short résumés (one to three pages), whereas their applications are very detailed. Academic résumés, or curriculum vitae, are typically fairly

C. Brenda Penburke, CNM, PhD
4 Yale Street
New Haven, CN 40511
Telephone: 203-455-1267

November 12, 2004

Dr. Lilly Sen
Walrus Woman's Center
4563 Utopia Way
Astoria, Oregon 46042

Dear Dr. Sen:

I am a certified nurse-midwife, presently employed at Planned Parenthood of New Haven, Connecticut. I am considering a move to Astoria and am very interested in the position of Advanced Practice Nurse in your family planning clinic.

I have twenty years' experience in all aspects of nurse-midwifery, most particularly in the areas of well-woman gynecology and family planning.

I have enclosed my résumé for your review. Please feel free to contact me if you require additional information or references. I am looking forward to hearing from you.

Sincerely,

C. Brenda Penburke, CNM, PhD

FIGURE 9–3   An example of a cover letter.

lengthy. The educational demands of an academic position are supported by previously given lectures, courses, and publications. Therefore, it is essential to list more fully all of these data.

There are two basic types of résumés:

1. The chronological résumé

2. The outcome or functional résumé

The chronological résumé provides a brief description of one's job history. This type is best used by those persons with a stable job history, with no more than a month between jobs. The outcome résumé does not describe the job history but rather focuses on areas of proficiency and expertise. This type is best used when an APN has changed fields or is reentering the job market.[30]

As a part of the networking process, sharing résumés with others in the nursing profession may give some perspective on how to support a job candidacy. In creating your résumé, consider the essential components of the job being sought, and present previous employment or education in this light. Be sure that the résumé describes your skills accurately and does not mislead a potential employer. Have a colleague read the résumé and job description for the position being sought. The colleague can comment on its accuracy and presentation.

The general components of a résumé include:

- Name
- Address, phone, fax, e-mail address
- Educational background and degrees
- Professional employment; other previous employment, if applicable
- Community service
- Research interests
- Grants written
- Publications
- Speaking engagements
- Honors and awards
- Consulting activities
- Professional memberships
- Military history

Keep demographic data (i.e., age, children, marital status, dates completed school) out of a résumé to avoid being screened out by any of these noncontributing factors.

The résumé is fundamentally an organized written communication of one's skills, education, and experience. To more effectively stress your previous experience, use action words to generate images of a "doer," a person who takes the initiative to get a job done. Some of these action words are "administered," "assumed responsibility," "supervised," "designed," "handled," "managed," "prepared," and "taught."

Consider reviewing specific health career résumé texts or using a professional résumé-writing service to increase the potential power of the document. Writing good résumés is like any other skill; it develops with good modeling and persistent practice. An excellent resource is *Résumés for Health and Medical Careers*.[30]

It is important to consider the online résumé services, such as Monster.com. This is a free information program that offers help with all aspects of résumé creation. The Monster Résumé Center can be reached by any Internet search engine. There is a specific section just for health care résumés.[31]

The Interview

The interview is the active phase of the exchange of information between an APN and a potential employer. The applicant and the interviewer create a purposeful relationship to exchange information about the persons involved in, and expectations of, a specific job. During this process, both parties have an opportunity to gather information to support the "correct fit" of the applicant to the position.

Simple cues such as one's attire, manner of speech, body language, demeanor, and timeliness create the first impression. If one is well groomed, comfortable, dressed appropriately in business attire, prepared to answer questions to support the skills and educational requirements for the job, and has arrived on time, the applicant will appear in a good light. The current trend toward a more casual work attire has made some impact on the expectations of dress for an interview. The best advice is to dress in business attire, suits or dresses, that have a professional appearance. Although pants are acceptable for women in most circumstances, leave the jeans and the casual shirts and sweaters at home. Whenever possible, attempt to dress in the manner that is considered the code for the office or institution you are interviewing with.

Prepare for the interview by finding out as much as possible about the position, the organization, the location, and the actual job requirements. Develop a list of questions to help clarify areas of concern. Review the personal mission statement, and ask questions related to issues that make job satisfaction high (i.e., salaries and benefits, educational support, vacation and holiday time, local professional networks, and personal relationship needs). Consider your strengths and weaknesses and how you can see yourself growing in the position. Ask what mutual benefits might be gained in this relationship. Be prepared to answer questions about educational background, human relationship skills, communication style, teaching skills, and leadership roles.

Do not be afraid to ask for some of the same information from a potential employer. Remember, the goal of the interview is to match people to positions and to other people. What one gives and what one gets are the basis for marketing as a voluntary exchange of goods and services.

Planning for the interview is the key to success. Consider these seven keys to getting a job offer as suggested by Dorothy Leeds in *Marketing Yourself*[32]:

1. Be prepared.

2. Be ready to turn negatives into positives.

3. Ask questions to keep control.

4. Listen actively to content and intent of questions asked.

5. Do not answer any questions not fully understood.

6. Ask for the job.

7. Follow up.

Practice enough to be relaxed and comfortable to allow your best self to shine through.[33]

After each interview, make a dated summary of the scope of questions, the perceived responses to the answers, and all promised follow-up. Finally, write a thank-you note that includes any follow-up information and a clear statement of your desire for the job. Tips to boost your interviewing success and excellent examples of thank-you notes for all interviewing situations can be found on the Monster Interview Center.[34]

EVALUATION OF JOB OPPORTUNITIES

When assessing a job offer, it is important to look at three factors:

1. The company
2. The position
3. The salary and benefits package

The Company

Many resources are available for research on companies that may be of interest. Local libraries have business directories that will provide detailed information about specific businesses. Included in these directories are the name of the business, names and titles of key personnel, complete address, phone number, number of employees, kind of business, type of location, and number of years in business.

The Position

It is helpful to get a written job description for any position negotiated. If the job description is available before interviewing, it can be a useful guide for questions and clarification of the position. If a job description is not available, request that one be written before accepting the position. Minimally, get a definition of what duties will be expected, who will supervise the position, and where the job will be performed. Find out what orientation or on-the-job training will be provided.

The Salary and Benefits Package

The salary offered or requested should meet or exceed the salary for similar positions in the area. It should be a salary with which one feels comfortable. Beware of salaries that are much higher or much lower than the norm for that area. If the salary is high, this may indicate a job that is undesirable for some reason and therefore hard to fill. If the salary is unusually low, this may indicate the lack of financial stability in the company or perhaps an undervaluing of the position by the company. A good benefits package is worth 20 percent to 40 percent of the salary. While successful negotiation is crucial to survival and growth in the profession, not many APNs possess these important skills.

Before beginning contract negotiations, it is important to have a clear goal. Negotiate from strength. Know the product. Know the negotiators, be familiar with the company, and reaffirm the personal mission statement previously devised.

Salary

Before beginning negotiations, know what salaries are typical for similar positions in the community. If a salary range is discussed, such as $55,000 to $60,0000, simply state that $60,000 would be acceptable. It is probably best not to quote a specific figure unless the limits of the salary range for the job are known. The employer might be willing to offer more than is requested. A counteroffer can always be made if the salary quoted is unacceptably low.

Benefits

Items to negotiate include:
- Full family medical and dental insurance
- Indemnity plan or managed care
- Acceptable panel of providers
- Point-of-service clause
- Pregnancy coverage
- Prescription plan
- Vision plan
- Orthodontics
- Preexisting conditions clause
- Vacation days
- Paid holidays
- Sick days
- Retirement benefits
- Time required for vesting
- Safety of investments in the pension plan
- Life insurance
- Long-term disability plan
- Optional short-term disability
- Optional long-term care insurance
- Dependent-care reimbursement account
- Health care reimbursement account
- Tax-deferred annuities
- Malpractice insurance
- Opportunities for advancement and career development
- Corporate cellular phone rates
- E-mail access
- Tuition waivers
- Continuing education: travel and registration fee
- Professional dues
- Subscriptions to professional journals

- Payment of consulting physician
- Provision of office space, supplies, personnel, and computers
- Payment of answering service and/or pagers

CLOSE OF THE DEAL

Contracts

Defining the parameters of the job through formal contracts, letters of agreement, memoranda, or even verbal agreements is a necessity. Employees without written contracts can legally be considered "at-will" employees. At-will employees are those who may be fired without cause at any time. Likewise, an at-will employee can quit any time.[23] A **contract** is defined as[16]:

- An agreement between two or more parties, especially one that is written and enforceable by law
- The writing or document containing such an agreement

An **employment agreement,** such as in Figure 9–4, is a type of contract describing an agreement between an employer and an employee that specifies duties and compensation as well as the rights and responsibilities of each party.

If not offered a contract by the prospective employer, another approach is to supply one. This may seem like a formidable task, but there are many sources of assistance. There are computer software programs, such as Family Lawyer by Quicken.[35] Basic contract forms can be purchased at many office supply stores. These resources provide a basic framework with which to begin. Most employment contracts are fairly straightforward. In negotiating phased-in compensation or a partial buy-in of a practice, have an attorney review the contract to ensure adequate protection. Contracts typically have similar areas of content. A basic employment contract should include date of agreement, name and address of the employee and employer, specific duties of the agreement, salary and fringe benefits, termination of employment agreement, and signatures of both the employer and employee.

Employment Confirmation Letter

Get the offer in writing for your own protection. If a verbal agreement is offered, request that the employer "clarify the job" in a written memorandum. If no written offer is made, it is advisable to send a letter to confirm the understanding. The letter should include a clause stating that the job will be defined by the letter unless the employer responds in writing.

Letter of Acceptance

A **letter of acceptance** is used by prospective employees to confirm the employee's understanding of the terms and conditions of the employer's offer of employment and to formally accept the offer.

EMPLOYMENT AGREEMENT

This Employment Agreement ("Agreement"), effective as of _____ (date), by and between _____ (name) of _____ (address), "the Employer," and _____ (name) of _____ (address), "the Employee."

1. EMPLOYMENT. Employee agrees to provide to Employer the services described in attached job description.

2. PAYMENT. The Employer agrees to provide Employee with an annual salary of $ _____.

3. MALPRACTICE. The Employer agrees to provide institutional malpractice insurance coverage for any duties performed within the scope of the Employee's job description. The Employee is not covered by this policy for any activities not specified in the job description.

4. VACATION/SICK DAYS. After completing the probationary period of not more than 90 days, each Employee accrues 0.8 sick days/month and 1.5 vacation days/month. Sick days may be accumulated up to 60 days. Vacation days must be used by the Employee's anniversary date each year.

5. CONTINUING EDUCATION. The Employer agrees to provide 7 days and $ _____ annually for continuing education, to be effective after completion of one year of employment.

6. COMMUNICATIONS. The Employer agrees to provide pagers and answering service to the Employee at no cost. Employee is entitled to corporate cellular phone rates (Employee provides cellular phone). Employee will be reimbursed for work-related calls by submitting an annotated monthly voucher.

This Agreement may be terminated for any reason by either party with a 14-day notice during the probationary period. After achieving Permanent Employee status, either party must give at least 30 days' notice prior to termination.

This Agreement is rendered null and void by falsification of information provided during the application process.

_____   _____
Signature of Employee   Signature of Employer

_____
Date

FIGURE 9–4   An example of an employee agreement.

Noncompete Agreement

A **noncompete agreement** is made by an employee (the noncompeting party) not to leave the current employer (the protected party) and become a competitor in the same market.[22] See Figure 9–5 for an example of a noncompete agreement. Frequently, these agreements specify an amount of time (e.g., 3 years) and a geographic area (e.g., within a 5-mile radius of the office of the protected party). In addition, these agreements may include a clause that prevents the noncompeting party from soliciting business (e.g., contacting patients to inform them of the new practice location). It is important to understand the terms of these agreements. Failure to do so may severely impair one's ability to relocate if the job does not work out.

MENTORS AND CAREER ADVANCEMENT

The final concepts for discussion are those of mentors and career advancement. **Mentoring** is a relationship between a novice and an expert in any given profession in which advice is shared toward a mutual goal of career advancement. This relationship has as its most important functions[36]:

NONCOMPETE AGREEMENT

This Agreement is effective as of _____ (date), by and between _____ (name and address), "the Employer," and _____ (name and address), "the Employee."

For a period of _____ (specify amount of time) after leaving the employment of _____, the Employee will not directly or indirectly engage in _____ (area of practice) within a _____ (specify a distance or specific geographical area) of _____ (address of employer).

In addition, the Employee agrees not to directly solicit transfer of care of any clients of Employer for a period of _____ (specify amount of time).

_____
Employer (Protected party)

_____
Employee (Non-Competing Party)

_____
Date

FIGURE 9–5   An example of a noncompete agreement.

- Preparation for the leadership role
- Promotion of career success and advancement
- Enhancement of self-esteem and self-confidence
- Increased job satisfaction
- Strengthening of the profession

Building a mentor relationship on a strong foundation of similar values, goals, and abilities is necessary for successful career advancement. The personal mission statement, which was discussed earlier, can help again in this relationship. Knowing oneself and knowing the character of the mentor become the cornerstones for a successful match.

The characteristics of good mentors consist of a set of behaviors that include guiding, supporting, and teaching as well as good communication skills, good judgment, appropriate use of power, well-honed people skills, an ordered personal life, and a good sense of humor.[37]

The novice professional who attracts a good mentor has been shown to possess six major character traits:

1. Good performance
2. Right social background
3. Striking appearance in a suit (either gender)
4. Social affiliation with the mentor
5. Flair for demonstrating the extraordinary
6. High visibility

The best age difference between mentor and protégé is said to be a half generation, or 8 to 15 years. A greater age difference may create a parent-child relationship. Prospective protégés in their late 20s and early 30s generally look for a match with mentors in their 40s.[38]

A single role model, or mentor, does not always meet the needs of every novice professional. An alternative to the traditional mentor model is proposed by Haseltine et al.[39] These authors have urged young professionals to actively participate in the creation of their professional identity by choosing advisors and considering multiple role models. The process of career goal attainment can be furthered, not just with a single mentor, but with a group of professionals who work at different levels of career advancement. The **patron system** is a continuum of benefactors whose roles are to guide, support, and advocate for the novice. It is composed of **peer pals**, **guides**, and **sponsors**.[39] The peer pals are people with whom you share information and strategies and, most important, who act as sounding boards for your new ideas. Guides offer invaluable information about the organizational structure and are able to offer suggestions for avoiding the wrong people or pathways as well as for pointing out the right people and shortcuts toward a goal. A guide may be a coworker or an administrative support person, such as a secretary or research assistant. The sponsor is a less powerful replacement for the mentor. Often, these three alternatives—peer pals, guides, and sponsors—are more attainable to the novice professional and may be available immediately. The perfect mentor relationship may be discovered during this networking process. This patron system functions on a more horizontal plane than the vertical, hierarchical mentor system. The advantage of this horizontal link is the wider range of contacts for information and career advancement. Remember that career advancement and support should be built on mutual trust and a fair exchange of information.

SUMMARY

Keep focused on your goals. Stay true to your well-conceived, carefully researched market plan. Having a simple philosophy of life can often work wonders in guiding you to your dream job. In his book, *The Four Agreements*, Don Miguel Ruiz offers a practical guide to personal freedom. He proposes that one will succeed in life by simply keeping these rules:

- Be Impeccable with Your Word.
- Do not Take Anything Personally.
- Do not Make Assumptions.
- Always Do Your Best.[40]

APNs must abide by their code of ethics. They must develop a philosophy that matches their own values and beliefs. The job is an extension of who we are and therefore should reflect these personal values. Taking the time to develop the personal mission statement may be the hardest and the most beneficial step toward marketing oneself.

The use of these marketing strategies allows APNs to present themselves and their role in the most effective manner. It also clarifies the major points of reference regarding the job for the employer as well as for the prospective employee, allowing each to make a decision regarding employment based on a foundation of well-defined facts.

SUGGESTED EXERCISES

1. A colleague of another discipline claims that APNs are not particularly cost–effective and that no evidence exists about how clients perceive the quality of care provided by these professionals. Relate the findings from major studies of the cost and quality of advanced practice nursing, and outline indicators that have been consistently evaluated to determine quality of APN care.

2. A physician colleague challenges you that one of the sources of resistance to APNs is that APNs compete with physicians' practices. Give examples of how nurses in advanced practice can substitute or compensate to provide medical care in underserved areas of health care. Recall that underserved can have several interpretations, such as insufficient numbers of providers, inadequate insurance system, poor geographic access, and so on.

3. **Résumé and cover letter**: Identify a hypothetical professional job opportunity for which you would like to apply. In response, write a cover letter, and enclose your professional résumé.

4 **Professional practice statement (PPS):** Develop your individual PPS (i.e., job description) for the hypothetical job sought. This assignment builds on the work of the cover letter and résumé. The PPS must include clinical, administrative, research, and education components. Although it will not be necessary to create supporting policy statements or clinical privilege lists, these considerations should help to frame the writing of the PPS.

5 Role-play an interview, including discussion of salary and benefits.

6 What analogies can be made to the characteristics and functions of a mentor? What concerns or cautions are frequently made regarding gender? Evaluate the logic of these assumptions, identify unstated assumptions, and propose solutions or conclusions. Identify the characteristics of a mentor you would select for your current position of the hypothetical job opportunity defined in Exercise 3.

7 Consider your present employment. Create a list of possible peer pals, guides, and sponsors. What made you choose these people? How could you introduce the idea of their cooperation in the patron system?

REFERENCES

1. McNeil, NO, and Mackey, TA: Unpublished material, 1995.
2. Woods, DK, and Cardin, S: Realizing your marketing influences: Part 2, Marketing from the inside out. J Nurs Admin 6 (32), 2002.
3. Crandall, R: Marketing Your Services: For People Who Hate to Sell. McGraw-Hill, New York, 2002.
4. Covey, SR: The Seven Habits of Highly Effective People. Simon and Schuster, New York, 1989
5. Fisher, R, and Brown, S: Getting Together: Building Relationships As We Negotiate. Penguin, New York, 1989.
6. Pearson, L: Fifteenth annual legislative update. Nurse Pract 1 (28), 2003.
7. Smith, K: Nursing economics. Capital Commentary 5 (15), 1997.
8. Gallagher, SM: Promoting the nurse practitioner by using a marketing approach. Nurse Pract 21:36, 1996.
9. McCormack, M: What They Don't Teach You at Harvard Business School. Bantam Books, New York, 1984.
10. Schweitzer, S: The relative costs of physicians and new health practitioners. In Staffing Primary Care in 1990: Physician Replacement and Cost Savings. Springer, New York, 1991.
11. Greenfield, S, et al: Efficiency and cost of primary care of nurses and physician assistants. N Engl J Med 298:305, 1978.
12. Brown, SA, and Grimes, DE: Nurse Practitioners and Certified Nurse-Midwives: A Meta-Analysis of Studies on Nurses in Primary Care Roles. American Nurses Publishing, Washington, DC, 1993.
13. U.S. Congress, Office of Technology Assessment: Nurse Practitioners, Physicians Assistants and Certified Nurse-Midwives: A Policy Analysis. US Government Printing Office, Washington, DC, 1986.
14. Crosby, F, Ventura, MR, and Feldman, MJ: Future research recommendations for establishing nurse practitioner effectiveness. Nurse Pract 12:75, 1987.
15. Gabay, M, and Wolfe, SM: Encouraging the Use of Nurse-Midwives: A Report for Policy Makers. Public Citizens Publication, Washington, DC, 1995.
16. Morris, W (ed): The American Heritage Dictionary of the English Language. Houghton Mifflin, Boston, 1981.
17. American Association of Colleges of Nursing: Position Statement: Certification and Regulation of Advanced Practice Nurses. Washington, DC, 1994.
18. American College of Nurse-Midwives: Essential Documents: Definition of a Certified Nurse-Midwife. Washington, DC, 1978.
19. Council on Accreditation of Nurse Anesthesia Education Programs: Standards for Accreditation of Nurse Anesthesia Education Programs. Park Ridge, IL, 1994.
20. Moloney, MM: Professionalization of Nursing: Current Issues and Trends, 2nd ed. JB Lippincott, Philadelphia, 1992.
21. Boyd, NJ: The merit and significance of clinical nurse specialists. J Nurs Adm 21:35, 1991.
22. Mallison, M: Nurses as house staff. Am J Nurs 93:7, 1993.

23. Collins-Fulea, C (ed): An Administrative Manual for Nurse-Midwifery Services. Kendall-Hunt Publishing, Dubuque, IA, 1996.
24. Puetz, BE: Networking for Nurses. Aspen Publishers, Rockville, MD, 1983.
25. Petras, K: The Only Job Hunting Guide You'll Ever Need. Poseidon Press, New York, 1989.
26. Kent, GE: How to Get Hired Today! VGM Career Horizons, Lincolnwood, IL, 1991.
27. Casey, R: How to Find a Job: Your 30 Day Action Plan. Thomas Nelson Publishers, Nashville, TN, 1993.
28. Crandall, R: Marketing Your Services: For People Who Hate to Sell. McGraw-Hill, New York, 2002.
29. Ibid.
30. Editors of VGM Horizons: Résumés for Health and Medical Careers. NTC Publishing Group, Lincolnwood, IL, 1996.
31. Monster.com Resume Center: Healthcare Resume Success Story—Multiple Resumes for Multiplied Success. http://resume.monster.com/restips/healthcare/successstory/. Accessed May 12, 2003.
32. Leeds, D: Marketing Yourself. HarperCollins, New York, 1991.
33. Fisher, R, and Ury, W: Getting to Yes: Negotiating Agreement Without Giving In. Houghton Mifflin, Boston ,1981.
34. Monster.com Interview Center: Ten Tips to Boost Your Interview IQ by Carole Martin. http://interview.monster.com/articles/challenge/. Accessed May 12, 2003.
35. Parsons Technology: Quicken: Family Lawyer. Intuit, Hiawatha, IA, 1995.
36. Vance, C: Is There a Mentor in Your Future? Imprint 36:41, 1989.
37. Alleman, E, et al: Enriching mentor relationships. Personal Guide J 62:329, 1984.
38. Hunt, DM, and Michail, C: Mentorship: A career training and development tool. Acad Manage Rev 8:475, 1983.
39. Haseltine, DP, Rowe, MP, and Shapiro, EC: Moving up: Role models, mentors and the patron system. Sloan Manage Rev 19:51, 1978.
40. Ruiz, Don Miguel: The Four Agreements. Amber-Allen Publishing Co, San Rafael, CA, 1997.

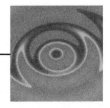

Caring for a Diverse Population: Ensuring Cultural Competency in Advanced Practice Nursing

CHAPTER 10

Pier Angeli Broadnax, PhD, RN

Pier Angeli Broadnax, PhD, RN, is Assistant Professor at Howard University in Washington, DC, teaching health promotion, research, and leadership in nursing. Her primary research interests are African American women experiencing breast cancer and community-based leadership development. Dr. Broadnax lived in Santiago, Chile, conducting research with Chilean women, including indigenous Mapuche Indian women. She also developed a leadership development model for the American Nurses Foundation, focusing on leadership in community settings. Dr. Broadnax graduated with a BS in nursing from Winston-Salem State University. She earned her MSN from Hampton University and Ph.D. from George Mason University. Dr. Broadnax has almost 20 years of nursing administrative experience in public health care institutions in urban areas.

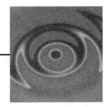

Caring for a Diverse Population: Ensuring Cultural Competency in Advanced Practice Nursing

CHAPTER OBJECTIVES

After completing this chapter, the reader will be able to:

1 Define the terms *culture, ethnicity, cultural competency, cultural incompetence, cultural diversity,* and *cultural sensitivity.*

2 Compare various cultural assessment models.

3 Discuss critical life events within specific ethnic groups.

4 Contrast family unit structures as an issue of diversity.

5 Discuss religious and spiritual diversity as it relates to health care.

Become comfortable with being uncomfortable.

—ANONYMOUS

Diversity, minorities, cultural competency, culture, ethnicity, race: these are terms that have frequently found their way into mainstream and professional media in recent years. They convey that groups of people are different from one another and that these differences carry critical meaning. The United States is a nation that has a rich mix of people from different racial, ethnic, and cultural backgrounds. When there are discussions about different groups of people, the discussions usually involve a comparison with European Americans as the standard for acceptable behavior, without regard for the values, beliefs, and practices of people who live in the United States. Our society is made up of people from different socioeconomic levels, from different racial and ethnic backgrounds, and with different sexual preferences. As people from other countries continue to immigrate to this country, the diverse fabric of society will increase and can add richness to both our personal and professional lives.

A provider who lacks cultural competency is one who is walking through a potential minefield of miscues. Cultural incompetence may result in miscommunication, noncompliance, and a lack of provider acceptance, contributing to health disparities. Although it is impossible for a health care provider to know all there is to know regarding all the cultures one might encounter, it is possible to develop a level of cultural competency so that one may enter into a therapeutic relationship with clients from different cultures.

The purpose of this chapter is to establish the extent of diversity in the United States, define terms pertinent to becoming culturally competent, to provide strategies for becoming culturally competent, and to identify areas of care that are most culturally identifiable.

DIVERSITY

According to the 2000 Census,[1] there were over 281,421,000 people living in the United States. Of these, 75.1 percent were White, 12.3 percent were African American, 12.5 percent were Hispanic or Latino, 3.9 percent were Asian, 0.9 percent were American Indian or Alaska Native, and 0.1 percent were native Hawaiian and Other Pacific Islander. Of the total population, 5.5 percent stated that they were some other race, and 2.4 percent stated that they were more than one race. Within each of the main racial groups are subgroups. African American subgroups include Caribbeans and recent African immigrants—West Africans, East Africans, South Africans, and various tribes within these countries. Asian subgroups include Japanese, Chinese, Filipinos, Koreans, Vietnamese, Asian Indians, Thai, Hmong, Indonesians, Pakistanis, Laotians, and Cambodians. Pacific Islanders include Polynesians (Hawaiians, Samoans), Micronesians such as Chamorros, and indigenous people of Guam and Melanesians such as Fijians. Latino/Hispanic subgroups include people from Mexico, Puerto Rico, Cuba, and Central and South

America. American Indians have hundreds of recognized tribes that vary by regions of the country. Some of the American Indian groups include the Sioux, Cherokee, Lakota, Choctaw, Hopi, Seminole, Navaho and Blackfoot tribes. Socioeconomic level, education attainment, acculturation, and level of linguistic isolation contribute to further divisions within the subgroups.

COMMONLY USED CULTURE-RELATED TERMS

Culture can be defined as patterned responses based on past experiences, values, and customs that are handed down from generation to generation. Giger and Davidhizar[10] state that culture is a "result of acquired mechanisms that may have innate influences but are primarily affected by internal and external environmental stimuli." Acquired mechanisms are shaped by values, beliefs, norms, and practices that are shared by members of the same cultural group (p. 3). Culture, according to Leininger[2-4] comprises the values, beliefs, and norms of a particular group that are learned and shared and guide the thinking, decisions, and actions in a patterned way. It also includes beliefs, habits, likes and dislikes, and customs and rituals learned from one's family.[2] Culture includes all human activities, taking on material and nonmaterial forms and expressions. It encompasses the political, economic, social, religious, philosophical, technological, and environmental context in which human beings live and function.

The Department of Health and Human Services[5] defines *cultural competency* not merely as receiving information regarding another culture but demonstrating attitudes, practices, and/or policies that respect other people and cultures. Cultural competency is the integration of practices into an organization to show respect for specific cultural practices. It is achieved by translating knowledge about individuals and groups of people into specific practices and policies applied in appropriate cultural settings.[6] Smith, Leake, and Kamekona[7] define cultural competency as a continuous process of skill, practice, and attitude attainment, seeking "to transform interventions into positive health outcomes." Cultural competency is measured by the development of positive helping relationships with clients, engaging the client in decision-making and seeking to improve the equality of services that are provided to particular groups.

There are generally three dimensions of cultural competency: surface, folk, and deep structures.[6] Surface structures are those activities that aim to match the content of the message to specific "superficial" characteristics of the target audience or culture. While the characteristics are labeled superficial, this is not intended to denote characteristics are of less importance. Surface structures include the methods for conveying the message as well as the setting that is most appropriate for delivery of the message.

Folk structures are customs or practices that help to identify a culture. These customs include notions of modesty, concepts of beauty, child-rearing practices, rules of descent, relationship to animals and nature, and courtship practices.

Deep structures refer to the sociodemographic and racial/ethnic differences as well as the cultural, social, environmental, and historical factors that affect specific behaviors.[6] Deep structures help determine the effectiveness of specific programs, whereas surface structures help to determine the feasibility of a program.

Cultural incompetence is a set of attitudes, practices, and/or policies that is designed to promote the superiority of the dominant culture and diminish other cultures because they are viewed as lesser, different, or distasteful.[7]

Cultural diversity is used to describe the differences between cultures. These differences are divided into primary and secondary characteristics. The primary characteristics are those that are the most obvious, such as nationality, race, color, gender, age, and religious beliefs. Secondary characteristics include socioeconomic status, education, occupation, length of time away from the country of origin, gender roles, and sexual orientation.

Cultural sensitivity or *cultural awareness* is knowing that cultural differences as well as similaritie exist, without assigning values of right or wrong or better or worse to the differences between cultures.[7,8] It is the process of developing an understanding of another ethnic group. This process usually involves self-examination and internal changes in attitudes and values. Sensitivity and awareness also refer to qualities of openness and flexibility in relations to people from other ethnic groups. To be effective, cultural awareness must be combined with cultural knowledge.

Cultural knowledge is familiarization with selected cultural characteristics, history, values, belief systems, and behaviors of other ethnic groups.[9]

Ethnicity is the grouping of people who share a common language, nationality, geographic origin, customs, traditions, and values, and who pass this heritage down through successive generations. The term ethnicity has commonly been used interchangeably with race as an identifier of people. In comparison, *race* is used to distinguish groups of people based on genetic or biological characteristics.[10,11] Among these characteristics are skin color, bone structure, and blood groups. The characteristics are also used as a classification system according to visible physical characteristics.

PRINCIPLES OF CULTURAL COMPETENCY

It is essential that health professionals work to achieve cultural competence in nursing practice. They must work to incorporate cultural knowledge, values, beliefs, and technical abilities to deliver the highest quality care possible to clients from other cultures. According to Stanhope and Lancaster,[12] it is imperative that nurse practitioners become culturally competent because:

- The nurse's culture is different from the client's culture.
- Care that is not culturally competent may be more costly.
- Care that is not culturally competent may be ineffective.
- Healthy People 2010 objectives for persons in different cultures need to be met.

The goal of culturally competent care is to provide nursing care that is consistent with the client's cultural needs. The American Academy of Nursing (AAN) Expert Panel[13] on culturally competent care suggested the following four principles:

1. Care is designed for the specific client.
2. Care is based on the uniqueness of the person's culture and includes cultural norms and values.
3. Care includes empowerment strategies to facilitate client decision-making in health behavior.
4. Care is provided with sensitivity to the cultural uniqueness of the client.

The AAN Panel also recommended the following principles regarding cultural competence be included in graduate nursing education:

- Nurses must learn to appreciate intergroup and intragroup cultural diversity and commonalities in racial/ethnic minority populations.
- Nurses must understand how social structural factors shape health behaviors and practices in racial/ethnic minorities; for example, nurses must avoid a "blaming" and "victim" pattern.
- Nurses must understand the dynamics and challenges of biculturalism and bilingualism.
- Nurses must confront their own ethnocentrism and racism.
- Nurses must begin implementing and evaluating service provided to cross-cultural populations.

CULTURAL ASSESSMENT MODELS

Advanced practice nurses (APNs) who work in a society as diverse as the United States must be adept at appropriately assessing behaviors of clients from other cultures. To assess cultural factors that influence health-related decision-making, APNs must be able to accurately assign meaning to the behaviors. If the behaviors are not interpreted correctly, appropriate interventions cannot be implemented.

The first cultural assessment models were non-nursing models developed by anthropologists conducting ethnographic studies.[14] Murdock's Model[14] is a well-designed and comprehensive model, but it was not intended for use by APNs It contains 88 categories of assessment, but it does not provide for the "systematic use of the nursing process."[10] Brownlee[15] also developed a model to assess culturally diverse communities with a special emphasis on health care. The Brownlee assessment model, although not a nursing model, focuses on three components of assessment: what to find out, why it is important, and how to do it. This model generally is considered too complex, too difficult, and too detailed for use with individual clients.

Leininger,[16] a nurse, developed a transcultural theory and assessment model known as the Sunrise Model. The model depicts the rising sun with four levels of foci. This model includes the social structure and worldview that influence health care through language and environment. It also includes the assessment of cultural phenomena on the micro, middle, and macro levels. Leininger's work is the basis for the development of other nursing cultural assessment models. They include models developed by Bloch,[17] Branch and Paxton,[18] Orque,[19] and Tripp-Reimer.[20] In an analysis by Giger and Davidhizar[10] of nursing models, two common limitations were identified. The models contained too much cultural content and lacked the ability to distinguish the ethnic client data from data obtained from mainstream clients.

The Transcultural Assessment Model[27] incorporates six phenomena to assess cultural factors: communication, space, time, social orientation, environmental control, and biological variations.

The communication component includes language differences, verbal and nonverbal behaviors, and the meaning of silence. An inability to accurately communicate and interpret nonverbal behaviors is one of the greatest obstacles to providing care in a multicultural environment. The Asian client may nod in agreement with health care instructions because it is important to agree with persons in authority. In actuality, the person may not understand the instructions or have any intention of complying with them. Eye contact during verbal communication also varies among cultures. Euro-Americans value direct eye contact; however, African Americans and Native Americans may avoid direct eye contact during conversations.

Space refers to one's attitude and comfort level regarding the personal space around one. Performing a physical examination may cause a level of discomfort in clients who are not comfortable with strangers being in the intimate zone of 0 to 18 inches between provider and client. Asians do not believe that touching by strangers is appropriate. Hispanic clients may be more comfortable being in close proximity to the provider because of a tendency to touch the person to whom they are speaking.[12]

Time orientation is viewed in terms of past, present, or future. Considering time orientation is important when engaging in health teaching, especially regarding medication schedules. Clients who view the past as more important than either the present or the future may make decisions that are more consistent with the views of their ancestors rather than those of the health care provider. Asian clients may not make being on time for appointments a priority because time is not important. Clients who view time in the present "relish the day" and only move or make decisions when the time is right. People who are future-oriented focus on long-range planning and engage in health behaviors in the present to prevent future illnesses.

Social orientation refers to the family unit, whether it is a nuclear family, single-parent, or extended family and the religious or ethnic groups with which the family identifies. The concept of family is variously defined across cultures. Families may include persons who are closely related, distantly related, or not related at all. The family unit is generally whomever the client identifies as family. In African American cultures, a mother or grandmother may be the major decision maker, especially for health-related decisions. In Asian cultures, the male makes the health care decisions.[12]

Environmental control refers to a particular culture's perceived ability to control nature or the environment. Some cultures perceive they have mastery over nature and believe in the effectiveness of medications, surgery, or other treatments to cure illness. Those who believe that they have little control over nature or the environment have a fatalist view of illness and believe that whatever happens to them is their destiny. African Americans and Hispanics tend to follow this second perspective on illness. Cultures that perceive illness as being in disharmony with nature tend to use natural remedies, herbs, or hot and cold applications to effect a cure for illnesses. A culture's perspective of its relationship with nature affects the group's utilization of health resources.

Biological variations include body build and structure, skin characteristics, eye color, shape of ear lobes, adipose tissue deposits, genetic differences, and susceptibility to disease. African Americans have denser bones than Euro-Americans, resulting in decreased incidence of osteoporosis.[12] Some Asian cultures have lower incidences of cardiovascular disease than Euro-Americans but higher levels of stress-related diseases, such as ulcers, colitis, psoriasis, and depression. Native American women have the highest incidence of diabetes. Mexican Americans also have higher rates of diabetes and obesity than the general population.

The Heritage Assessment Tool (HAT), designed by Spector,[11] builds on the foundation of the Giger and Davidhizar[10] model. The HAT combines the six cultural phenomena and provides a quick reference to assess groups of people from a variety of cultures.

Camphina-Bacote[21] proposed a framework for delivering culturally competent care. The constructs within this framework are cultural awareness, cultural knowledge, cultural skill, cultural encounters, and cultural desire. The purpose of this model is to aid in the development of culturally responsive interventions.

Purnell's Model of Cultural Competence[33] contains 12 domains of cultural competence: addressing the part of the world from which the patient originated, communication patterns, family roles, workforce issues, biological variations, high-risk behaviors, nutrition, pregnancy, childrearing practices, death rituals, spirituality, health care practices and health care practitioners. Although the model is lengthy, it provides the nurse with a method of understanding the client's world.

Other medical cultural assessment models include the LEARN Model and the Eliciting the Patient's Explanatory Model. The LEARN Model[23] is an acronym used to guide patient assessment:

L—Listen with sympathy and understanding to the patient's perception of the problem.

E—Explain your perceptions of the problem.

A—Acknowledge and discuss the differences and similarities.

R—Recommend treatment.

N—Negotiate agreement.

The Explanatory Model[24] is a series of nine questions used to discern the client's perception of what leads him or her to seek health care. The Explanatory Model also includes questions regarding the client's opinion on how severe the illness might be and what treatments he or she should receive. Clients are also asked about the most important result they wish to see and what they fear most about treatment. This model may be beneficial in gaining the cooperation of clients. Initially, however, some clients may not be comfortable with this level of collaboration because they are accustomed to being told by the health care provider what is going on or what needs to occur.

HEALTHY PEOPLE 2010

The U.S. Department of Health and Human Services has developed a guide to improve the nation's health, *Healthy People 2010: Understanding and Improving Health.*[5] Healthy People 2010 has set two major goals for this effort:

- Increase quality and years of healthy life
- Eliminate health disparities

The goals are supported by specific objectives in 28 focus areas. The need for cultural competence is addressed in the objective "Access to Quality Health Care." The goal for this specific objective is to improve access to comprehensive high-quality health care services. Differences in culture and language have been identified as one of the barriers to accessing quality health care.

CULTURALLY SENSITIVE LIFE EVENTS

When providing health care to clients from other cultures, certain life events are sensitive to specific cultural mores and beliefs. These life events include birth, pain, death, and spiritual and religious events. Culturally sensitive life events will be discussed from a broad cultural perspective of specific ethnic groups: African American, Hispanic/Latino, Middle Eastern, and Asian. This chapter is not meant to be an all-inclusive discussion of ethnically bound practices, but rather it is meant to create a recognition that differences are found in different cultures. This discussion of life events and practices reflects the traditional cultural beliefs of a group; they are not universally accepted or practiced. Variations may occur within subgroups of the culture and are dependent on a variety of factors, a primary one being the extent of the client's acculturation.

Birth Practices

African American

The acceptance of pregnancy in the African American community is dependent upon economic status. Because pregnancy is considered a "state of wellness," lower-income African American women may delay seeking prenatal care. Women, especially those whose families migrated from the southern United States to other sections of the country, may experience pica, the craving for certain nonfood items such as starch, clay, or dirt. Self-medicating for various pregnancy-related discomforts is also very common. These problems may include constipation, nausea and vomiting, headache, and heartburn. Men view pregnancy as a measure of virility. There are many old wives' tales relating to pregnancy in the African American community. The more common ones include the belief that having your picture taken during pregnancy can cause stillbirth or that reaching above the mother's head will cause the cord to strangle the baby. It also is considered taboo to buy clothes before the baby's birth. Some African American women may use home remedies to induce labor. These remedies include riding over a bumpy road, drinking castor oil, eating a heavy meal, or sniffing pepper. During the postpartum period, the African American mother is advised to avoid cold and to get adequate rest. The infant may have the umbilical area wrapped with a bellyband, a coin taped to the umbilicus to prevent the navel from protruding.

At birth, African American infants generally weigh less than Euro-American infants. The differences in weight persist even when socioeconomic status, maternal age, parity, and smoking are factored out.[25] A recommendation has been made to change the limits of prematurity from 2,500 g to 2,200 g to address the size of African American infants.[26]

Hispanic/Latino

Hispanic couples desire pregnancy soon after marriage. Men desire a large number of children as evidence of their virility. The only acceptable methods of contraception for traditional Hispanics are abstinence and the rhythm method. Condoms are seen as a method of disease control and should only be used with prostitutes.

Because pregnancy is perceived as natural, prenatal care is either obtained late in the pregnancy or discouraged altogether. The pregnant woman is supported and influenced by her mother and mother-in-law. Hispanic or Latino women also experience pica on occasion, craving ashes or dirt. They may use herbs to treat common complaints of pregnancy and to facilitate labor. Milk is usually avoided because it is believed to contribute to a difficult labor and to having large babies. A woman who has just delivered will not sit upright while she still has stitches. Hispanic women may resist and may refuse to have a pelvic examination by a male health care provider.

Middle Eastern

High fertility rates for Middle Eastern women are encouraged. It is the belief that "God will decide the family size." Birth control use is discouraged but not forbidden. Pregnant women are indulged, and cravings are satisfied to prevent the development of birthmarks in the shape of the craved food. Because male children are preferred, the mother may feel extreme stress during the pregnancy to bear a male. During Ramadan, pregnant women are excused from fasting, but some women may choose to engage in the practice despite the threat to her and her baby's health.

According to the Muslim culture, birth activities are considered women's work. Traditionally, Muslim women have had their babies at home with a midwife, known as a dayah, because of limited financial resources, modesty, and a lack of access to hospitals.[22] However, Muslim women now deliver in hospitals at the same rates as other women. During labor, women tend to be very expressive and emotional during contractions.

Several customs pertaining to newborns also exist in the Muslim culture. Newborns have their stomachs wrapped immediately after birth to prevent cold from entering the body. The Muslim call to worship is whispered in the newborn's ear at birth. Males are required by their religion to be circumcised.

Mothers delay bathing during postpartum because of the belief that being exposed to air will make the mother ill and that washing the breast "thins the mother's milk." Infants are not breast-fed until the third day because of the belief that "colostrum makes the baby dumb."[22] The postpartum diet includes lentil soup to increase milk production and tea to cleanse the body.

Asian

For Asian women, pregnancy is viewed as a natural process. Pregnancy is a time when the mother "has happiness in her body." Milk is usually excluded from the diet because of the belief that it causes gastric distress, but more meat is added to the diet to strengthen the blood for the fetus. Shellfish is usually avoided during the first trimester to prevent the development of allergies. Soy sauce may also be eliminated to prevent having a dark-skinned baby.[12] Excessive sleeping and inactivity are believed to contribute to a difficult labor. Mothers believe in the benefits of hot and cold applications. Women may not go outside or bathe during the first postpartum month because of the belief that cold may cause illness in the mother. Some women may dress in layers, even in summer, to prevent exposure to the cool air. Soup is made with ginseng roots to strengthen the mother. Asian women may also prefer a female health care provider.

Pain Management

Pain management, which is known as the "fifth vital sign," is one of the most culturally diverse behavioral responses. To intervene appropriately, expressions of pain must be assessed and interpreted within a cultural framework. Although cultural frameworks give guidance to ethnic group behaviors, each client must be assessed and treated as an individual. Some clients may respond to analgesics, others to comfort measures such as therapeutic touch, heat applications, or spiritual support. The health care provider may need to encourage the acceptance of pain medication, explaining that it assists in the process of recovery. The following is a short discussion of guidelines to ethnic responses to pain.

African American

African Americans associate pain with illness or a diseased state. If the person is not experiencing pain, then a medical regimen that includes routine medications may not be followed. Because of their spiritual and religious beliefs, some African Americans may accept that pain and suffering are inevitable and must be endured. This helps to explain what appears to be a high pain threshold. Instead of pain medicine, some patients may request prayer from a church member or spiritual leader or the "laying on of hands" in seeking relief from pain and suffering. Those who continue to experience pain may be thought to have little faith.

Hispanic/Latino

Hispanics consider an absence of pain, an ability to work, and spending time with family as indicators of good health.[28] Pain is perceived as a necessary part of life that must be endured. Men see pain as a test of strength and will tolerate it as long as possible. As long as the person is able to work, the pain will be tolerated. This attitude to pain may result in a delay in seeking treatment. Villarruel and Ortiz de Montellano[29] identified six themes that describe Mexican Americans' experience with pain:

- Mexicans accept and anticipate pain as a necessary part of life.
- They are obligated to endure pain in the performance of duties.
- The ability to endure pain and suffer stoically is valued.
- The type and amount of pain a person experiences is divinely predetermined.
- Pain and suffering are a consequence of immoral behavior.
- Methods to alleviate pain are directed toward maintaining balance within the person and the surrounding environment.

These themes may help the health care provider with the development of culturally appropriate interventions.

Middle Eastern

Patients of Middle Eastern descent regard pain as unpleasant and something that must be controlled. The client may be very expressive and vocal about his pain in front of the family and become restrained in his expressions in front of the health care provider. The exception is during childbirth when the client will be very expressive in the presence of the provider. The family may become insistent that the provider medicate the client based on what the family has observed. The actual level of pain may be somewhere in the middle. Although they believe in the superiority of Western medicine, Middle Eastern clients may not always trust it and may use home remedies in conjunction with prescribed treatments.[31] These remedies may be herbs, hot/cold foods, or concentrated sugar preparations. They also put more faith in invasive measures than in noninvasive ones, intravenous medicines than in oral, colored pills rather than white ones, or injections rather than pills. The health care provider must ensure that the patient is not overmedicated as a result of the intense emotional expressions of pain.

Asian

Asian clients rarely express pain and may appear stoic to Western health care providers. Children are taught early in life to minimize their reaction to injury and illness. Bearing pain is a virtue and a sign of family honor. The use of analgesics is less in Asian countries than in the United States. Patients may have to be convinced that treating pain enhances their recovery rather than contributing to addiction, which is a taboo. One recommendation for health care providers is to medicate Asian patients on an established schedule rather than on an as-requested basis.

Family Units and Lifestyle Diversity

In many cultures, the family unit will take on different forms. In simplest terms, the definition of a family is the basic unit for personality development and the development of parent-child relationships.[10] The Western ideal of the nuclear family is fading as the norm of family structures. The nuclear family unit is composed of a father, mother, and non-adult biological children living in a single household and interacting with the larger society.[10] The traditional family is recognized as the couple who have been joined together by marriage.

Other forms of the nuclear family include the nuclear dyad family and the skip generation family. The nuclear dyad family consists of a couple without children. The skip generation family is one in which grandparents assume primary responsibility for raising grandchildren. With many parents deeply involved in substance use or dying of AIDS and single parents unable to assume the parenting role, more grandparents are finding themselves in this primary role.[30]

The extended family is a multigenerational unit and consists of relatives joined by birth, marriage, or adoption. The family group may include parents, grandparents, in-laws, brothers, sisters, children, nieces, nephews, and cousins.

The single parent family may be either a mother or father living with a biological or adopted child or children. There may be another adult living in the household who is a partner in the relationship but not legally joined to the primary caregiver.

Other family forms include blended families, same sex families, communal families, and single households. Blended families, also known as reconstituted families, are those that are formed by "putting together parts" from previously existing families to form a new nuclear family. A single person may marry a person with children, and the couple may have other children together. Another form of blended family occurs when both partners have children from previous relationships, and the couple has children together. This type of family can become very complicated and stressful as the people involved try to work out relationships between stepbrothers and sisters, half-brothers and sisters, stepparents and stepgrandparents. It has been estimated that the number of children living in blended households is increasing by 3 percent annually.[1]

Same sex families may consist of two persons and function as a nuclear dyad. The families sometimes include the biological children of one partner, children adopted into the union, or those born to the union through artificial insemination or surrogate parenting. A study of nurses' attitudes toward sexual orientation[32] found the attitudes to be skewed. Frequently, gays and lesbians report being treated with insensitivity, antagonism, and discrimination during their health care encounters.

Communal families are multigenerational units of husband-wife, parent-child, and brother-sister types of relationships who have chosen to live together in a single household or adjacent housing. Generally, there are rules and expectations that govern the behavior of members. A commune may be formed when groups of people have common goals such as religious, philosophical, or political. They also may share common needs, such as economic, social, or physical needs. Some examples include retirement homes, religious cults, Israeli kibbutzim, or adults who live together to share expenses.

Single family households are becoming more common as people divorce, delay marriage, become widowed, or never marry.

Religious Diversity

Health care practitioners have shown an increased interest in the relationship between religion and health. As individuals go through stages of the life cycle, such as childbirth, illness, recovery, or death, they may seek spiritual support. The APN may be called to assist in finding or providing this support. Although nurses cannot purport to know all about the world's religions or spiritual practices, basic knowledge of the major religions can be expected. If the APN is not familiar with practices of a religion, one excellent resource is to ask the client or family member.

In a discussion of religion, a few definitions help to lend clarity to the discussion. First, religion and spirituality are not the same. Religion is defined as a specific system of and values and beliefs and a framework for ethical behavior that its members must follow.[22,30] Religion also is viewed as a belief in a supernatural or divine force that has power over the universe and commands worship and obedience. It signifies that a "group of people have established and organized practices that are related to spiritual concerns."[31] Being identified as religious usually means being affiliated with a specific religious denomination.

Spirituality is a more individualized approach or search for internal harmony. Spirituality entails a sense of transcendental reality that draws strength from inner resources, living fully for the present, and having a sense of inner knowing.[30] Spirituality is a set of beliefs and values that influence the way people conduct their lives. It focuses on an individual's relationship with a Supreme Being who is sometimes known as God. The concept of hope is central to spirituality. Being grounded in spirituality does not necessarily denote a religious affiliation.

Prayer is a critical component of both religion and spirituality. It is viewed as communicating with a Higher Power or Supreme Being. All of the world's major religions have some form of prayer in that they communicate with someone greater than themselves in a search for healing, guidance, or peace.[10,22]

Two other terms associated with religion are concerned with nonbelievers: agnostics and atheists. Agnostics are incapable of knowing God exists. They want tangible proof of God's existence. Atheists do not believe that God exists. They do not believe in any higher power or supreme being.

All of the major religions of the world are practiced in the United States. These religions are Hinduism, Buddhism, Shinto, Confucianism, Taoism, Judaism, Christianity, and Islam.[22,31]

Hinduism

Hinduism is thought to be the oldest of the world religions. The largest sect of Hindus is found in India. Hindus believe in the Divine Intelligence, the Supreme Reality. The purpose of life is enlightenment through a union with Brahman, or God. Focus is directed toward uniting the inner and real self. Hindus believe that the universe is in constant change but that there is order and meaning in the constant change.[10] One must participate in this process of constant change to find health and well-being. Believers adhere to moderation in eating and other activities. They practice yoga, which strives for self-control, self-discipline, cleanliness, and contentment. Hinduism teaches the living how to die well. It is believed that health occurs when consciousness and body function are in harmony. Disease is thought to be a result of disharmony in these two activities. In the United States, an outgrowth of this movement is the Hare Krishna sect.[31]

Buddhism, Shintoism, Confucianism, and Taoism

People of mostly Asian descent practice Buddhism, Shintoism, Confucianism, or Taoism.[10] The Buddha or Enlightened One was thought to be a reformer of Hinduism. There are many different sects of Buddhism, but one prominent belief that is common to most of the sects is the promotion of happiness, profit, goodness, and beauty. A goal of Buddhism is to reach Nirvana, which is the removal of ignorance. To reach Nirvana, a person must follow a strict moral code that prohibits the use of intoxicants; lying; and killing of any kind, including meat for food, leading to a large percentage of followers being vegetarians. Buddhism also includes the Zen sect. Those who follow the Zen movement may spend hours in meditation, contemplation of word puzzles, and in consultation with a Zen Master.

Shintoism is a religion that focuses on affirmations and positive effects. Those who follow Shintoism feel a strong connection to Japan and all of the ancestral beings there. There is also a great focus on cleanliness.

Confucianism is considered a way of life using a code of ethics rather than a religion. Confucius is viewed as more of a teacher than a god. His sayings, which are short proverbs, were written by his disciples. In following Confucianism, there is an emphasis on family relationships, the hierarchy of society, respect for ancestors and the elderly, and maintaining wellness.

Taoism, or "The Way," emphasizes that when things are allowed to follow their natural course, they will move toward harmony and perfection. Tao also uses the symbol of Yin and Yang to explain the importance of harmony. Yin is the feminine or negative sign, representing wet, bold, passive, restful, and empty. Yang is the masculine or positive sign and represents dry, hot, active, moving or activity, and light.

Judaism

Judaism is a religion that is over 3,000 years old. Judaism believes in one God and one creator. The spiritual leader is the rabbi, who is responsible for interpreting Jewish law. Judaism in America recognizes three denominations, Orthodox,

Conservative, and Reform. The Orthodox branch is the most traditional and adheres closely to the Code of Jewish Law, or halakhah.

Orthodox Jews pray three times a day. They wash their hands and say a prayer upon awakening and before meals. The Conservative branch is not as strict in its adherence to halakhah. Conservative Jews may keep a kosher home but may not follow all of the dietary laws outside of the home. Men and women sit together during the religious service. The Reform branch is known as the progressive or liberal movement. Reform Jews practice fewer rituals; men and women share full equality and engage in many social action activities. Clients in the hospital may request to see a rabbi or spiritual leader and to have their prayer items close by. Because one of the tenets of Judaism is to care for the physical, emotional, psychological, and social well-being of others, the client may have many visitors.[22] Unless the Orthodox client is in a life-threatening condition, any procedures should not be performed on the Sabbath or on the high holy days Rosh Hashanah and Yom Kippur.

Christianity

Christianity is based on the belief that Jesus Christ is God's son. Christianity is divided into three branches: Roman Catholic, Eastern Orthodox, and Protestant. Christians observe four major days representing key days in Jesus' life: Christmas, Ash Wednesday—the beginning of Lent, Good Friday, and Easter. The focus of this religion is personal responsibility for one's own soul, spirituality, and aiding the spiritual needs of others.

Roman Catholics believe in the dignity of the person as a social, intellectual, and spiritual being in the image of God. Sacraments are given to help follow the example of Christ's life. A hospitalized client may want to attend Mass, have a priest visit, or receive the Eucharist at bedside. A dying client may be administered the last rites by a priest. The use of extraordinary or artificial measures may not be seen as necessary.

The Orthodox Church is divided into groups by nationality. It is similar to Catholicism but does not have a Pope. Its religious practices include the giving of sacraments and baptism. If an infant is dying and no religious leader is available, a symbolic baptism by the health care provider is acceptable. This is done by placing a small amount of water on the infant's forehead three times.

Protestantism is divided into many denominations. The belief that God has not given any one person or group of persons sole authority to interpret His truth to others has led to the development of multiple denominations. New groups come into being as they believe they are interpreting God's word in a new and more enlightening way. The minister or pastor is the Protestant spiritual leader. There are two major sacraments common to most denominations, baptism and Communion. Most believe in the healing power of prayer, whereas others request the addition of anointing oil to aid healing. Some denominations view death as a penalty and punishment. Others see death as a transition from an earthly body to an eternal reward. Still others believe death to be the absolute. With so many varieties of Protestantism with different beliefs and practices, it is important to ask what practices the client pursues.

Other religions include Seventh Day Adventists; Church of Jesus Christ of Latter Day Saints (Mormon); and Church of Christ, Scientist (Christian Scientist). Seventh Day Adventists rely on the teachings of the Old Testament. Seventh Day Adventists may refuse procedures or medical treatment on their Sabbath, from sundown Friday to sundown Saturday. They also adhere to a restricted diet, eliminating fish without scales or fins, tea, and coffee. They eat milk and eggs but no meat.

The Church of Jesus Christ of Latter Day Saints embraces most teachings of the Book of Mormon. Every Mormon is seen as an official missionary of the Church. There is no official congregational leader. Mormons believe that the dead are able to hear the gospel and can be baptized by proxy. They also believe that diseases are a result of a failure to obey the laws of health and a failure to keep other commandments. They have established programs of health that include diet, exercise, family life, and work that help to maintain the body as the "temple of God."

Two denominations, Jehovah's Witnesses and Church of Christ, Scientist (Christian Scientist), hold beliefs that do not accept some types of medical treatments. Jehovah's Witnesses refuse to accept blood transfusions. This refusal is based on the commandment given to Moses that no one from the House of David shall eat blood or they will be cut off from their people.[31]

A member of the Church of Christ, Scientist, believes totally in spiritual healing except for setting of broken bones, provided no medication is used during the procedure. Children are not allowed to have physical examinations for school; to have eye, ear or blood pressure screenings; or to receive immunizations. Mary Baker Eddy's *Science and Health with Key to the Scriptures* published in 1875 provides a basis for the Christian Scientists' religious practices. Comfort measures are provided to residents of their nursing homes and sanatoriums. These facilities are staffed with Christian Scientist nurses who provide first aid and spiritual guidance.[31] These health care workers are trained in nursing arts, care of the elderly, cooking, bandaging, nursing ethics, care of reportable diseases, and obstetrics. Principles of care and comfort are taught without teaching the administration of medications.

Islam

Islam is the youngest of the world's religions. It is practiced mostly in Middle Eastern countries, but not all Arabs are Muslim. Followers of Islam believe in Allah and that Muhammad is His Prophet. There is no priest, but each individual's relationship is directly with God. Followers adhere to the Quran (Koran) and Hadith (traditions) for thinking, devotions, and social obligations. Devotees pray five times a day and wash with running water over the face, arms, top of head, and feet before each prayer. A prayer rug and water are required for each prayer ritual. For the ill, bedridden client, pouring water out of a receptacle is acceptable. During each prayer, the believer must face toward Mecca unless that direction is in line with the in-room bathroom, then the person must adjust accordingly. Each Muslim follows Ramadan, fasting for a month. During this time he or she eats or drinks nothing from sunrise to sunset; after sunset, nourishment is taken in moderation. In keeping with the teachings of the Quran, Muslims do not eat pork or pork-containing products, gamble, drink intoxicants, use illicit drugs, or engage in religiously unlawful sexual practices such as premarital sex, homosexuality, or infidelity. One sect that is growing in the United States is the Black Muslims, or Nation of Islam. The Nation of Islam has attracted a large following among young African American men because of its focus on self-help and building self-esteem.

Even when Muslims are ill they may want to participate in the religious rituals as much as possible. They do not discuss death because it may cause the sick person to give up hope. When death appears imminent, the family will prepare for death. After death, the body is washed with running water, and the hands are folded in prayer. Muslims do not perform autopsies, embalm, or use caskets for burial. The body is instead wrapped in a white linen cloth and placed into the ground facing Mecca.

SUMMARY

Cultural competency is a multifaceted, all-encompassing concept that cannot be taught in a few paragraphs. Health care needs do not come in a "one size fits all" package. Clients have a right to be respected, understood, and treated as individuals, regardless of their ethnic identity. Clients have a right to expect APNs acknowledge their perspectives on their health care needs and respect them as legitimate. The APN who is practicing in today's society must make a commitment to becoming culturally sensitive and competent in cultural concepts. APNs who have specific cultural knowledge can maximize therapeutic interventions by becoming co-participants and client advocates in diverse health care environments. Becoming culturally competent is a lifelong learning process. Multicultural education is a critical component of personal as well as professional development and cannot be overemphasized. Even with continuous learning, the APN must become comfortable with being uncomfortable, not knowing everything about multicultural populations.

SUGGESTED EXERCISES

1 Mr. Yun, an 81-year-old Asian American, has lived in the United States for the past 50 years. He was brought to the emergency room by his son with whom he now resides. His wife of 55 years died a year ago. The son states that his father suddenly stopped eating and talking 3 days ago. Mr. Yun has a history of diabetes, controlled with oral agents and anemia. He is a devout Buddhist. His vital signs are T-99, P-120, R-18, B/P-92/70. How would you proceed with Mr. Yun?

2 Kathy Brown, a 28-year-old Caucasian, has been admitted to Labor and Delivery in active labor. This is her first pregnancy. Her partner, Mary Green, a 32-year-old African American, arrives later to support Kathy during her labor. The two held a commitment ceremony last year to publicly demonstrate their lives as a couple. Jose Ramos, a 21-year-old Mexican American, who is the donor father, comes to await the arrival of "his" baby. An argument ensues because Jose now wants to claim his parental rights. His family and friends are pressuring him to assume control of the situation and to "get his baby back from those weird women."

As the health care provider attending this birth, what are your feelings/biases about the relationships? How are you going to counsel the parties involved?

3. Yazi Ibrahim, a 45-year-old Iranian, is admitted to the unit for abdominal pain, nausea, and vomiting. The family states that she is in extreme pain and needs some medicine. When you make rounds, the patient is calmly looking out of the window. When you ask whether she needs anything for pain, she says no, she is feeling fine. Five minutes later the family again states that she is having terrible pain, rolling around in bed, and crying. When you arrive in the room, the patient is asleep, slightly diaphoretic, with an elevated B/P and pulse. An empty container with dried powder on the lid is open on the bedside table.

How would you proceed with this patient and family? Would you medicate this patient? Discuss why or why not.

4. Select a cultural assessment model. Conduct an assessment of a person who is from a culture different from your own. Analyze the data. Identify areas that you are least familiar with in that culture. Propose appropriate interventions.

REFERENCES

1. U.S. Department of Commerce, Bureau of Census, American Fact Finder: Profile of General Demographic Characteristics. Washington, DC, 2000.
2. Leininger, ML: Transcultural nursing: The study and practice field. Imprint, 38:22, 1991.
3. Leininger, M: Qualitative research methods in nursing. Grune & Stratton, Orlando, FL, 1985.
4. Leininger, M: Transcultural care, diversity and universality: A theory of nursing. Nursing Health Care, 6:209, 1985.
5. U.S. Department of Health and Human Services: Healthy People 2010: Understanding and Improving Health, 2nd ed. Government Printing Office, Washington, DC, November 2000.
6. Administration on Aging: Achieving Cultural Competence: A Guidebook for Providers of Services to Older Americans and Their Families: http://www.aoa.dhhs.gov/minorityaccess/guidebook2001/default.htm
7. Nickerson, KJ: Valuing Diversity: Key Components to Ethical Health Care Administration, Service and Research. Presentation at Howard University, School of Medicine, August 29, 2001.
8. National Maternal and Child Center for Cultural Competency: Georgetown Center for Child and Human Development, Washington, DC: www.georgetown.edu/research/gucdc/nccc/cultural5.html
9. Adams, DL, ed: Health Issues for Women of Color: A Cultural Diversity Perspective. Thousand Oaks, CA, Sage Publications, 1995.
10. Giger, JN, and Davidhizar, RE: Transcultural Nursing: Assessment and Intervention, 3rd ed. St. Louis, Mosby, 1999.
11. Spector, RE: Cultural Diversity in Health and Illness, 5th ed. Upper Saddle River, NJ, Prentice-Hall, 2000.
12. Stanhope, M, and Lancaster, J: Community Health Nursing, Promoting the Health of Aggregates, Families and Individuals. St. Louis, Mosby, 1996.
13. American Academy of Nursing Expert Panel on Culturally Competent Health Care: Culturally competent health care (1992) Nurs Outlook 40:277, 1992.
14. Murdock, GP, et al: Outline of Cultural Materials, 4th ed. New Haven, CT: Human Relations Area, 1971.
15. Brownlee, AT: Community, Culture, and Care: A Cross-Cultural Guide for Health Workers. St Louis: Mosby, 1978

16. Leininger, M: Transcultural Nursing: Concepts, Theories and Practices. New York, Wiley, 1978.
17. Bloch, B: Bloch's assessment guide for ethnic/cultural variations. In Orque, MS, Bloch, B, and Monroy, LSA (eds.): Ethnic Nursing Care: A Multicultural Approach, pp. 49–75. St. Louis, Mosby, 1983.
18. Branch, MF, and Paxton, PP (eds.): (1976). Providing Safe Nursing Care for Ethnic People of Color. Englewood Cliffs, NJ, Prentice-Hall, 1976.
19. Orque, MS: Orque's ethnic/cultural system: A framework for ethnic nursing care. In Orque, MS, Bloch, B, and Monroy, LSA (eds.): Ethnic Nursing Care: A Multicultural Approach, pp. 5–48. St. Louis, Mosby, 1983.
20. Tripp-Reimer, T: Cultural Assessment: A Multidimensional Approach, pp. 226–246. Monterey, CA, Wadsworth, 1984.
21. Camphina-Bacote, J: The Process of Cultural Competence in the Delivery of Heathcare Services: A Culturally Competent Model of Care, 3rd ed. Cincinnati, Transcultural Care Associates, 1998.
22. Purnell, LD, & Paulanka, BJ: Transcultural Health Care: A Culturally Competent Approach. Philadelphia, FA Davis Company, 2003.
23. Berlin, EA, and Fowkes, WC: Teaching framework for cross-cultural care: Application in family practice. West J Med 139:934, 1983.
24. Kleinman, A, Eisenberg, L, and Good, B: Culture, illness, and care: Clinical lessons from anthropologic and cross-cultural research. Ann Intern Med 88:251, 1978.
25. Hulsey, TC, Levkoff, AH, and Alexander, GR: Birth weight of infants of black and white mothers without pregnancy complications. Am J Obstet Gynecol 164:1299, 1991.
26. Morton, NE: Genetic aspects of prematurity. In Reed, DM, and Stanley, FJ (eds.): Epidemiology of Prematurity. Baltimore: Urban & Schwarzenberg, 1977.
27. Giger, JN, and Davidhizar, RE: Transcultural nursing assessment: A method for advancing practice. Int Nurs Rev 37:199, 1990.
28. Zoucha, RD: The experiences of Mexican Americans receiving professional nursing care: An ethnonursing study. J Transcultural Nurs 9:34, 1998.
29. Villarruel, AM, and Ortiz de Montellano, B: Culture and pain: A Mesoamerican perspective. Adv Nurs Sci 12:21, 1992.
30. Catalano JT: Nursing Now: Today's Issues, Tomorrow's Trends, 2nd ed. Philadelphia, FA Davis Company, 2000.
31. Murray, RB, and Zentner, JP: Health Assessment and Promotion Strategies: Through the Life Span. Stamford, CT, Appleton & Lange, 1997.
32. Misener, T, Sowell, R, Phillips, K, and Harris, C: Sexual orientation: A cultural diversity issue for nursing. Nurs Outlook 45:178, 1997.
33. Purnell, LD, and Paulanka, BJ: The Purnell model for cultural competence. In Purnell, LD, and Paulanka, BJ (eds.): Transcultural Health Care: A Culturally Competent Approach. Philadelphia: FA Davis Company, 1998.

ADDITIONAL RESOURCES

1. Adminstration on Aging: Achieving Cultural Competence: A Guidebook for Providers of Services to Older Americans and Their Families: http://www.aaoa.dhhs.gov/minorityaccess/guidebook2001/default.htm
2. American Nurses Association: Position Statements: Cultural Diversity in Nursing Practice: http://www.nursingworld.org/readroom/position/ethics/etcldv.htm
3. The California Endowment: http://www.calendow.org
4. The California Endowment: Resources in Cultural Competence Education for Health Care Professionals. 21650 Oxnard Street, Suite 1200, Woodland Hills, CA 91367.
5. Camphina-Bacote, J: A model and instrument for addressing cultural competence in health care. J Nurs Education 38:203, 1999.
6. The Center for Health Professions, University of California, San Francisco: http://futurehealth.ucsf.edu/cnetwork/resources/curricula/diversity.html
7. Smith, DC, Leake, DW and Kamekona, N. (1998). Effects of a culturally competent school-based intervention for at-risk Hawaiian students. Pacific Educational Research Journal 9 (1), 3–15.
8. Diversity Home Page: http://www.diversityrx.org/HTML/MOCPT1.htm
9. Kleinman, A, Eisenber, L, and Good, B. Culture, illness and care: Clinical lessons from anthropologic and cross-cultural research. Ann Intern Med 88:251, 1978.
10. Office of Minority Health Resource Center: http://www.omhrc.gov/clas/ds.html

11. Rooda, L: Knowledge and attitudes toward culturally different patients: Implications for nursing education. J Nurs Education 32:209, 1993.
12. Stewart, M, Brown, JB, Weston, WW, McWilliam, CL, and Freeman, TR: Patient-Centered Medicine: Transforming the Clinical Method. Thousand Oaks, CA: Sage Publications, 1995.
13. Transcultural C.A.R. E. Associates, 11108 Huntwicke Place, Cincinnati, OH 45241
14. Zoucha, R, and Zamarripa, C: The significance of culture in the care of the client with an ostomy. J Wound Ostomy Continence Nurs 24:270, 1997.

CHAPTER 11

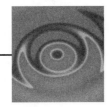

Clinical Research in the Advanced Practice Role

CHAPTER 11

Julie Reed Erickson, PhD, RN, FAAN
Christine Sheehy, PhD, RN

Julie Reed Erickson, PhD, RN, FAAN, is Associate Professor of Nursing at the University of Arizona College of Nursing. After completing her master's degree, Dr. Erickson practiced for 5 years as a pulmonary clinical nurse specialist in pediatrics. After completing her doctorate, Dr. Erickson received federal grant funding to study the implementation and outcomes of community-based interventions for AIDS risk reduction among adult intravenous drug users, treatment of homeless adult drug users, substance abuse prevention among high-risk youth, teen pregnancy prevention, and violence prevention among Native American youth. She teaches undergraduate role development courses and graduate statistics courses at the University of Arizona.

Christine Sheehy, PhD, RN, has a doctoral degree in public policy from Virginia Commonwealth University. Between 1989 and 1990, she taught in the master's and doctoral programs and was project director for the master's level geriatric nurse practitioner option at the University of Arizona College of Nursing. After a 2-year period as director of health services research for the Maricopa Health System, she returned to the academic setting at Arizona State University in Tempe. In her current position, she is the Chief, Quality of Care and Program Monitoring for Geriatrics and Extended Care, in the Veterans Health Administration in Washington, DC. Dr. Sheehy's substantive expertise is in the area of health policy analysis, quality-of-care and health-outcome measurement, and chronic illness and aging. She has also worked as a temporary consultant for the World Health Organization in the Western Pacific Region.

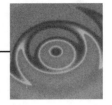

Clinical Research in the Advanced Practice Role

CHAPTER OBJECTIVES

After completing this chapter, the reader will be able to:

1 Analyze the influence of the "research-practice gap" on advanced practice nurses (APNs) as consumers of research and the implications for clinical care.

2 Compare and contrast the research experiences and characteristics of the four APN groups, including their respective strengths and limitations.

3 Delineate strategies for one's own APN role to enhance utilization of research findings in clinical practice and relate these to other topics in this text, such as critical thinking, change and leadership theories, and excellence in practice.

4 Synthesize information about research priorities for APNs and the relevance to APNs as researchers.

According to Diers,[1] decision-making is what most characterizes advanced practice, and underlying decision-making are clinical judgment, scholarly inquiry, and leadership. Clinical judgment includes systematic data gathering, ordering of phenomena, and discriminating analysis of observations. Scholarly inquiry involves performing logical analysis of findings, raising interpretation beyond the facts to higher levels of conceptualization, and reinforcing clinical judgment. Both clinical judgment and scholarly inquiry use the scientific method and should reflect the rigor of the research process. The work of advanced nurses is practice, and the product is patient care; therefore, leadership in the advanced practice role supports the scientific processes by[1]:

- Interpreting the context of practice
- Demonstrating influences on care
- Leading changes in practice

Nurse clinicians use research methods every day to evaluate patient outcomes and responses to treatments, to solve problems, and to answer questions about delivery of care.[2-5] Knowledge of research enables one to read critically, to evaluate published research, and to function as a change agent in planning, implementing, and sustaining innovation in practice (Fig. 11–1).

The scientific orientation of clinical nursing practice was formed by Florence Nightingale, who instructed nurses to use objective, sound observations, not just as information or interesting facts, but to save lives and to increase the comfort and safety of those for whom they cared.[6,7] As far back as the 1890s, this mandate heralded the need to relate interventions methodically to desired improvement in outcomes. Her use of the scientific approach to practice led Nightingale to claim the profession as a "science of nursing."[8]

The scientific process is inherent in the clinical decision-making of advanced practice nursing and in the achievement of high-quality patient care. Research must be an integral part of the advanced practice role:

- To support APNs in becoming more influential in determining health care policy
- To provide a common language that encourages sharing of information
- To enhance the bridging of medical and nursing perspectives in provision of health care
- To support and improve quality of health care

Nursing will become increasingly influential in health care policy formulation to the extent that nurses can demonstrate competence in their knowledge and actions.[9] To justify advanced practice roles in a rapidly changing and competitive health care market, APNs must address accountability by measuring and evaluating outcomes of their care. Research provides a critical component of what legitimizes nursing as a health care profession.[10] According to Hawkins and Thibodeau[9]:

> Research is the means by which outcomes can be validated, the value of nursing management demonstrated, and the practice quantified as unique and, in some cases, superior to that of other health care professionals. (p. 112)

"Advanced-practice nurses also engage in a variety of activities consistent with the goals of the profession. These activities include. . . participation in research and utilization of scientific findings to improve patient outcomes" (American Nurses Association [ANA], *Nursing: A Social Policy Statement*, 1994 Revision, p. 17).[14]

"As a leader or change agent, the nurse-midwife demonstrates: . . . The ability to evaluate, apply and collaborate in research. . . " (American College of Nurse Midwives [AANM], *Core Competencies for Basic Nurse-Midwifery Practice*, 1993, p. 5).[15]

One of the primary roles of the Clinical Nurse Specialist is research, and implementing it can be done by the conduct of research or its utilization (Stetler, Bautista, Vernale-Hannon & Foster, *Nursing Clinics of North America*, 1995).[16]

"Nurse practitioners are committed to seeking and sharing knowledge that will promote quality health care and improve clinical outcomes by conducting research and applying the research findings of others" (American Academy of Nurse Practitioners [AANP], *Scope of Practice for Nurse Practitioners*, 1993, p.1).[17]

"The nurse practitioner uses research findings as a basis for practice and improves health care through participation in research" (American Nurses Association [ANA], *Standards of Practice for the Primary Health Care Nurse Practitioner*, 1987, p.8).[18]

"The purpose of research at the master's level is to prepare a practitioner for the utilization of new knowledge to provide high-quality health care, initiate change, and improve nursing practice....Course work should provide graduates with the knowledge and skills to:. . . access current and relevant data. . . analyze the outcomes of nursing interventions. . . utilize information systems. . . initiate a line of inquiry into comprehensive data bases in order to utilize available research in the practice of nursing" (American Association of Colleges of Nursing [AACN], *The Essentials of Master's Education for Advanced Practice Nursing*, 1996, pp. 6–7).[19]

FIGURE 11–1   Defining the role of research in advanced practice.

Research also provides essential information to policy makers about health care options.[11] Research provides a common language for communicating with other health professionals about the contributions of nursing to patient care[2] and disseminates information about nursing's effectiveness that is crucial to survival of the APN role.[12] In addition, because APNs work with interdisciplinary colleagues whose training required research,[1] using scientific methods provides a standardized vocabulary for exchanging findings and interpreting clinical information. Finally, because the advanced practice role typically bridges nursing and medical functions, APNs are ideally situated to share research findings, evaluate care plans, and contribute to the scientific basis of care.[13]

The research function of APNs can be operationalized as both a consumer of research findings and as a researcher. Both orientations, consumer and researcher, are consistent with expectations enumerated in policy statements and standards of practice directed at the four APN groups: clinical nurse specialist (CNS), nurse practitioner (NP), certified nurse midwife (CNM), and certified registered nurse anesthetist (CRNA).[14-19]

Research methods are the proper subject for research courses in advanced practice training. Macnee[20] and Fonteyn[21] discuss two approaches to teaching research for advanced practice. The purpose of this chapter is not to undertake an exhaustive and likely duplicative description of methods but rather to provide insights into selected dimensions of operationalizing research in the APN role. Among the four groups of APNs, many research concerns and issues are shared. However, differences arising from the historical development of each role and the context in which care occurs may be a strength or limitation for research in one group or another. Elucidation of the development and care associated with a role can alert the APN to pitfalls and emphasize areas of potential research optimization. The chapter also addresses practical ways that the research component of APN roles can be actualized as well as broad areas of research priority.

APNs AS CONSUMERS OF RESEARCH

Research utilization implies that the consumer[6,22–24]:

- Reads the literature
- Makes critical judgments on the purpose, methods, results, and conclusions of a research study
- Evaluates the clinical applicability of the research
- Uses relevant findings in clinical practice
- Evaluates the effects of the new treatment on clients
- Disseminates the findings to others providing care to patients

The Research-Practice Gap

The literature has repeatedly confirmed that research findings with important implications for care are not widely used in clinical settings, despite clear evidence that use of the findings would improve patient care.[2,25,26] That is to say, a research-practice gap exists. Although the fundamental reason for doing nursing research is to develop a body of knowledge relative to practice,[27] research has little value unless it is applied.[28] Titler and Goode[27] suggested that "the conduct of research is essentially unfinished unless the findings are synthesized and applied in practice to improve patient outcomes" (p. xv).

Many authors attest that a key responsibility of APNs is to help close the research gap by implementing research findings in practice settings.[11,29–34] Several barriers have been identified as contributing to the research-practice gap:

- The belief that research holds an "ivory tower" mystique
- A preference for research investigation as superior to utilization of research findings
- Inadequate personal and administrative empowerment
- Lack of clinically relevant studies in the research literature
- Insufficient skill and/or experience in interpreting studies

The Ivory Tower Mystique

Perhaps because of the perceived complexity of research methods, a mystique has evolved about research and researchers. Hawkins and Thibodeau [9] viewed the major barrier to inclusion of research in advanced practice as the belief that research is separate and magical. However, nurses collect data every day, make hypotheses on desired outcomes of care, evaluate their clinical judgments for each patient encounter, write up their findings, and discuss their observations with others in clinical conferences. Ferrell, Grant, and Rhiner[2] believed that involvement in research means abandoning research as an ivory tower–academic activity and viewing research as clinical problem-solving using scientific methods. Research cannot be limited to the few nurses who have doctoral degrees or to nurses in research positions in clinical settings.[2, 35]

Investigation as Superior to Utilization

Graduate education often understates the importance of research utilization because "the emphasis in educational settings has for many years been conduct of research"[11] (p. 457). Although efforts have been made to increase the research utilization training of nurses, research application remains minimal,[36] and investigations are infrequently replicated in clinical settings.[17] APNs frequently articulate the conduct of research to be the gold standard of the research role.[11]

APNs need to understand and be skilled in study design, sampling, reliability, and statistics.[1,37] However, the emphasis on learning and practicing these skills should be balanced by an equally endorsed orientation toward the use of such skills to interpret and apply findings reported in the research literature. Replication studies, in addition to original research for honor's and master's degree theses, would reinforce the importance and value of research utilization.[36] Knowledge of research is necessary to read critically, to evaluate published research, and to function as change agents capable of planning, introducing, and sustaining innovation in a practice setting.[28] The publication of clear and intelligible reports would help APNs to better use research findings. Many of the published reports suffer from[11,36]:

- Use of research jargon
- Emphasis on measurement instead of measures
- Focus on statistical methods rather than their meaning
- Presentation of statistical analyses that are not easily understood
- Failure to explore fully the clinical implications of the findings

Research communications need to be carefully examined by nurse researchers and research journals.[25]

Inadequate Personal and Administrative Empowerment

There is some evidence that APNs have a poor self-image; that is, they do not see themselves as capable of shaping their own practice.[9] As an extension, APNs and nurses in general have expressed concern that they do not have enough power or authority to change patient-care practices even if research supports such initiatives.[25,36] Inadequate time due to heavy workload and competing priorities has been identified as discouraging research efforts in clinical settings.[11,22,25,36] Other barriers to research among APNs include[11,22,25,36,38,39]:

- Inadequate facilities and organizational infrastructure for research
- Lack of administrative incentives
- Resistance and lack of cooperation in the work setting by administrators, other health care professionals, and nursing staff
- Practice changes recommended from the findings that may be too costly to implement
- Previous negative experiences with research
- Isolation from knowledgeable colleagues

Hawkins and Thibodeau[9] suggested that greater clinician-researcher interaction is critical to overcoming the self-image barrier. As described later in this chapter, many collaborative arrangements can be instituted to increase this interface and to foster mentoring relationships. To counter the authority barrier, Funk et al.[25] advocated for increased nurse control over practice through decentralization and shared governance. Administrators can help create time for research activities by incorporating these activities into staff job responsibilities, allowing time for literature reviews, exploration of new ideas, and pilot projects on new practices.[25] Administrative backing in the form of supporting attendance at conferences and continuing education opportunities, funding to support studies, providing access to library and consultative services, photocopying, and funding of pilot projects is also greatly needed.[11,22,25,36,40] Additional strategies include instituting research journal clubs, forming research committees, promoting research presentations, subscribing to journals that emphasize research implementation in practice such as *Applied Nursing Research* and *Clinical Nursing Research*,[36] and developing formal mechanisms for incorporating research findings.[25]

All nurses must contribute to making research utilization a reality. According to Titler and Goode[27]:

> Advanced practice nurses must embrace the pivotal leadership role they play in the synthesis and implementation of research findings. Staff nurses are essential in making the practice changes a reality at the bedside. ... Nursing administrators at all levels of the organization must create practice environments that support and reward use of research. ... Nurse educators must teach students the "hows" and "whys" of research utilization (p. xv).

Lack of Clinically Relevant Studies

The lack of clinically relevant studies inhibits research utilization.[22,36,41] Hawkins and Thibodeau[9] found that the nursing journal with the largest number of readers publishes few, if any, research studies. Often, years lapse between the start of a clinical study and the publication of results in nursing research journals.[38] Until recently, the paucity of clinically relevant and well-designed studies was due to the historical development of several APN roles.

Nurse Practitioner

There were three fairly distinct phases in development of the NP role[42]:

1. The "precursor period," during which the expanded role was initially conceived

2. The subsequent phase of progressive role definition, legitimation, and competencies

3. Role consolidation and maturation

Because some momentum for the NP role came from concern about shortage of physicians and the problem of access, underlying early research was the "unstated assumption that primary care services as defined and provided by physicians were adequate in every respect except quantity." (p. 71)[43]

The emphasis on "access" led researchers to study patient outcomes in terms of the extent to which access was achieved (e.g., number of visits), comparing NPs with physicians (MDs), and considering medical care to be standard and/ or uniform.[43] Diers and Molde[43] stated: "The overwhelming majority of research on nurse practitioners has not dealt with a conceptual understanding of the practice; rather, the independent variable has been conceived of as the practitioner" (p. 74).

Further, because NPs were often seen as a subset of medical practice, the dependent variable, or patient outcome, was also cast or defined in traditional medical terms, and when other measures were included, they typically were patient satisfaction and acceptance.[43]

Most original studies:

- Evaluated the roles of NPs in relation to physicians

- Assessed client acceptance

- Were descriptive in design

- Were conducted by investigators with limited research expertise

- Used retrospective analysis that suffered from incomplete data retrieval[40]

According to Stanford,[40] one notable exception was the study by Lewis and Resnik,[44] which employed randomized assignment of patients to control and experimental groups, follow-up, and multiple outcomes, including satisfaction with care, patients' knowledge about their illnesses, and system variables about the number of missed appointments and the utilization of hospital services.

After these early efforts, studies of NPs were done mostly by physicians, sociologists, and program evaluators (i.e., non-nurses); used primarily questionnaires for data collection; did not use longitudinal designs; and lacked rigor in pretesting of instruments for reliability and validity and appropriate statistical analyses.[40,42,43,45] Not all studies suffered from these weaknesses, however. A well-known exception was the Burlington randomized trial, which employed randomized controlled design, psychometrically tested instruments, and specification of patient outcomes.[40,46]

Recent studies[40]:

- Have greater sophistication in methods

- Have more NPs involved in the investigations

- Address analysis of nursing components of practice pursued, including process and outcomes and factors that influence NP performance (e.g., scope of the extended role, patient assignment, economic issues)

The fact that many clients of NPs are chronically ill poses a substantial challenge to research. Selecting measures and relating interventions to outcomes of care are more difficult when studying persons who have multiple and complex health care needs.[43] Conversely, the fact that NPs frequently work in primary care settings is clearly an advantage. The practice population and setting usually include a wide range of health maintenance and illness problems that afflict persons from infancy to old age, support ongoing relationships between patients and nurses that are needed for prospective and longitudinal studies of interventions and outcomes, and support collaborative research between nurses and other health care providers.[47]

Clinical Nurse Specialist

Similar to the case for NPs, the literature before 1990 offers more information about the "role" of the CNS than about the "effectiveness" of these practitioners in patient care.[48] Most published reports describe what a CNS "does" but say little about what this advanced practice role "achieves."[49]

Perhaps the CNS has an advantage in length of experience and clarity of expectations about research because the entry-level requirement for practice has always been the master's degree. However, the tasks of documenting CNS practice and delineating the effects of interventions on patient outcomes are hampered by the complexity of the role and wide variation in its implementation.[50] Thus, it is difficult to identify which of the activities are most effective in achieving outcomes.[50] In several studies where CNSs collaborated with other disciplines on patient outcomes, distinguishing the effects of individual team providers on outcomes is difficult.[50]

Certified Nurse Midwives

Of all the advanced practice groups, CNMs appear to have had the greatest leverage in documenting and reporting their contributions. Many clinically relevant and well-designed studies are available. Among the explanations for this success are:

- The availability of data on effectiveness
- Establishment of linkages between data on effectiveness and health policy issues and/or concerns
- Well-defined and sensitive outcomes measures

From inception of the role, the CNM was encouraged to keep statistics, and since 1972, this requirement has been formally acknowledged.[51] The statistics were primarily intended for self-evaluation of clinical programs but were drawn on as data from which effectiveness studies were reported.[51] "Effectiveness" usually meant program effectiveness, linked to the reason the nurse midwife was brought into a situation, which usually was to improve access to health care for childbearing women and babies who were not receiving adequate services.[51] Many data on infant and maternal mortality, as well as improvements in access for women in rural areas, were collected from studies done by the Metropolitan Life Insurance Company for the Frontier Nursing Services between 1925 and the mid-1950s.[51]

In the mid-1950s, midwifery made a "deliberate" and "successful" attempt to provide services in hospitals, because most women were delivering in that setting.[51] Effectiveness had been documented in rural and underserved populations. Once CNMs were practicing in hospitals, effectiveness included comparison of care given by CNMs and physicians, using such medical criteria as amount of analgesia given, duration of stages of labor, type of delivery, and complications. These effectiveness studies helped to justify the CNM's role not only to the public but also to other professionals.[51]

By the 1960s and 1970s, effectiveness meant reduction of mortality rates, evidence of medical efficacy, quality of life, and cost-effectiveness. In the early 1970s, CNMs expanded into the private sector, and studies focused on patient acceptance and physician receptivity in addition to the effectiveness questions.[51] The effectiveness evaluations were largely conducted so CNMs would be accepted by the professional community and have access to childbearing women. Diers and Burst[51] stated: "Thus the effort was to prove being 'as good as' physician care, to prove being 'safe,' to prove being 'acceptable,' and to prove being 'cost-effective'" (p. 72).

According to Diers and Molde,[43] the practice of CNMs was developed more through accreditation mechanisms, professional association positions, and legal parameters than through other nursing expanded roles. Therefore, greater standardization exists, and it has been possible to study much about nurse midwifery practice.

> For example, investigators have clearly examined both the effect of nurse-midwifery practice on medical or obstetrical outcome (morbidity, mortality, complications) and the effect of the nursing component in nurse midwifery on compliance (with postpartum recommendations, prenatal visits, or diet advice). (p. 79)

Nurse midwifery has been very successful in influencing health policy about changes in care, reimbursement, and other policy agendas.[51] This influence is explained partly by the quantity and quality of the effectiveness data.[51,52] The data sets were more complete than usual record-keeping because many of the data collected were required for public health statistical reports, had procedures for verifying reliability, and were collected repeatedly longitudinally.[51] The primary reason for collecting and analyzing the data in the studies was to support a clinical position, not to build a body of knowledge; hence findings were closely tied to policy issues rather than to a theory base.[51] Although many studies were based on retrospective analysis, the integrity of those data is likely more robust than data collected in other areas of advanced practice nursing. Further, CNM findings are relevant to practice problems,[17] variables are easy to understand, outcomes are self-explanatory, and implications are obvious, connecting data to issues policy makers worry about.[51] The nurse midwifery literature has, to a great extent, avoided obstacles to policy creation, including isolated research findings, disjointed investigations, and infrequent replication resulting in several strong studies that provide support for the role.[17]

Nurse midwives have had fewer problems in defining patient outcomes because of the obvious validity of the dependent variables (e.g., neonatal mortality), and the dependent variables (e.g., infant birth weight) are fairly sensitive to different practice interventions (e.g., nutritional counseling).[43,51] According to Diers and Molde[43]:

> Because the normal obstetrical situation is relatively less complicated methodologically (though not necessarily clinically) than internal medicine, considerable progress has been made in devising measures of the effect of nurse midwives and in describing the independent variable. (p. 79)

Numerous studies reported in the 1980s and early 1990s provide support for the positive outcomes of nurse midwives.[53,54] Anderson and Murphy[55] described the outcome of planned home births (N = 11,788), over a 5-year period, including hospital transfers, practice protocols, risk screening, and emergency preparedness. Beal[56] evaluated the nature of nurse midwifery care and the relationship of clinical practice to outcomes in order to identify differences in intrapartum management between CNMs and physicians. Variables included patterns of administration of intravenous fluid, amniotomy, electronic fetal monitoring, pain medication, pitocin augmentation, lengths of the three stages of labor, total hospitalization time from labor until delivery, mode of delivery, incidence of episiotomy and laceration, and Apgar scores.[56] Yeates and Roberts[57] studied the relationship between nutritional intervention by CNMs and the outcome of birth weights. Corbett and Burst[58] investigated the relationship between CNM interventions of bearing-down technique in second stage of labor and energy expenditure, mean duration of the second stage, and Apgar scores. Although the last two studies had small samples,[57,58] the second did employ random assignment to control and intervention groups.

Certified Registered Nurse Anesthetist

Research on CRNAs is scant. Gunn[59] calls on the CRNA community for greater accountability in practice, a move toward evidence-based practice, and identification of best practices. According to Waugaman[60]:

> There has been little incentive to conduct outcome studies in anesthesia since the Centers for Disease Control & Prevention (CDC) has asserted that the incidence of adverse outcomes, morbidity and mortality is too low to justify a nationally conducted study. (p. 51)

Cowan, Vinayak, and Jasinski[61] found that only a small percentage of CRNAs were involved in research at any level, that most CRNAs conducting research did not receive educational preparation for research, and that a significant relationship existed between working in a teaching hospital and conducting research.

The majority of CRNAs and anesthesiologists practice in an interdisciplinary care team, yet little research exists on this practice model.[60,62] The medical direction ratios (that is, the number of nurse anesthetists per physician) for delivery of anesthesia care in the anesthesia care team model have not been substantiated in outcome research.[60] Horton[63] examined the provision of culturally congruent nursing care by CRNAs. McAuliffe and Henry[64] studied nurse anesthetists in 94 countries and concluded the following:

1. Nurses were the main administers of anesthesia in many countries.

2. Most duties were performed inside operating rooms, contributing to lack of visibility of the profession.

3. Nurse anesthetists must document their practice.

4. Nurse anesthetists should participate in collaborative research at the local, regional, national, and international levels.

Using the AANA Foundation closed malpractice claims database, Kremer, Faut-Callahan, and Hicks[65] found that use of cognitive biases and inaccurate probability estimates were associated with adverse outcomes.

Insufficient Skill and/or Experience in Interpreting Studies

The inability of clinicians to understand research reports limits research utilization.[22,41] APNs often lack adequate knowledge and an explicit set of criteria for judging the applicability of research findings to practice. APNs may recognize the term "research utilization," but few are formally educated in use of a specific model for utilization.[11] Models for research utilization are helpful in incorporating research findings into practice[25,66] and in increasing knowledge about application of those findings.

Three major models for research utilization in clinical settings were developed and tested in nursing. The models are quite similar in many respects but are distinguished by their intended goals. The first project for nursing research utilization began in 1975 by the Western Interstate Commission for Higher Education (WICHE) Regional Program for Nursing Research Development.[32] Five components were described as necessary for nurses in order to achieve the goal of change in practice[32,67]:

1. Access to research findings

2. Ability to evaluate studies critically

3. Competence in change theory and strategies

4. Approaches to managing risk taking

5. A plan for implementation and criteria by which to evaluate the effects

One outgrowth of the WICHE model was the formation of information systems, including a list of nurse researchers by areas of interest and/or expertise, a compendium of nursing instruments, a compilation of funding sources, and a list of research priorities derived from a Delphi survey.[32,68]

Developed in the late 1970s, the Conduct and Utilization of Research in Nursing (CURN) model delineated six phases to achieve the goal of putting research knowledge into nursing practice.[6,16,69] The six phases are:

1. Creating an atmosphere for change by identifying specific patient-care problems

2. Evaluating current scientific knowledge of the clinical problem, institutional policies, and potential costs

3. Determining the fit of the nursing practice innovation

4. Carrying out clinical trials

5. Deciding to accept, reject, or change the innovation

6. Disseminating the innovation to other nursing practice units

The collaboration of nurse clinicians and nurse researchers was critical in all six phases of the CURN model.

The Stetler/Marram[70] Model for research utilization has been tested and refined into six phases. The six phases are:

1. Reviewing the literature of a clinical problem

2. Critiquing the research

3. Evaluating its clinical applicability

4. Determining the potential use of the research findings

5. Translating the findings into practice

6. Evaluating the expected outcomes

Stetler's approach to the goals of enhancing knowledge and increasing use of research findings reflects a model of critical thinking that has been applied many times and in different settings.[11,71] In particular, the 1995 article by Stetler et al[16] demonstrates the functioning of a research utilization interest group, contains a worksheet to apply the model and strategies, and suggests strategies and/or tips to help ensure success of such a forum.

Bridging the Research-Practice Gap

Many strategies have been suggested to bridge the research-practice gap in advanced practice. Evidence-based practice and collaboration are at the forefront.

Evidence-Based Practice

Since the 1990s, evidence-based practice (EBP) has been advanced as a strategy to link best scientific findings, clinical judgments, clinical expertise, clinical reasoning skills, and the patient's unique characteristics to inform clinical practice.[72-74] Pravikoff and Donaldson[75] report that EBP should result in consistent up-to-date nursing practice and the most effective patient outcomes. APNs have the educational background, clinical expertise, and critical thinking skills to lead discovery of and incorporation of EBP into prevention and treatment settings.[76] Soukup[77] reports on one EBP model for advanced practice. The process of EBP includes[21,75,76]:

1. Formulating a clear, precise clinical question to answer

2. Searching for evidence

3. Applying clinical guidelines for improving clinical practice

4. Critiquing/validating the evidence

5. Putting evidence into practice

6. Evaluating the results of the EBP.

Search for evidence has focused primarily on use of the Internet. Commonly used databases include MEDLINE, CINAHL, PubMed, and PsycINFO. Searching the World Wide Web is challenging. APNs need skills to find the best resources, select useful sites, evaluate sites, and sort through the evidence found. The literature describes basic and advanced strategies for using the Internet and validating the evidence.[76,78–81] Online journals are another source for evidence-based practice. Table 11–1 provides a directory of online sources for evidence.

TABLE 11–1. Online Sources of Information

Online Databases and Sources of Data

1. Clinical Performance Measure Database: Available through the Agency for Health Care Policy and Research. The database is in Access 1.0, and the documentation (which is voluminous) is in WordPerfect 6.0 and up. This database comprises data from JCAHO, HEDIS, HCFA, and Rand. Go to http://www.ahcpr.gov/query.idq

2. Healthcare Cost and Utilization Project (HCUP-3): National Inpatient Sample Release (NIS) 2, 1993, data available May 1996. The 1993 NIS data include: (a) 6.5 million inpatient stays in 900 hospitals from 17 states; (b) clinical and resource use variables usually found on discharge abstracts; (c) weights to produce national estimates; (d) hospital identifiers to link with American Hospital Association's Survey of Hospitals. This 6-CD set can be purchased for $160 from National Technical Information Service or on the Internet at hcupnis@cghsir.ahcpr.gov.

Online Sources of Grant Funding

- For health grants: National Institutes of Health at nih.gov
- For mental health grants: National Institute of Mental Health at nimh.nih.gov
- For nursing grants: National Institute of Nursing Research at ninr.nih.gov
- Sigma Theta Tau International at nursingsociety.org
- For substance abuse grants: National Institute on Drug Abuse at nida.nih.gov
- National Institute on Alcohol Abuse and Alcoholism at niaaa.nih.gov
- Substance Abuse and Mental Health Administration at samhsa.gov

Online Sources for Information

- Evidence-based practice: Joanna Briggs Institute for Evidence-Based Nursing and Midwifery at joannabriggs.edu.au
- University of York Centre for Evidence-Based Nursing at http://www.york.ac.uk/healthsciences/centres/evidence/cebn.htm
- Sarah Cole Hirsh Institute at hirshinstitute.com
- Cochrane Library at hiru.mcmaster.ca/cochrane/
- Centers for Disease Control and Prevention at cdc.gov
- TRIP (Translating Research Into Practice) at tripdatabase.com
- WHO (World Health Organization) at who.ch

(Table continued on following page)

TABLE 11–1. **Online Sources of Information** (Continued)

Online Sources for Information (Continued)

- Healthfinder at healthfinder.gov
- Health Touch at healthtouch.com
- Mayo Clinic at MayoClinic.com
- Merck Manual at merck.com
- Virtual Hospital at vh.com
- Virtual Nurse at virtualnurse.com
- Sigma Theta Tau International at nursingsociety.org
- CNN Interactive Health at cnn.com/HEALTH

Online Journals

- Graduate Research Journal
- Health Informatics Europe
- International Electronic Journal of Health Education
- International Journal of Advanced Nursing Practice
  Journal of Advanced Nursing
- NLM (National Library of Medicine) Technical Bulletin
- Nurse Beat
- Online Journal of Clinical Innovations
- Online Journal of Issues in Nursing
- Online Journal of Knowledge Synthesis for Nursing
- Online Journal of Nursing Informatics
- Research for Nursing Practice

Collaboration

Collaboration must be encouraged between academic and clinical institutions for mutual support in establishing programs for research utilization.[19,38,82] Blending of research resources is critical to providing a scientific basis for advanced nursing practice and providing answers to clinical questions that arise every day.[82]

Dufault[38] examined a model of collaboration among nurse researchers, staff nurses, clinical managers, clinicians, and nurse administrators to enhance research utilization and development. Sprague-McRae[13] advocated either a collaborative intradisciplinary or interdisciplinary team to validate clinical practice and to support NPs as primary investigators in the research process. More research by clinical practitioners, in collaboration with academic researchers, could overcome the barrier of finding relevant literature on clinical problems. The American Nurses Association Cabinet on Nursing Research[83] endorses the partnership of clinicians and researchers in research utilization.

There are many barriers to the utilization of nursing research to effect change in clinical practice and improve clinical outcomes. These barriers include the ivory tower mystique about research, the perception that the conduct of research is superior to the application of research findings, inadequate personal empowerment, lack of administrative support, lack of clinically relevant studies for some APN groups, and insufficient skill among APNs to access, critique, and interpret studies. On the positive side, many strategies for overcoming the barriers exist. Ultimately, overcoming barriers to effective research utilization is accomplished by developing intellectual curiosity, by thinking reflectively about one's actions, by promoting and valuing innovation,[28] and by creating an environment that supports questioning, evaluating current practice, and seeking and testing of research-based solutions.[36]

APNs AS RESEARCHERS

Scientific inquiry (i.e., research) and the continuing discovery of new knowledge are crucial to a profession[2,84] and have as their goal the generation of knowledge for science-based clinical practice.[15] As mentioned earlier in this chapter, research contributes to the validation of nursing outcomes, the explanation and quantification of the unique nature of advanced nursing practice, and the documentation of the superiority of nursing care when higher quality exists.[9] Krywanio[3] stated that the NP is critical to identifying issues that are important in clinical research as well as in providing firsthand insight into the research process. This unique perspective and insight into care processes and care outcomes are held by all APNs across a variety of clinical settings.

Hawkins and Thibodeau[9] suggested that not every APN has the array of research skills needed to carry out a clinical research study. Diers[1] stated that a major advantage for an APN is to complete a research thesis that can be integrated into clinical practice and that can serve as a model for future clinical investigations. However, a difference of opinion exists on the need for a research thesis in a graduate program. The American Association of Colleges of Nursing[19] concluded that in a professional master's degree program, a research thesis is not an appropriate mandatory requirement.

APNs can assume many roles in the conduct of research. Hawkins and Thibodeau[9] suggested the roles of subject, research assistant, consultant, content expert, nursing expert, collaborator, or principal investigator.

Collaboration

Collaboration is advantageous to the conduct of clinical nursing research.[85,86] The collaborative approach pools complementary talents, research skills, and clinical experiences from among its members,[87] and may be interdisciplinary or intradisciplinary. For example, in one interdisciplinary interpretation, an NP might consult with a clinical nurse researcher on the design of the study protocol, sources of funding, and implementation.[3] Sprague-McRae[13] suggested that intradisciplinary research collaboration occurs between nurse researchers–nurse clinicians, nurse researchers–nurse researchers, or nurse clinicians–nurse clinicians. Havelock and Havelock[88] recognized intradisciplinary collaboration as building on the strengths of practice-based and academic-based models of clinical research. Dufault[38] used a model of reciprocity between nurse clinicians and nurse scientists. In Dufault's model, clinicians learn research methods and gain an appreciation of research, whereas scientists learn about clinically relevant problems and the challenges of conducting clinical investigations.

The interdisciplinary research team can involve nurse clinicians, nurse researchers, physicians, finance officers, psychologists, sociologists, anthropologists, attorneys, nutritionists, statisticians, and other health care professionals. The chosen mix of disciplines depends on the clinical problem being investigated, the setting of the study, the desired talent pool of team members, and the goals of collaboration. Sprague-McRae[13] suggested that interdisciplinary research collaboration increases the visibility of nurse clinicians as uniquely skilled and contributing members of the health care team, promotes positive working relationships among health disciplines, and distributes the workload of a clinical investigation. Consulting with experts, formally or informally, and piloting of studies are always advisable.

Identification of Researchable Topics in Clinical Practice

Whatever collaborative arrangement APNs choose, another important decision concerns identifying what should be investigated. Research ideas arise from one's own interests, observation of a recurring problem or unexplained phenomenon, suggestions of colleagues, and published results that recommend areas of further study.[89] The study topic should be of great interest to the researcher because the implementation of a study is long and involved and because it is necessary to sustain motivation to carry out the project.[89]

General Areas of Research Priority

Although the term *outcome* has recently been popularized, the need to study the impact of nursing interventions on client response has been espoused for years.[7,90–94] Gurka[91] and Peglow et al.[92] insisted that to document effectiveness, clinical research must focus on both the process and outcome of the activities of APNs. Health care costs, cost-effectiveness, and financing[15,92,95]; health care delivery; interdisciplinary dynamics and the interface of nurses with other disciplines[15,40]; and quality of care[92] are other aspects that must be woven into study designs. Lengacher et al.[96] reported an acute need for outcome research on the design and use of nursing practice models. It is reasonably well accepted that "risk adjustment" is important to measurement of outcomes. However, the research method by which that is accomplished and the variables contributing to risk adjustment formulas are still being debated and therefore are not fully established. Examples of variables that may be included are measures of severity (e.g., diagnosis, comorbidity, complications) and additional case mix modifiers, such as age, the contribution of depression, and other patient characteristics that influence outcomes, such as functional level and cognitive status.[52,97,98] Case mix differs in measurement depending on the setting in which patients are seen. For example, diagnosis-related groups apply to hospital settings, whereas ambulatory-care groups are under development for outpatient settings. A comprehensive discussion of risk adjustment is not possible within the context of this chapter, but its rapid growth in development suggests that the reader may wish to pursue independent reading more fully. Resources on this subject and sources of measurement are included in the bibliography of this chapter.

Crummer and Carter[99] suggested studying the critical pathway model for its ability to define current practice and to meet the goals of nursing case management. Lusk and Kerr[100] saw increased hazards facing employees in the work site as important to study. Prichard et al.[90] encouraged exploration of the influence of technology because nursing practices may be eliminated or altered as technological advances occur. Examination of the evaluative component of the Stetler-Marram research utilization model, implementation of research findings in an interdisciplinary manner, and research utilization competencies are also needed.[11] Qualitative studies about styles of practice are also increasingly important.[40]

It should also be noted that research questions can be examined using existing data. For example, birth certificate data provided by the Natality, Marriage, and Divorce Statistics Branch of the CDC contain information on mother's age, parity, starting date of prenatal care, birth weight, and 1-minute Apgar score, which can be used as was the case in the midwifery study.[53] Nurse midwives have used existing data for many years in studies of CNM effectiveness.[51,52] Molde and Diers[52] suggested that patient-care charts provide data and that encounter forms are another good source. NP research would be improved if existing data were systematically tabulated in each setting.

Sources of data could be greatly increased and comparability and benchmarking across APN patient groups improved by the routine collection of assessment data by means of using standardized assessment instruments. Valid and reliable instruments assessing coping, functional status, quality of life, stress, and other variables of interest to APNs are available in the literature. An APN planning a research study should carefully consider using established instruments to avoid the exacting, tedious process of instrument development and, more importantly, to allow comparisons with published findings. APNs should also look to existing taxonomies for standardized nursing language, performance measures, decision-making, and classification of nursing interventions.[101-104]

Selected Research Priorities Specific to APN Groups

With regard to NPs, Stanford[40] suggested the following areas as warranting continued investigation:

- Development of theoretical models to help link research, theory, and practice
- Improvement in methods, including sampling and defining comparison groups and target populations

- Implementation of longitudinal studies
- Refinement and extension of findings that can be generalized
- Determination of more appropriate instrumentation

Diers and Molde[43] recommended that if NP care is defined to encompass dimensions of nursing in addition to medical criteria, many more dependent measures can be identified for patients, such as outcomes for persons with chronic illnesses, measures of counseling and patient knowledge, standards of care, and appropriate units of study for cost analysis. Gerace[47] expanded on the preceding theme of selecting outcome measures for study. Gerace stated that because much of the practice of NPs is based on meaningful interactions with patients, qualitative rather than quantitative research may be more appropriate. Clinical practice domains might include nutritional assessment and counseling, the patient's perspective of chronic illness and associated self-care needs, family systems, patient education, the NP role in team interaction and telephone encounters,[47] and the influence of differences in practice patterns.[40]

Outcome studies should be designed to improve rather than merely evaluate styles of practice, including the helping relationship, and with a policy framework in mind.[52] Molde and Diers[52] caution:

> Explaining the outcomes, however, requires a systematic search of the characteristics of the care, the provider, the context, the relationship of patient to clinician, and the resources broadly conceived in the setting. (p. 364)

For CNSs, Rizzuto[50] urged formal documentation of the process of consultation and further investigation of patient outcomes and the type and frequency of outcomes achieved. Hamric[95] suggested that studies are needed on cost-effectiveness of CNSs and their role in improving patient outcomes.

Areas for research by CRNAs appear to be wide open and fertile. Waugaman[60] advised outcome research to provide necessary evidence for state and federal governments to make decisions about health care reform. Elements of such research might include:

- Provider data
- Paradigms of cost equality and efficiency relative to case management technique application in a variety of institutional settings
- Participation of CRNAs in continuous quality improvement programs that can be maintained individually and in a national data bank

Cromwell[105] added two important avenues to pursue. First, in the "team model" of physician anesthesiologist–CRNA practice, there is substantial regional variation in the number of CRNAs supervised (i.e., the ratio of physicians to CRNAs), and little is known about the impact. As a result, significant opportunities exist to demonstrate possible improvements and differences in cost and outcomes. Second, anesthesia is an ideal laboratory for studying substitution effects. According to Cromwell: "Anesthesia, therefore, provides an excellent example of what can go wrong with the workforce mix when you pay for inputs (i.e., types of providers) rather than outputs (i.e., the services delivered)" (p. 220).

Despite all their accomplishments, CNMs still have many interesting research topics to pursue and challenges to overcome. Ament[11] reported that CNMs still face barriers to practice in many areas of the country, including difficulty with reimbursement from state and private sources, denial of hospital privileges, uncertain access to malpractice insurance, and lack of uniform prescriptive authority. Hence, much more documentation of outcomes and dissemination of findings to policy makers are needed. Positive outcomes of midwifery provide support for increased use of midwives and suggest the need for systematic studies of the cost savings associated with midwifery care.[53,54]

Mead[106] suggested study of the fit between the theory of research and the practicalities of everyday midwifery. Lehrman[107] examined a theoretical framework for nurse midwifery. Declerc[53] stated that further research into the content of midwifery care is recommended.

SUMMARY

Every professional nurse must contribute to the flow of information from one organization to another, from academia to practice, and from written journals to bedside caregivers.[27] For nursing, it is critically important that clinical research influence health policy.[17]

The scope and standards of practice for APNs mandate utilization of research in clinical practice as well as a role in generating research to build the scientific base of nursing. The demands for time and skills to meet these research expectations are enormous. However, the APN should confront the challenge using models of research utilization and research collaboration already in the professional literature. APNs are in the unique position to expand nursing practice, to prove the value of advanced practice, and to build knowledge for future generations of nurses.

SUGGESTED EXERCISES

1 Consider your current or most recent place of employment.
  a. Make a list of general areas of opportunity for conducting collaborative research or collaborating on research utilization and the discipline(s) likely to participate.
  b. Determine whether there are any critical pathways for the researchable area, what questions might be examined using existing data, and identify the database(s) where such data reside.
  c. Propose the measures, perhaps process and outcome, and sources of instrumentation.
  d. Identify some funding sources to support the project.

2 Quality management, health policy-making, and research are related concerns for APNs.
  a. Consider the features of each of these three and how they characterize the interrelationship.
  b. Construct a potential sequence as to how one (i.e., quality management, policy-making, research) might contribute to the other in terms of improving client and/or patient outcomes.

c. For each of the three, propose indicators for evaluating access, costs, effectiveness, utilization, and practice patterns.

d. For your particular advanced practice area of study (e.g., CNM, CNS, CRNA, NP), relate these three to priorities for program evaluation and/or research.

REFERENCES

1. Diers, D: Preparation of practitioners, clinical specialists, and clinicians. J Prof Nurs 1:41, 1985.
2. Ferrell, B, Grant, M, and Rhiner, M: Bridging the gap between research and practice. Oncol Nurs Forum 17:447, 1990.
3. Krywanio, M: Integrating research into private practice through consultation. Nurse Pract 19:47, 1994.
4. Kleinpell-Nowell, R, and Weiner, T: Measuring advanced practice nursing outcomes. AACN Clin Issues 10:356, 1999.
5. Whitman, G: Outcomes research in advanced practice nursing: Selecting an outcome. Crit Care Nurs Clin North Am 14:253, 2002.
6. McGuire, D, Walczak, J, and Krumm, S: Development of a nursing research utilization program in a clinical oncology setting: Organization, implementation, and evaluation. Oncol Nurs Forum 21:704, 1994.
7. Nightingale, F: Notes on Nursing: What It Is and What It Is Not [commemorative 1992 edition]. JB Lippincott, Philadelphia, 1859.
8. Nightingale, F: Notes on Nursing: What It Is and What It Is Not. New York, Dover Publications, 1969.
9. Hawkins, J, and Thibodeau, J: The role of research in advanced practice. In Hawkins, J, and Thibodeau, J: The Advanced Practitioner: Current Practice Issues. New York, Tiresias Press, 1993.
10. Huber, G: Clinical nurse specialist and staff nurse colleagues in integrating nursing research with clinical practice. Clin Nurse Specialist 8:118, 1994.
11. Ament, LA: Strategies for dissemination of policy research. J Nurse Midwifery 39:329, 1994.
12. Papenhausen, J, and Beecroft, P: Communicating clinical nurse specialist effectiveness. Clin Nurse Specialist 4:1, 1990.
13. Sprague-McRae, J: Nurse practitioners and collaborative interdisciplinary research roles in an HMO. Pediatr Nurs 14:503, 1988.
14. American Nurses Association: Nursing: A Social Policy Statement. Kansas City, MO, American Nurses Association, 1994.
15. American College of Nurse-Midwives: Core Competencies for Basic Nurse-Midwifery Practice. Washington, DC, American College of Nurse-Midwives, 1993.
16. Stetler, CB, et al.: Enhancing research utilization by clinical nurse specialists. Nurs Clin North Am 30:457, 1995.
17. American Academy of Nurse Practitioners: Scope of Practice for Nurse Practitioners. Austin, TX, American Academy of Nurse Practitioners, 1993.
18. American Nurses Association: Standards of Practice for the Primary Health Care Nurse Practitioner. Kansas City, MO, American Nurses' Association, 1987.
19. American Association of Colleges of Nursing: The Essentials of Master's Education for Advanced Practice Nursing. Washington, DC, American Association of Colleges of Nursing, 1996.
20. Macnee, C: Integrating teaching, research , and practice in a nurse-managed clinic: A nonrecurvise model. Nurse Educator 24:25, 1999.
21. Fonteyn, M: Teaching advanced practice nursing students how to use the Internet to support an evidence-based practice. AACN Clin Issues 12:509, 2001.
22. Pettengill, M, Gillies, D, and Clark, C: Factors encouraging and discouraging the use of nursing research findings. Image J Nurs Scholarship 26:143, 1994.
23. American Nurses Association: Guidelines for the Investigative Function of Nurses. Kansas City, MO, American Nurses Association, 1981.
24. Nunnelee, J, and Spaner, S: Research utilization. J Vascular Nurs 20:68, 2002.
25. Funk, S, et al.: Barriers to using research findings in practice: The clinician's perspective. Appl Nurs Res 4:90, 1991.
26. Heater, B, Becker, A, and Olson, R: Nursing interventions and patient outcomes: A meta-analysis of studies. Nurs Res 37:303, 1988.
27. Titler, MG, and Goode, CJ (eds.): Preface. Nurs Clin North Am 30:xv, 1995.

28. Sleep, J: Research and the practice of midwifery. J Adv Nurs 17:1465, 1992.
29. Briones, T, and Bruya, M: The professional imperative: Research utilization in the search for scientifically based nursing practice. Focus Crit Care 17:78, 1990.
30. Edwards-Beckett, J: Nursing research utilization techniques. J Nurs Adm 20:25, 1990.
31. Kirchhoff, K: A diffusion survey of coronary precautions. Nurs Res 31:196, 1982.
32. Phillips, L: A Clinician's Guide to the Critique and Utilization of Nursing Research. Norwalk, CT, Appleton-Century-Crofts, 1986.
33. Rogers, E: Diffusion of Innovations. New York, The Free Press, 1983.
34. Melnyk, B, and Fineout-Overholt, E: Putting research into practice. Reflections Nurs Leadership 28:22, 2002.
35. Martin, M, and Forchuk, C: Linking research and practice. Int Nurs Rev 41:184, 1994.
36. Funk, SG, Tornquist, EM, and Champagne, MT: Barriers and facilitators of research utilization. Nurs Clin North Am 30:395, 1995.
37. Chochesy, J: Research designs for advanced practice nursing outcomes research. Crit Care Nurs Clin North Am 14:293, 2002.
38. Dufault, M: A collaborative model for research development and utilization: Process, structure, and outcomes. J Nurs Staff Dev 11:139, 1995.
39. Jastremski, C: Using outcomes research to validate the advanced practice nursing role administratively. Crit Care Nurs Clin North Am 14:275, 2002.
40. Stanford, D: Nurse practitioner research: Issues in practice and theory. Nurse Pract 12:64, 1987.
41. Miller, J, and Messenger, S: Obstacles to applying nursing research findings. Am J Nurs 78:632, 1978.
42. Edmunds, MW: Evaluation of nurse practitioner effectiveness: An overview of the literature. Eval Health Professions 1:68, 1978.
43. Diers, D, and Molde, S: Some conceptual and methodological issues in nurse practitioner research. Res Nurs Health 2:73, 1979.
44. Lewis, CE, and Resnik, BA: Nurse clinics and progressive ambulatory patient care. N Engl J Med 277:1236, 1967.
45. Shamansky, SL: Nurse practitioners and primary care research: Promises and pitfalls. In Werley, H, and Fitzpatrick, J (eds.): Annual Review of Nursing Research. New York, Springer, 1985.
46. Spitzer, WO, et al.: The Burlington randomized trial of the nurse practitioner. N Engl J Med 290:251, 1974.
47. Gerace, TM: Primary care nursing: A model for research. In Norton, PG, et al. (eds.): Primary Care Research: Traditional and Innovative Approaches. Newbury Park, CA, Sage Publications, 1991.
48. Lipetzky, P: Cost analysis and the clinical nurse specialist. Nurs Manage 21:25, 1990.
49. Beyerman, K: Making a difference: The gerontological CNS. J Gerontological Nurs 15:36, 1993.
50. Rizzuto, C: Issues in clinical nursing research: Documenting clinical nurse specialist role functions and outcomes. West J Nurs Res 17:448, 1995.
51. Diers, D, and Burst, HV: Effectiveness of policy related research: Nurse-midwifery as case example. Image J Nurs Scholarship 15:68, 1983.
52. Molde, S, and Diers, D: Nurse practitioner research: Selected literature review and research agenda. Nurs Res 34:362, 1985.
53. Declerc, ER: The transformation of American midwifery: 1975 to 1988. Am J Public Health 82:680, 1992.
54. Rooks, J, et al.: Outcomes of care in birth centers. N Engl J Med 321:1804, 1989.
55. Anderson, RE, and Murphy, PA: Outcomes of 11,788 planned home births attended by certified nurse-midwives: A retrospective descriptive study. J Nurse Midwifery 40:483, 1995.
56. Beal, MW: Nurse-midwifery intrapartum management. J Nurse Midwifery 29:13, 1984.
57. Yeates, DA, and Roberts, JE: A comparison of two bearing-down techniques during the second stage of labor. J Nurse Midwifery 29:3, 1984.
58. Corbett, MA, and Burst, HV: Nutritional intervention in pregnancy. J Nurse Midwifery 28:23, 1983.
59. Gunn, I: Evidence-based practice, research, peer review, and publication. CRNA 9:177, 1998.
60. Waugaman, WR: Outcome research: The gold standard for professional practice. Nurse Anesth 4:51, 1993.
61. Cowan, C, Vinayak, K, and Jasinski, D: CRNA-conducted research: Is it being done? AANA J 70:18, 2002.
62. American Society of Anesthesiologists: Statement to the Committee on Finance, US Senate (Position on FY 93 Budget Proposals). Park Ridge, IL, February 18, 1992.
63. Horton, B: Nurse anesthetists' perspectives on improving the anesthesia care of culturally diverse patients. J Transcultural Nurs 9:26, 1998.

64. McAuliffe, M, and Henry, B: Nurse anesthesia practice and research: A worldwide need. CRNA 11:89, 2000.
65. Kremer, M, Faut-Callahan, M, and Hicks, F: A study of clinical decision making by certified registered nurse anesthetists. AANA J 70:391, 2002.
66. Mackay, M: Research utilization and the CNS: Confronting the issues. Clin Nurse Specialist 12:232, 1998.
67. Kruegar, J, Nelson, A, and Wolanin, MO: Nursing Research: Development, Collaboration, and Utilization. Germantown, MD, Aspen Systems, 1978.
68. Lindeman, CA, and Krueger, JC: Increasing the quality, quantity, and use of nursing research. Nurs Outlook 25:450, 1977.
69. Horsley, J, Crane, J, and Bingle, J: Research utilization as an organizational process. J Nurs Adm 8:4, 1978.
70. Stetler, C: Refinement of the Stetler/Marram model of application of research findings to practice. Nurs Outlook 42:15, 1994.
71. Hanson, JL, and Ashley, B: Advanced practice nurses' application of the Stetler model for research utilization: Improving bereavement care. Oncol Nurs Forum 21:720, 1994.
72. Glanville, I, Schirm, V, and Wineman, N: Using evidence-based practice for managing clinical outcomes in advanced practice nursing. J Nurs Care Quality 15:1, 2000.
73. Hawkins, J: Evidence-based practice: A new name for an old concept. Clin Excellence Nurse Pract 4:261, 2000.
74. Sebastian, J, et al.: Evidence-based practice and the advanced practice nurse: A curriculum for the future. Semin Perioperative Nurs 9:143, 2000.
75. Pravikoff, D, and Donaldson, N: Online journals: Access and support for evidence-based practice. AACN Clin Issues 12:588, 2001.
76. Morrisey, L, and DeBourgh, G: Finding evidence: Refining literature searching skills for the advanced practice nurse. AACN Clin Issues 12:560, 2001.
77. Soukup, M: The center for advanced nursing practice evidence-based model: Promoting the scholarship of practice. Nurs Clin North Am 35:301, 2000.
78. Bagshaw, B, and Neill, K: Nurse practitioners and the Internet. Clin Excellence Nurs Pract 4:245, 2000.
79. Conrick, M: Looking for a needle in a haystack: Searching the Internet for quality resources. Contemp Nurse 12:49, 2002.
80. Graves, J: Electronic access to scientific nursing knowledge: The Virginia Henderson International Nursing Library. Semin Oncol Nurs 17:62, 2001.
81. Morris, M, Scott-Findley, S, and Estabrooks, C: Evidence-based nursing web sites: Finding the best resources. AACN Clin Issues 12:578, 2001.
82. Duffy, M: Strengthening communication signals to build a research-based practice. Nurs Health Care 6:238, 1985.
83. American Nurses Association Cabinet on Nursing Research: Guidelines for the Functions of Nurses. Kansas City, MO, American Nurses Association, 1989.
84. McClure, M: Promoting practice-based research: A critical need. J Nurs Adm 11:66, 1981.
85. Oberst, M: Integrating research and clinical practice roles. Topics Clin Nurs 7:45, 1985.
86. Barnard, K: Knowledge for practice: Directions for the future. Nurs Res 29:208, 1980.
87. Engstrom, J: University, agency and collaborative models for nursing research: An overview. Image J Nurs Scholarship 16:77, 1984.
88. Havelock, R, and Havelock, M: Training for Change Agents. Ann Arbor, MI, University of Michigan, 1973.
89. Biddle, W, et al.: An introduction to research: A primer for the nurse anesthetist. AANA J 59:421, 1991.
90. Prichard, L, et al.: The natural connection: The clinical nurse specialist and bedside nursing research. Clin Nurse Specialist 8:307, 1994.
91. Gurka, A: Process and outcome components of clinical nurse specialist consultation. Dimensions Crit Care Nurs 10:169, 1991.
92. Peglow, D, et al.: Evaluation of clinical nurse specialist practice. Clin Nurse Specialist 6:28, 1992.
93. Bloch, D: Evaluation of nursing care in terms of process and outcome: Issues in research and quality assurance. Nurs Res 24:256, 1975.
94. Ford, L: A nurse for all settings: The nurse practitioner. Nurs Outlook 27:520, 1979.
95. Hamric, A: Creating our future: Challenges and opportunities for the clinical nurse specialist. Oncol Nurs Forum 19:11, 1992.
96. Lengacher, C, et al.: Effects of the partners in care practice model on nursing outcomes. Nurs Economics 12:300, 1994.

97. Iezzoni, LI (ed.): Risk Adjustment for Measuring Health Outcomes. Ann Arbor, MI, Health Administration Press, 1994.

98. American Nurses Association: Nursing Care Report Card for Acute Care. Washington, DC, American Nurses Association, 1995.

99. Crummer, M, and Carter, V: Critical pathways: The pivotal tool. J Cardiovasc Nurs 7:30, 1993.

100. Lusk, S, and Kerr, M: Conducting worksite research: Methodological issues and suggested approaches. AAOHN J 42:117, 1994.

101. Corrigan, J, and Nielsen, D: Toward the Development of Uniform Reporting Standards for Managed Care Organizations: The Health Plan Employer Date and Information Set. The Joint Commission Journal on Quality Improvement 19:566, 1993.

102. Delaney, C, et al.: Standardized nursing language for healthcare information systems. J Med Syst 16:145, 1992.

103. Martin, K, Leak, G, and Aden, C: The OMAHA system: A research-based model for decision making. J Nurs Adm 22:47, 1992.

104. McCloskey, J, and Bulechek, G: Validation and coding of the NIC taxonomy structure: Iowa Intervention Project. Image J Nurs Scholarship 27:346, 1995.

105. Cromwell, J: Health professions substitution: A case study of anesthesia. In Osterweis, M, et al. (eds.): The US Health Workforce: Power, Politics and Policy. Washington, DC, Association of Academic Health Centers, 1996.

106. Mead, M: Research: A professional responsibility. Midwives 108:322, 1995.

107. Lehrman, E: A theoretical framework for nurse-midwifery practice. University of Arizona Doctoral Dissertation, 1988. Dissertation Abstracts International, 49–173:5230.

BIBLIOGRAPHY

Quantification and Measurement of Variables
Iezzoni, LI: Risk Adjustment for Measuring Health Care Outcomes. Ann Arbor, MI, Health Administration Press, 1994.
Journal of Nursing Measurement. 536 Broadway, New York, NY 10012, Springer Publishing Co.
Spilker, B (ed.): Quality of Life Assessments in Clinical Trials. New York, Raven Press, 1990.
Waltz, CF, and Strickland, OL (eds.): Measurement of Nursing Outcomes, vols. 1–4. New York, Springer, 1988.
Improved Discrimination in Interpreting Hospital Readmission Data
Farmer, RG, et al.: Hospital readmissions: A re-evaluation of criteria. Cleveland Clin J Med 56:704, 1989.
Case Mix in Ambulatory Care Settings: Ambulatory Care Groups
Parkerson, GR, Broadhead, WE, and Tsa, C-K: Quality of life and functional health of primary care patients. J Clin Epidemiol 45:1303, 1992.
Smith, NS, and Weiner, JP: Applying population-based case mix adjustment in managed care: The Johns Hopkins ambulatory care group system. Managed Care Q 2:21, 1994.
Weiner, JP, et al.: Development and application of a population-oriented measure of ambulatory care case-mix. Med Care 29:452, 1991.
Depression as a Risk Adjustment
Hays, RD, et al.: Functioning and well-being outcomes of patients with depression compared with chronic general medical illnesses. Arch Gen Psychiatry 52:11, 1995.
Mulrow, CD, et al.: Case-finding instruments for depression in primary care settings. Arch Intern Med 122:913, 1995.
Simon, GE, VonKorff, M, and Barlow, W: Health care costs of primary care patients with recognized depression. Arch Gen Psychiatry 52:850, 1995.
Sturm, R, and Wells, KB: How can care for depression become more cost effective? JAMA 273:51, 1995.
Short Forms 12 and 36
McHorney, CA, Kosinski, M, and Ware, JE: Comparisons of the costs and quality of norms for the SF-36 health survey collected by mail versus telephone interview: Results from a national study. Med Care 32:551, 1994.
McHorney, CA, Ware, JE, and Raczek, AE: The MOS 36-item short-form health survey (SF-36): Psychometric and clinical tests of validity in measuring physical and mental health constructs. Med Care 31:247, 1993.
Medical Outcomes Trust, 20 Park Plaza, Suite 1014, Boston, MA 02116–4313; e-mail: motrust@delphi.com
Ware, JE, and Sherbourne, CD: The MOS 36-item short-form health survey (SF-36): Conceptual framework and item selection. Med Care 30:473, 1992.

Measurement of Home Health Outcomes

Adams, CE, Kramer, S, and Wilson, M: Home health quality outcomes: Fee-for-service versus health maintenance organization enrollees. J Nurs Adm 25:39, 1995.

Ellenbecker, CH: Profit and non-profit home health care agency outcomes: A study of one state's experience. Home Health Care Services Q 15(3):47, 1995.

Harris, MD: Clinical and financial outcomes in patient care in a home health care agency. J Nurs Quality Assurance 5:41, 1991.

Martin, KS, Scheet, NJ, and Stegman, MR: Home health clients: Characteristics, outcomes of care, and nursing interventions. Am J Public Health 83:1730, 1995.

Williams, JK: Measuring outcomes in home care: Current research and practice. Home Health Care Services Q 15(3):3, 1995.

General Chapter Support

Phillips, LRF: A clinician's guide to the critique and utilization of nursing research. Norwalk, CT, Appleton-Century-Crofts, 1986. (Note: The author uses the term consumer.)

Titler, MG, and Goode, CJ (eds.): Research utilization. Nurs Clin North Am 30:xv, 1995.

CHAPTER 12

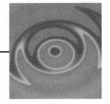

Publishing
Scholarly Works

CHAPTER 12

Suzanne Hall Johnson, MN, RN,C, CNS

Suzanne Hall Johnson, MN, RN,C, CNS, is the Editor Emeritus of *Nurse Author & Editor* and *Dimensions of Critical Care Nursing.* She is Director of Hall Johnson Consulting, where she presents seminars and provides audiotaped courses on professional development topics such as publishing, presenting, consulting, and entrepreneurship for advanced practice nurses. Her e-mail is NurseAuthormail@aol.com

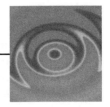

Publishing Scholarly Works

OBJECTIVES

After completing this chapter, the reader will be able to:

1 Differentiate elements of style typically used in papers written to meet academic requirements from those style characteristics of papers composed for publication.

2 Examine opportunities to publish using different formats.

3 Appropriately target and plan an article for publication.

Nurses in advanced practice roles are the clinical leaders who are developing new nursing strategies and knowledge through their clinical research and practice. Chapter 11 emphasized the importance of conducting research on clinical questions and the effectiveness of the advanced practice nurse (APN). However, answers to clinical questions and visions of the valuable aspects of the APN role could remain a secret if the nurse does not publish these results.

In addition to publishing research findings, the APN can publish other types of manuscripts based on clinical practice. Even though quantitative studies are needed to develop nursing theory, qualitative studies have a place in scholarly writing as well. Dr. Kathleen Dracup wrote that "a case study can be considered a study with an 'n' size of one"[1] (p. 2). Indeed, even case study reports can be valuable scholarly work because clinical observations often lead to researchable questions.

Nurse practitioners (NPs), clinical nurse specialists (CNSs), certified nurse midwives (CNMs), and certified registered nurse anesthetists (CRNAs) should consider writing for advanced practice journals as well as for specialty journals. While editing the "Interviews with Editors" column for *Nurse Author & Editor* over the past few years, I have noticed a proliferation of new journals targeted to APNs. All of these journals will be vying for authors.

Also, many specialty journals are looking for articles on the new roles for APNs. For example, *Dimensions of Critical Care Nursing* has published articles about expanded APN roles, such as NPs in intensive care units, CRNAs in postanesthesia units, and CNSs in nurse-run clinics for recently discharged acute care patients. Similarly, the *Journal of Perinatal & Neonatal Nursing* has requested articles on advanced practice roles. APNs who have developed new roles, like those in Chapter 9, could publish these accomplishments in one of many different journals.

All APNs have the same publishing challenge: how to develop a manuscript that will be accepted by the publication. Whether the APN is interested in publishing clinical observations or research, there are two main problems to avoid:

1. Using a school paper style

2. Submitting a thesis

Dr. Florence Downs, a previous editor of *Nursing Research,* mentioned the latter when she advises, "Use the journal style; do not assume the editor will rewrite your thesis to their [sic] style"[2] (p. 160).

You can avoid these two common problems and improve your manuscript's chance of acceptance by:

1. Recognizing the difference between the style for a school paper and the style for a publication

2. Adapting a thesis report to a more concise manuscript style before submitting it

The following sections of this chapter describe specific strategies on what the APN can do to make this transition from school to professional writing. The sections include tips to help the APN make the transition from being a graduate student to a published author. APNs in several roles can use these guidelines for scholarly publication:

- Graduate students can use the publication guidelines to negotiate the style with a course instructor for their next paper. This way, they will gain experience in a professional publication style during their graduate work.
- Faculty members can use the guidelines to teach APN students the publication format so that these students will be able to make the transition to professional publication after graduation.
- APNs in clinical practice can use the guidelines to develop their manuscripts for publication.

AVOIDING THE "SCHOOL PAPER" STYLE REJECTION*

Papers written in a "school paper" style are frequently rejected. As a matter of fact, this is probably the most common reason for rejection when a manuscript is received in the editorial office. Because the school paper problem is obvious on a quick review by the editor, many manuscripts with this problem are rejected outright by the editor. Worse yet, some potential manuscripts are declined at the query letter stage, because it is obvious that the paper will be in a school paper format.

The problem is not that the paper comes from school work; rather, it is the style in which the paper is written. Many papers rejected for school paper style problems were not written for a class; they were written for publication by a nurse who used the last known style—that of school work. New authors are not the only ones who encounter this problem; even experienced authors revert to this past style on occasion.

The school paper style rejection is more serious than it might appear at first. School paper style problems cause frustration for both the author and the editor. It is a major cause of wasted time for the author and of author-editor interpersonal problems. Because a school paper style is very different from most publication styles, the author of a rejected manuscript must take considerable time for a major revision. In addition, when the author does not understand the difference in the publication styles and believes the work is good because of good grades in school, the author can resent the rejection or request for revision.

There are good reasons for the style differences between a school paper and a professional manuscript. One is that the purpose of the school paper is different from that of the professional publication. The purpose of the school paper is for the students to demonstrate their knowledge of theories and work done by previous nursing leaders. This is appropriate for the classroom because part of becoming a professional is to build your ideas on the nursing theory base and to quote professionals' ideas. In more advanced school papers, the students are encouraged to develop their own ideas; still, the paper usually starts with a summary of basic information on that topic.

Another reason for the style differences between the school paper and profes-

---

sional manuscript is that in the school paper, the author is the student, whereas in the professional publication, the author is the expert. The author's goal in a professional publication is to communicate something new (an idea, technique, theory, or research project) that the nurse-reader can use. For a paper on "developing an APN outpatient clinic," the expert is the APN who developed this technique. For a paper on "qualitative research on the experience of family members of patients with Alzheimer's disease," the nurse investigator is the expert. This switch in perspective from student to expert is what makes this style change difficult for most authors.

I often wonder exactly how many new nurse authors with excellent ideas and potential are lost each year because they get a rejection due to this problem and never write again. My experience with CNSs and graduate students indicates that we are losing reports of excellent research because the investigators are not certain how to adapt their theses into articles.

If you have experienced any of the following, you probably had a problem because of a school style:

- A "please-do-not-send it" response (or no response) to a query letter where you mentioned a school paper or a project that you did as a student.

- A quick rejection where you suspected the manuscript did not get through the first review.

- A rejection response with a notation that the paper looked like it was a school project.

- An acceptance with suggestions for revision that included taking out basic information, omitting long quotations, shortening the extensive literature search, reducing the number of references, or editing the style of the references.

- An acceptance, but a surprise at page-proof stage that the editor added a new introduction, took out some material, edited the literature review, changed sentence structure, or rearranged sections.

- A rejected book proposal in which the sample of the author's writing was in a school paper style.

If you have had one or more of these experiences, you are in good company. As all of us learned this paper style first in nursing school, all successful authors have learned how to adapt their style to that used by the professional publications. Most of us learned the hard way, and I was no exception.

Fortunately, I was one of the lucky ones. My first lesson about the difference between school and publication styles came early in my career. My first research-based paper was accepted but revised by the editor. I was fortunate the editor was willing to put in this time to help convert the paper from school to publication style. My paper was from graduate work and was titled "Premature Infant's Reflex Behaviors: Effect on the Mother-Infant Relationship."[3]

Although I knew to adapt the paper to publication style, some school paper style still remained, and it needed editing. My original 15 pages of literature summary on bonding theory from a research grant, which I had already shortened to an introduction of 3 pages in the manuscript, was reduced to 1 paragraph for print.

From that experience, I was determined to learn how to write better so the editor would not have to edit heavily the next time. I knew if the editor revised the paper, it was because I did not write it to the publisher's style in the first place. After the initial shock, I went back and asked myself, Did the editing make my paper better? The answer was, Yes, it did. The paper was more concise, focused on my points better and, to my surprise, I really was the expert on this topic.

Unfortunately, most authors are still learning the hard way, because most editors and experienced authors have not clarified what makes the professional style different. Table 12–1 provides a comparison of school and professional styles.

Every journal and book publisher's style is different, and it is important to follow each one's format. If you have questions about whether an article or book project is appropriate for a particular publication, query the editor about it, and suggest how it would fit into the journal. You can even query the editors directly from a Web site sponsored by *Nurse Author & Editor*. The Web page (http://members. aol.com/suzannehj/hello.htm) will guide you to the ONLINE Nursing Editors'™ page, where you can query many nursing editors.

Some general components of professional writing are similar among all professional nursing publications. These basic similarities apply for clinical or research articles as well as for book or journal formats. Following these eight steps can help convert your paper from school writing style to professional publications style.

Eliminate Basic Material

School papers usually start with a review of basic information. In a professional publication, you do not need to review basic material before you present your key

TABLE 12–1. Comparison of School Paper and Professional-Publication Styles	
School Paper Style	**Professional-Publication Style**
Basic material is covered first.	Content is specific to the level of reader.
Many long quotations are used.	Quotations are rare; when used, are short.
Long literature search is presented in summary form in one section	References are spaced throughout to highlight author's ideas.
Subject of sentence is the name of a person.	Subject of sentence is a key point.
Reference list is exhaustive.	Reference list is selective.
Reference list is in the school's style.	Reference list is in the publication's style.
Research format is used regardless of method.	Research format is used only if author has reliable, valid research.
Main idea is introduced at the end.	Main idea is stated clearly in the first paragraphs.

point. A good policy is to omit all material that the target reader of the journal already knows. For example, if your target audience is the CNS, do not start your paper describing a new independent study course with a discussion about independent study; this audience already knows what that is. Instead, start with the uniqueness of your project because this reader wants to know about the new independent study project you completed. In an article on an ethical dilemma, do not start with a definition of ethics; start with the dilemma. Writing at the audience's level is true for books and articles of all types. For research articles, include key definitions critical to your project or sample selection, but avoid the tendency to include definitions of common terms not specific to your research. For example, if you were describing a statistical test seldom used in nursing studies, you would provide more detail on why it was selected and more references to support it than if you were describing a test frequently used in nursing research and familiar to the audience.

Avoid Long Quotations

Avoid using long quotations in your paper. Although teachers want to make sure you know and can quote authorities, readers want to know what you think. Remember, your readers are busy, experienced nurses who are APNs, clinicians, educators, managers, or researchers, depending on the journal you pick. They probably have already read the primary sources from which you want to quote. Long quotes rarely fit into your point anyway and take the reader off in another direction.

Yes, in professional publications, do build on the work of others, and do give credit to nursing leaders for their initial ideas and material. However, rather than quote them, put your ideas in your own words, and then reference the authorities who agree. Remember, you are the expert, and the readers want to know what *you* think. If they want more detail on what the other nursing leaders said about your topic, they can refer to that person's work in your reference list.

Of course, exceptions to the rule do exist, and sometimes quotations do fit nicely with your topic. For example, short quotations of actual clinical incidents or cases described in the literature would fit well in an article on humor in nursing. However, avoid the tendency to spend the first half of your paper quoting others.

Use Selected References

School papers frequently have long reference lists. It is important for students to research and read all of the publications in their topic area, but you do not need to put all these publications in your paper. Some graduate students believe, because they did that much work, they should at least let their teachers know. Fortunately, faculty are starting to require more of students by requesting that they select only key references. Selecting pertinent references, deciding which are the best ones and determining which ones are valid, can be difficult. It is a higher level of learning than just repeating reference after reference, because it requires selection of key references.[4]

Remember, the audience for professional publications is different from that for school papers. You are writing for the readers, not a teacher. The readers are busy and want you to do some of the work for them; therefore, they are relying on you to refer them to the best references. Authors want guidance for finding the best references when they are seeking additional information on your topic. Even readers of research articles want help in finding the most relevant articles on the problem, instrument, or methods. A list of 150 references after an article is not as helpful as a selected list of the best 50 or even the best 20 references.

One strategy for avoiding the use of too many references is to check on the average number of references used in similar articles, so you know the style of that publication. General clinical journals frequently use only a few references per article, whereas specialty, academic, and research journals may list 50 or more references. However, in most cases, professional articles include fewer references than most school papers or theses.

Synthesize the Past Literature

In addition to having too many references, school papers frequently have a different style for using literature support. School papers usually have a separate literature review section where past publications are summarized one after another. However, most clinical articles and research reports do not have a separate literature section; instead, the authors weave the key concepts that support their ideas throughout the entire paper. In research reports, use references that support the problem, conceptual framework, research methods, and data analysis technique throughout the respective sections of the article rather than create a separate section for a discussion of the literature.

Analysis is the key word here. For almost all professional publications, the author analyzes the literature to show how it fits the idea or research.[5] This subtle change from literature review to synthesis demonstrates the transformation of the author from student to expert.

Use the Reference Style of the Publication

Learning to use precise reference styles is painful. Faculty appropriately take off points on papers for reference lists not in the school's accepted format. This is an important lesson, but sometimes the point behind this practice is unclear. The point is that you must follow a particular reference format precisely, not that you should always use your school's format or that there is only one format.

In fact, there are many formats for references, including the formats of the American Psychological Association (APA)[6] and the American Medical Association (AMA).[7] To determine which format is the right one, study past publications to determine what style they used. Then, use that style as precisely as you did in school.[2]

Avoid Proper Names as Sentence Subjects

Because of the need in school writing to review nursing leaders' work, the subjects of many sentences in school papers are the names of past nursing leaders. For example, one manuscript I recently read had a style similar to this:

Brice suggests that decision-making authority is a key retention factor for APNs. Vandance believes that APNs who participate in decision-making are more likely to stay. Cervente found that 9 out of 10 APNs wanted more decision making. ...

In this example, the subjects are Brice, Vandance, and Cervente. This is appropriate in a literature section of a research report but not in a clinical or project type of article. The main problem is that the writer's idea never surfaced, so the reader is uncertain of the writer's point of view.

In a clinical or project description article, write so that the main point is the subject of the sentence. For example, the sample paragraph above is trying to express some very important (but hidden) points that might be clearer by using "participation" and "projects" as the subjects:

The APN's participation is a key retention factor (Brice, Vandance). Because 9 out of 10 APNs want more decision-making (Cervente), projects that involve delegating decisions can save recruitment and orientation costs by increasing retention.

There are rare exceptions when you want to focus on the person, not the concept. For example, if the person is the main point, then focus on the person by making him or her the subject; otherwise, use the key word from your idea as the subject.

Select the Research Format Carefully

School papers, which are intended to teach the research format, are written with research headings. However, sometimes the research is not reliable or valid, and the author mistakenly tries to publish it in the same research format. Use the research format when the research is reliable and valid, but select a clinical or project type of format when it is not.

For example, if an NP interviewed 10 family members of sudden-death patients in the Emergency Department, selected the family members while working, and had no consistent interviewing tool, then the author should not write the report in a research format. However, this could still be valuable information, and the author might consider selecting one significant case and using a case-study format. Research is a strong format and is essential to building the practice and theory base of nursing, but it should not be used when the project does not meet acceptable research criteria.

I remember that the first article I rejected as a journal reviewer was because of this problem. I empathized with the author because I knew that she had done an interesting project, but she used the wrong format for the paper. I suggested revising using a case study approach, but as commonly happens when a school paper error occurs, the revision was major, and the paper was never revised.

Make Your Idea Clear

Making your idea clear from the start is probably the hardest step in converting to professional writing. Most of us remember writing graduate papers Sunday evening before the Monday class when it was due. Usually, I wrote and wrote and wrote.

When it was about long enough, I ended with the main point as the conclusion. I know that is still done, because I see these papers submitted for publication. They are often rejected because the APN reader does not want to, nor has time to, wander around the subject before getting to the point.

In professional writing, make the point clear from the start. Make sure all paragraphs relate back to that same point. If they do not, omit those paragraphs. Readers should feel they have a good grasp of the main point and that the main point builds throughout the paper. Avoid the tendency to put some new point in a conclusion at the end; instead, reinforce the same key point at the end with which you began. The conclusion should reinforce for the readers that they did indeed understand the main point.

Each journal and book publisher handles these aspects of style differently, so investigate how they are handled in your target publication. By following these steps and the advice of the target journal's editor, APNs can develop a professional style that communicates their professional ideas and reflects their expertise.

ADAPTING THE THESIS STYLE FOR PUBLICATION†

Some APN authors are uncertain what to do with all the information they uncover in their research projects. Some try to put all the information into one manuscript, thus making the manuscript 50 or more pages long with more than 200 references and more than 10 illustrations. These thesis-style articles are usually rejected or, at best, returned for revision.

Probably the reason APNs use thesis style is that it is the most common research style taught to them in their advanced practice work in graduate school. Although this style is excellent for developing a thesis, it is not the style of most research articles published in nursing journals.

Editors and editorial board members can tell quickly when authors have tried to put every detail about their project into one publication. In addition to length, some typing items are a sure sign: very narrow margins, single spacing, and small typeface. When struggling with the problem of getting a 100-page thesis into a publication, some authors try to "squeeze" as much text into as small a space as possible. Those manuscripts are usually rejected.

An even greater problem for the nursing profession is the number of good research projects that are never published. I find more researchers who admit they did not write a manuscript after their project because of a prior rejection. These researchers tell me there are several reasons for this problem, including:

- Loss of interest, often after graduating from school and needing time "away" from the thesis topic
- Wanting to just retype the long thesis report "as is" for publication without having to reorganize the content

---

†Adapted and reprinted with permission from Johnson, SH: Getting your research published: Adapting the thesis style. *Nurse Author & Editor* 2(1):1–4, Winter 1992. Copyright 2004 EBSCO Publishing, Inc. All rights reserved.

- Not knowing where to start to break down the voluminous information to a manageable size for publication

- Failing to plan manuscript development time during the research project

If you are one of these researchers who finds it hard to convert your research project into a publication, the following advice can help. By dividing your topic into sections of manageable size and selecting the right research-based article style for your topic, you will find it easier to write the article and will have a greater chance of acceptance.

Avoid the "All-in-One" Syndrome

First, avoid the feeling that you need to put everything about your project into one manuscript. Most research projects take considerable time to complete, often years. They go through many phases, from development of concept through collection of data to determination of results and consideration of implications. By the time the researcher is finished, she or he knows so much about the topic, it is very difficult to put all the information into an article.

Although journals vary in the lengths of articles, the range is 10 to 20 double-spaced, manuscript pages for most research-based articles. For example, the author guidelines for the *Journal of Gerontological Nursing* recommends 16 pages.[8] That corresponds to approximately 3,200 words at 200 words per page.

When you have accumulated important information, such as a new conceptual framework from your literature review, a valuable research instrument shown to be reliable and valid, or significant results in a comparative study, these items need to be communicated. Publish as you progress through each research phase. Figure 12–1 shows you how to divide a long thesis into parts.

Avoid Duplicate Publication

You should not duplicate articles or even parts of articles; instead, write each one as an original manuscript. The analysis of a new conceptual framework, data on reliability and validity of a new research instrument, and the results of a controlled study all make excellent articles, as long as you do not duplicate information, data, results, or conclusions among them.[9]

This does not mean you "milk" the project for multiple publications by publishing the same research report multiple times or by splitting three hypotheses from one project into three separate articles. These tactics are considered duplicate publication and are unacceptable in nursing publications.

Bailey[10] suggested that there are five levels of duplication, which reflect a range of duplication from identical articles or identical paragraphs (the worst level) to articles with the same message for different disciplines (the least offensive, but still duplication). Davidhizar and Giger [11] suggest authors disclose any type of duplication and seek the advice of the editors of the involved publications.

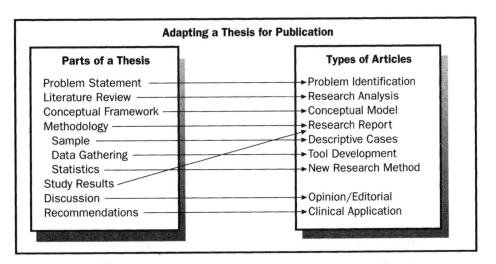

FIGURE 12–1   Model showing how a thesis project has various parts. Arrows show how various steps of a large, unique project might result in different, but not duplicate, publications. Publish articles on valuable steps as they occur, and avoid duplication in later publications.

Identify Valuable Aspects

Identify the truly valuable aspects of your research. Some research projects have several key parts; unfortunately, others have none. A project that included in-depth validity and reliability testing of an instrument plus a descriptive study using that instrument could be developed into two articles: one on the research tool and one on the descriptive study. A project using an already available research instrument on a sample size that is too small or a questionable methodology should not be submitted for publication at all.

Consider Many Article Formats

There are many different types of articles you can write. Review the current journals for articles based on research projects to identify examples of the many different formats. The most common types of articles written from research projects are listed in the following sections.

Problem Identification

Some projects do an excellent job of identifying a problem that was not previously recognized or understood. If your research project highlights a new problem, consider writing a descriptive report about it. For example, one APN wrote about the problem of providing health care to residents in rural settings.

Conceptual Framework and Theory Development

Some early steps in research projects result in new theoretical frameworks. If you analyzed the literature and developed or adapted a new conceptual framework or theory, write an article about it. For example, in the article "Empirical Development of a Middle Range Theory of Caring" in *Nursing Research,* the authors described and validated a new theory of caring.[12] If you applied a theory like one of those in Chapter 4 in a new way, consider writing about this theory application.

Research Analysis

Unique synthesis and analysis of past research are valuable. If you analyzed other research reports on a specific topic in the literature review step of your research, consider writing an article that analyzes that body of research. The article "Continuous S_VO_2 Monitoring" in *Dimensions of Critical Care Nursing* is one of several in the ongoing research-analysis section that includes charts comparing the methods and results of published research reports from acute-care clinical nurse specialists.[13]

Most advanced practice journals publish reports of research. Most even include specific authors' guidelines for articles using the research format. Search the journals, and review descriptions of journals on the Web for their interest in research articles. For example, research formats are mentioned on the Web pages for *Clinical Excellence for Nurse Practitioners: The International Journal of Nurse Practitioner Associates for Continuing Education* at http://www.npace.org/publicat.htm; *The Journal of Midwifery & Women's Health* at http://www.acnm.org; and *The Nurse Practitioner* at http://www.nursingcenter.com (all retrieved April 2004).

Reliable and Valid Instrument

Articles on tool development can be even more valuable than studies using the instrument, because they provide tools for future research. If you demonstrated or confirmed the reliability and validity of a new or classic research tool, write an article as soon as you complete this work. A recent article by Reigel et al. describing the sensitivity of "The Minnesota Living With Heart Failure Questionnaire," which was published in *Nursing Research,* shows how amenable these articles are to publication.[14]

Descriptive Cases

Qualitative studies are a valuable addition to the literature because they add descriptive details about a situation and help identify new research questions. If you have significant descriptive cases, develop an article that includes these case reports. Quotations from case reports of patients in a rehabilitation program regarding the difficulties in making lifestyle changes were used very effectively in the *Nursing Research* article "Empowering Potential: A Theory of Wellness Motivation."[15]

Articles that analyze case situations are not only acceptable, they are requested by most advanced practice journals. Scan the journals, and look for author guidelines that request this format. For example, "scholarly papers" are requested in the author guidelines of the *Australian Journal of Advanced Nursing.*

Research Method

When you have refined a research method, write an article on that procedure. For example, Regina Lederman described how to develop a coding procedure for content analysis in "Content Analysis: Steps to a More Precise Coding Procedure" in *MCN.*[16]

Research Report

One of the most important types of articles for the nursing profession and for building your credibility as a researcher is the research report. The research report describes your research methods and results. If your research project uses credible research methods, write in the format. Usual headings include Introduction, Theoretical Background and/or Literature Review, Hypotheses, Methods, Results, and Discussion and/or Implications.

Although these headings are similar to those used in a thesis, the article covers a different amount of detail in each section. Most articles include extensive details in the Methods and Results sections but use summaries in the other sections and fewer tables than a thesis.

To adapt your research report to a specific journal's style, check the headings and the length of each section in the journal for which you would like to write. Avoid the common misconception that it is best to include all details and tables because the editor can pick what he or she wants; most likely the editor will reject it instead. If you conducted the research in a partnership, and you are coauthoring a report, discuss the research format guidelines with your partner.[17,18]

Research Implications and Clinical Applications

Research projects that have significant implications for nursing practice can result in publications in clinical, education, administration, and research journals. If you have completed a research project similar to those described in Chapter 11, write a detailed article describing the clinical recommendations based on your study. After writing the research report article, consider expanding your recommendations in an article written specifically for the practicing nurse.

Research application articles are printed in most nursing journals. Although they should not duplicate material from your published study, the clinical strategies can reference your previous publication.[9]

Select a Specific Journal

There are many journals focused specifically on advanced nursing roles for which the APN might target a manuscript. Some examples of journals for the nurse practitioner, clinical nurse specialist, nurse midwife, and nurse anesthetist, which are listed in the Cumulative Index to Nursing and Allied Health Literature (CINAHL), are:

- *AACN Clinical Issues: Advanced Practice in Acute and Critical Care*
- *British Journal of Midwifery*
- *Clinical Excellence for Nurse Practitioners*
- *Clinical Nurse Specialist*
- *Complementary Therapies in Nursing and Midwifery*
- *CRNA: The Clinical Forum for Nurse Anesthetists*
- *Current Reviews for Nurse Anesthetists*
- *International Midwifery Matters*
- *Journal of Nurse-Midwifery*
- *Journal of the American Academy of Nurse Practitioners*
- *MIDIRS Midwifery Digest*
- *Midwifery*
- *Midwifery Matters*
- *Midwifery Today* with *International Midwife*
- *Midwives*
- *Nurse Practitioner Forum*
- *Nurse Practitioner: The American Journal of Primary Health Care*
- *Patient Care Nurse Practitioner*

These are examples only, so search for journals in your area, and consider writing for journals that you or your colleagues read; make sure you have the format and target audience that matches your manuscript's plan.

In addition, there are hundreds of clinical, research, theory, administration, education, and review journals in nursing, medical, or health fields for which the APN might target a manuscript. Consider writing for specialty journals as well. For example, an FNP might write an article for the *Journal of School Nursing,* or a CNM might write for *MCN, The American Journal of Maternal Child Nursing.* It is essential to evaluate the style of articles in several recent issues before writing for a journal. Target the article for the audience of the selected journal, and follow the journal's author guidelines. You can find direct links to author guidelines of many nursing journals on the ONLINE Nursing Editors' Web Page, which can be found through a Web search service like www.google.com

Write as Your Project Develops

One of the mistakes of many nurse researchers is to wait until their projects are finished to start thinking about communicating the project. Plan your publications as the project evolves. This way, you will avoid the major problems of being "too tired" from your project to publish it later or seeing it as an "after-the-fact" step in your project. Use project proposals to request time and support for writing. I was granted funding for extra secretarial time for manuscript development in several projects. Many funding sponsors want you to disseminate the information, so they consider the publication step as a legitimate part of the project.

In fact, many articles need to be developed as the project unfolds. For example, if you were doing a project on retention of NPs, you could write an article after each major step in the project. Here are some of the articles:

- After you developed a new model of various NP retention factors based on the literature, you could write the new concept article describing this innovative model.

- When you have analyzed 15 published research studies to determine significant NP retention factors identified in past projects, you could write the research analysis article.

- After testing the validity and reliability of an employee satisfaction tool used in other industries that you applied to NPs, you could write the research instrument article.

- After completing the study showing increased satisfaction of NPs who run their own clinics, you could write the research methods article.

- Finally, after refining your strategy further, you could write a detailed application article with strategies for NP retention for an advanced practice nursing or administrative journal.

Write a Research-Based Book

If your research projected is comprehensive and all phases of the project are valuable for clinicians and researchers, consider writing a book. If you have strong answers to questions like "why this book" and "what makes this book special," you can use these answers to draft a book proposal.[19] The popular book *Coping with Reality Shock* by Claudia Schmalenberg and Marlene Kramer was based on experiences from a research project.[20]

When I wanted to publish a new family assessment tool, detailed case examples, and multiple strategies for working with high-risk families from experiences in a research project, I chose to combine them in a book. I had already published the research report article, but I wanted to share the clinical cases and intervention tools, which would not fit in an article. These original sections based on research might have contributed to the book, *High-Risk Parenting: Nursing Assessment and Strategies for the Family at Risk* (JB Lippincott, Philadelphia, 1994), being selected by the *American Journal of Nursing* for the Book of the Year award.

APNs have many ideas, clinical experiences, and research scenarios that might fit into a book. If you select the book format, you still need to reorganize your work, because even research-based books seldom use the thesis format.

Writing a research-based book is similar to the research experience; both processes have many distinct steps. Break your research project into parts, and convert key accomplishments into chapters as you complete each milestone in the project.

SUMMARY

APNs have valuable clinical experiences to share with colleagues and have findings from research projects that can help build nursing theory. By distinguishing between school and publication formats and adapting the thesis style to a journal or book format, APNs can succeed in publishing their work and help build advanced practice nursing theory.

SUGGESTED EXERCISES

All of the following suggested exercises lend themselves to student peer review. Students can perform blind peer review by selecting a special code number and having their papers refereed by other students or faculty. Students review according to criteria developed for the assignment. Students can be evaluated not only on their written products but also on their ability to provide constructive critique to others and by developing criteria for the peer-review process.

1 From the published theses or dissertations available in the library, select one on a topic that is of interest to you. The literature section constitutes an entire chapter.
   a. Rewrite the literature review, consolidating it into two to three double-spaced pages.
   b. Develop the focus (that is, the purpose and article title) for two to three individual articles, with content that does not duplicate each other, which could be constructed from the thesis or dissertation.

2 Select multiple examples of direct quotations (preferably something in block form or a section of text that employs extensive use of direct quotations) from published source documents, and paraphrase the citation, giving appropriate credit using your school's publication style guidelines or author guidelines from a selected journal.

3 Plan a paper in the format of an article to be submitted for publication.
   a. Locate the ONLINE Nursing Editors' Web Page or similar listing of nursing journals on the Web. Use a search engine to find the Web page.
   b. Select a journal that you would target for the article, justifying why it is appropriate. Obtain that journal's Guidelines for Authors from the Web.
   c. Conduct a review of the article topics that appeared in the previous year of the selected journal, and draw conclusions about the timeliness, fit, and style of your topic in comparison with the articles already printed.
   d. Write a cover letter, abstract, biographical sketch, or similar elements as dictated by the guidelines, and develop a topical outline or draft of your article to submit to the class or faculty for review.

REFERENCES

1. Johnson, SH: Strengthening your case study approach. Nurse Author Editor 2:2, 1992.
2. Johnson, SH: Adapting a thesis to publication style: Meeting editors' expectations. Dimens Crit Care Nurs 15:160, 1996.
3. Johnson, SH: Premature infant's reflex behaviors: Effect on the mother-infant relationship. J Obstet Gynecol Neonatal Nurs 4:15, 1975.

4. Brooks-Brunn, JA: Tips on writing a research-based manuscript: The review of literature. Nurse Author Editor 1:1, 1991.
5. Heinrich, KT: Slant, style, and synthesis: 3 keys to a strong literature review. Nurse Author Editor 12:1, 2002.
6. American Psychological Association (APA): Publication Manual of the American Psychological Association, 5th ed. Washington, DC, American Psychological Association, 2001.
7. Iverson, C, et al: American Medical Association Manual of Style, 9th ed. Baltimore, Williams & Wilkins, 1997.
8. Information for authors: Journal of Gerontological Nursing. Thorofare, NJ, Slack Inc. Retrieved July 18, 2002, from http://www.slackinc.com/allied/jgn/jgninfo.htm
9. Johnson, SH: Duplicate publication part 2: A case analysis. Nurse Author Editor 12:7, 2002.
10. Bailey, BJ: Duplicate publication in otolaryngology (abstract). In Proceedings of the First International Congress on Peer Review in Biomedical Publication. Chicago: IL, American Medical Association, May 1989.
11. Davidhizar, R, and Giger, JN: Duplicate publication part 1: Consideration of the issues. Nurse Author Editor 12:1, 2002.
12. Swanson, K: Empirical development of a middle range theory of caring. Nurs Res 40:161, 1991.
13. Copel, LC, and Stolarik, A: Continuous S_VO_2 monitoring. Dimens Crit Care Nurs 10:202, 1991.
14. Riegel B, et al: The Minnesota living with heart failure questionnaire: Sensitivity to differences and responsiveness to intervention intensity in a clinical population. Nurs Res 51:209, 2002.
15. Fleury, JD: Empowering potential: A theory of wellness motivation. Nurs Res 40:286, 1991.
16. Lederman, RP: Content analysis: Steps to a more precise coding procedure. MCN 16:275, 1991.
17. Engebretson, J, and Wardell, DW: The essence of partnership in research. J Prof Nurs 13:38, 1997.
18. Giefer, C: Publication of a thesis: The relationship between graduate student and thesis advisor. Nurse Author Editor 6:7, 1996.
19. London, F: Writing a book proposal: Using a question approach. Nurse Author Editor 12:7, 2002.
20. Schmalenberg, C, and Kramer, M: Coping with reality shock. Gaithersburg, MD: Aspen Publishers Inc., 1979.

(Note: All product, journal, company, Web, and other names are the trademark or registered trademark of the respective company, and all are the responsibility of the respective company. Journals listed are for examples only and are not intended to be the exhaustive list of possible journals for which the APN can write. Contact the editor of the target journal for guidance on your specific idea.)

CHAPTER 13

Legal and Ethical Aspects of Advanced Practice Nursing

Linda Callahan, PhD, CRNA
Mary Jeanette Mannino, JD, CRNA

Linda Callahan, PhD, CRNA, received her nursing education at Rockingham Community College, Wentworth, North Carolina, and her anesthesia education at the Anesthesia Program for Nurses, North Carolina Baptist Hospital, Bowman Gray School of Medicine, in Winston-Salem, North Carolina. Dr. Callahan received her bachelor of science in biology from Guilford College, Greensboro, North Carolina, as well as a master of arts in education and a master of science in nursing from California State University in Long Beach. She completed her doctorate in educational research and evaluation at Florida State University in Tallahassee. Dr. Callahan has a broad base of practice experience as an educator, clinician, administrator, and consultant. She has written numerous publications and is widely known as a continuing education lecturer in anesthesia and the sciences. She is past president of the American Association of Nurse Anesthetists (1993–1994). Dr. Callahan is Associate Professor in the Department of Nursing, California State University, and remains active as a clinical anesthetist.

Mary Jeanette Mannino, JD, CRNA, combines an independent anesthesia practice with medical-legal and business consulting. She is a graduate of George Washington University in Washington, DC, with a bachelor of science in anesthesia, and Irvine University School of Law. Ms. Mannino's professional activities include having served as a president of the American Association of Nurse Anesthetists in 1987–1988. She has been recognized for outstanding contributions to the profession, as the recipient of the Agatha Hodgins Award in 1996. She has written two books, *The Nurse Anesthetist and the Law* and *The Business of Anesthesia: Practice Options for Nurse Anesthetists*. She has also been editor of several journals and publications for nurse anesthetists. Her professional career has included work as an educator, manager, and clinical anesthetist. Ms. Mannino currently practices anesthesia in ambulatory surgery in her own corporation, The Mannino Group.

Legal and Ethical Aspects of Advanced Practice Nursing

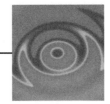

CHAPTER OBJECTIVES

After completing this chapter, the reader will be able to:

1 Interpret components of his or her state's nurse practice act, which define the legal scope of practice, need for collaboration, and prescriptive authority for a specific type of advanced practice.

2 Articulate the concepts of duty, standard of care, causation, and damage as applied to professional negligence in advanced practice nursing.

3 Demonstrate techniques for ethical decision-making by application of a specific decision model as well as by analysis of the process of model application.

4 Discuss ethical issues currently of concern to advanced practice nurses (APNs).

5 Incorporate knowledge about caring as an ethical concept into the development of personal moral agency within a managed care setting.

As advanced practice nursing has continued to evolve to new and exciting heights, legal issues have become increasingly important to the practitioner, the state, and, of course, the patient. The expansion of nursing practice into areas once considered the exclusive domain of medicine and the independence of APNs lead to questions of legality, standards of practice, and the legendary "turf battles." Unfortunately plaintiffs' attorneys have already recognized nonphysician providers as fair game. For example, even the best prepared midwives may become involved in cerebral palsy/fetal asphyxia cases, and nurse practitioners are targets for failure to diagnose various cancers.[1] The law, including statutory, regulatory, and case law, moves independently from science; therefore, it may be years before a concept becomes law and legal rulings become precedent. With that in mind, APNs should look at rulings in other related fields to better understand the legality of their practices.

Nurse anesthesia has set some legal trends for other APNs. Although obvious differences exist between nurse anesthetists, nurse midwives, clinical nurse specialists, and nurse practitioners, most of the case law that sets precedent has been from the anesthesia portion of advanced practice nursing. The legal aspects of nurse anesthesia practice have been an area of discussion, myths, political activity, and clinical concerns for as long as the profession has existed. The legal definition of nonphysician anesthesia practitioners, the role of advanced practice nursing, state nurse practice acts, and federal legislation continue to be debated in legal and political arenas. Likewise, medical malpractice concerns and the issue of vicarious liability accompany the nurse anesthetist to the operating room (OR) every day.

Even though nurses have been administering anesthesia for more than 100 years, there have been constant legal challenges to the practice, for example, whether nurse anesthesia constitutes the illegal practice of medicine. These challenges continue in various formats and have been expanded to encompass all APNs.

The American legal system functions at several levels, including laws enacted by the state and federal legislative branches, regulations at the executive levels, and the common-law system based on precedent. The legal authorization for all of nursing practice is found in nurse practice acts; state health and safety codes; other professional practice acts, including those of medicine, dentistry, and podiatry; and federal medical laws and cases that interpret those laws. Judicial decisions on vicarious liability and professional negligence are important in identifying the standards of practice of the profession and set a precedent for future decisions.

It is important for the reader to understand that each state has the constitutional right to set its own laws and legal process. The cases presented in this chapter and elsewhere should be evaluated with that understanding. However, to complicate the issue, one state's courts will review similar rulings in other states when formulating its opinions.

NURSE PRACTICE ACTS

Each state has the obligation to protect the health and safety of its citizens. By various statutes, the state attempts to assure the public that a professional who is granted a license has met the qualifications and scope of practice as defined by the legislature. The nurse practice act is the prevailing state law that defines the practice for registered professional nurses. In recent years, recognition has been given to APNs based on education, skills and, frequently, certification. The majority of the states recognize advanced practice nursing, but there is no uniformity to their laws, with every state using different or unique language in framing its law. Generally, the advanced practice portions of the nursing statutes contain:

- Definition of advanced practice
- Legal scope of practice
- Educational requirements
- Collaboration and consultation requirements

Prescriptive authority may also be codified in this area of the nurse practice act, but this practice varies from state to state (Tables 13–1 and 13–2).

Historically, many states have considered advanced practice nursing to encompass nurse anesthetists, nurse midwives, and nurse practitioners, but a recent trend in advanced practice nursing has been the formal recognition and definition of scope of practice of the clinical nurse specialist (CNS) in state laws. The implementation of the role is subject to any number of interpretations and refinements. The traditional academic preparation of the CNS includes preparation as a clinician in a

TABLE 13–1. Summary of Legal Authority for the Scope of Practice of the Nurse Practitioner

	Specific States
States with NP title protection through the Board of Nursing: 1. Board of Nursing has sole authority in scope of practice 2. No requirement for physician collaboration, direction, or supervision	AK, AR, AZ, CO, DC, HI, IA, KS, KY, ME, MI, MT, ND, NH, NJ, NM, OK, OR, RI, TX, UT, WA WI, WV, WY
States with NP title protection through the Board of Nursing: 1. Board of Nursing has sole authority in scope of practice 2. Physician collaboration requirement is present	CT, DE, IL, IN, LA, OH, MD, MN, MO, NE, NV, NY, VT
States with NP title protection through the Board of Nursing: 1. Board of Nursing has sole authority in scope of practice 2. Physician supervision requirement is present	CA, FL, GA, ID, MA, SC
Scope of NP practice is authorized conjointly by the Board of Nursing and the Board of Medicine	AL, MS, NC, PA, SD, VA
State without NP title protection where APN functions under a broad nurse practice act	TN

Note: Each state should be contacted to ascertain varying requirements, if present, for other APNs (clinical nurse specialists, certified nurse midwives, and certified registered nurse anesthetists) (Adapted from Pearson, L. [2002]. Fourteenth Annual Legislative Update. The Nurse Practitioner 27[1]: 12.)

TABLE 13–2. Summary of Prescriptive Authority Legislation for Nurse Practitioners	
States where nurse practitioners can prescribe: 1. Including controlled substances, and 2. Independent of requirements for physician involvement in prescriptive authority	***Specific States*** AK, AZ, DC, IA, ME, MT, NH, NM, OR, UT*, WA, WI, WY
States where nurse practitioners can prescribe: 1. Including controlled substances, but 2. Requiring some amount of physician involvement or delegation of prescriptive authority	AR, CA, CO, CT, DE, GA, HI, ID, IL, IN, KS, LA, MA, MD, MI, MN, NC, ND, NE, NJ, NV, NY, OH, OK, PA, RI, SC*, SD, TN, VA, VT, WV
States where nurse practitioners can prescribe: 1. Excluding controlled substances, and 2. Requiring some amount of physician involvement or delegation of prescription writing	AL, FL, KY, MO, MS, TX
States where nurse practitioners cannot prescribe and/or do not have authorized ability to receive and/or dispense pharmaceutical samples	None

*Schedule IV and V controlled substances only
Note: Each state should be contacted to ascertain varying requirements, if present, for other APNs (certified clinical specialists, certified nurse midwives, and certified registered nurse anesthetists). (Adapted from: Pearson, L. [2002]. Fourteenth Annual Legislative Update. The Nurse Practitioner. 27[1]: 15.)

specialized area: educator, administrator, consultant, researcher, change agent, and case manager. Although the educational level has been variable, master's degree preparation is supported by the Federal Balanced Budget Act of 1997, which defines a CNS as a registered nurse who is licensed to practice nursing in the state in which the services are performed and who holds a master's degree in a defined clinical area of nursing from an accredited educational institution.[2] In addition to graduating from an appropriate educational program, completing the requirements for certification from a national specialty body and being recognized as an APN by a state agency, such as the Board of Nursing, are more frequently becoming prerequisites for employment and enjoyment of a full scope of practice. Managed care entities often use credentialing as a mechanism for establishing provider panel membership. Based on credentialing status, CNSs may be able to seek provider status for reimbursement purposes from public and private insurers.[3]

The desire for peer review, self-regulation, and assurance of quality patient care are all part of the motivation for credentialing and privileging processes. However, other forces also have led many states and professional organizations to attempt to validate practitioner qualifications and ongoing competence. One of these external forces is the National Practitioner Data Bank (NPDB), which was established in 1986 to collect and release information related to the competence and professional conduct of physicians, dentists, and "other healthcare practitioners." The NPDB is a federal repository for data related to malpractice settlements and adverse actions against licensure or clinical privileges. The purpose is to prevent health care practitioners from changing locations without disclosure of previous misconduct or incompetence. In the case of APNs, only medical malpractice payments must be reported to the NPDB. It is optional for a state board of nursing to report any action against the license of an APN. A practitioner may query the data bank, and although a report, if present, may not be deleted, the practitioner may request correction of any inaccuracies and submit a personal statement to be filed with the report. State licensing boards, hospitals, and other health care institutions have access to information in the data bank. Under certain circumstances, plaintiffs' attorneys may obtain data bank information, but members of the public, medical malpractice insurers, and defense attorneys may not. The data bank helpline may be reached at 1-800-767-6732. States vary in their requirements for submission of similar information on APNs for storage in state data banks.[4,5]

PROFESSIONAL NEGLIGENCE (MALPRACTICE)

If a patient suffers harm from the actions of an APN or any other health care professional, the legal theory that usually applies is the tort concept of negligence. Tort law recognizes the responsibility of an individual to act in the way an "ordinary, reasonable person" would under similar circumstances. A deviation from, or breach of, this reasonable person standard is considered actionable under the rules of negligence. The term *malpractice* has been used to encompass all liability-producing conduct by professionals.

For an action to be considered negligent, the following components must be present and established by the plaintiff:

- Duty
- Standard of care
- Causation
- Damages

Duty

To be held liable for professional negligence, it must first be established that the APN owed a duty to the injured party. This may be established under contract theory or, most frequently, by a professional-patient relationship. The legal issue is whether an APN has a legal duty to the patient, when this duty starts, and when it ends.

In *Ascher v Gutierrez,* the precedent was set for the time component of duty as it relates to anesthesia cases. There is not much direction from the courts on when the duty begins in anesthesia; however, it is generally considered to be when the anesthesia professional begins the continual care of the patient. When the legal duty ends has been addressed by the courts in the following case:

> The facts as reported in the court decision show that the patient was an 18-year-old female admitted to Columbia Hospital for Women in Washington, DC, for dilatation and

curettage. Thiopental was administered, and shortly thereafter the patient developed a laryngospasm. Attempts to relax the spasm manually and by injections were unsuccessful. An endotracheal tube was inserted, but the patient was cyanotic, hypotensive, and ultimately had severe disabling brain damage.

There was considerable dispute regarding the presence of the anesthesiologist in the OR at the time of the incident. The anesthesiologist claimed he left the OR shortly after injecting the thiopental but only after being relieved by another anesthesiologist. The plaintiff showed that the other anesthesiologist was administering an anesthetic in another section of the hospital when the incident occurred and could not have relieved on the case.

The court ruled that once a physician enters into a professional relationship with a patient, he is not at liberty to terminate the relationship at will. The relationship will continue until it is ended by one of the following circumstances: (1) the patient's lack of need for further care, or (2) withdrawal of the physician upon being replaced by an equally qualified physician. The court ruled that withdrawal from the case under other circumstances constitutes a wrongful abandonment of the patient and if patient suffers any injury as a proximate result of such abandonment, physician is liable.

The plaintiff was awarded $1,550,000.

Ascher v Gutierrez, 533 F2d 1235 (DC Cir), add 175 US 100 (1976)

Standard of Care

Negligence law, in general, presupposes some uniform standards of behavior against which a defendant's conduct is to be evaluated. Members of the health care professions are expected to possess skill and knowledge in the practice of their profession beyond that of ordinary individuals and to act in a manner consistent with that added capability.

Formulation of the standard of care by which an APN is evaluated is complex when it is considered that an identifying characteristic of any professional group is its inherent right to direct and control its activities.

The standards by which an APN will be judged usually come from expert testimony and standards established by the profession. The judicial system recognizes that juries are composed of lay people with limited or no knowledge of medical activities. For that reason, expert witnesses, who are members of the profession, are asked to testify about the standard of care. The rationale is that all professionals should be held to the same level of skill as their peers.

Most professional organizations have formulated and published standards of practice for the profession. It is likely that those standards would be admitted into evidence in a negligence action and, although not conclusive of the standards of practice, would carry some authority.

Locality Rule

Historically, the defined standards of care for the medical profession were limited to a specific geographic setting. This narrow ruling was interpreted to mean that one had to practice in terms of the standard of practice in one's community. However, the strict locality rule proved to be impractical and severely limited the pool of expert witnesses. The courts considered the fact that modern communications have expanded access to information and modified the rule to include practice in the "same or a similar locality."

In more recent years, the locality rule has undergone continued scrutiny by the courts, and in most jurisdictions the standard has been expanded from a local level to a national level. For that reason, it is imperative that APNs remain current in state-of-the-art practice for the entire country because they will be held accountable for practice consistent with a national standard.

Causation

In malpractice actions, the plaintiff must establish that the alleged negligent act of the defendant caused the injury. This element of negligence, called causation, is an important factor in malpractice cases. Proof of causation may be based on direct testimony, usually from expert witnesses.

The two most common tests to establish causation are classified as "but for" and "substantial factor." In the former, the plaintiff must prove that it was more probably true than not that the patient's injury would not have occurred but for the defendant's action. The latter test requires that the defendant's conduct was a substantial factor in producing the injury. The standard most commonly applied to causation requires that the patient's injury has been "more likely than not" the result of the defendant's conduct.

Multiple causation can present difficulties in malpractice cases. The cause of the injury frequently is not easily determined to be due to a single factor. An example of this can be seen in anesthesia cases in which a patient dies from hypovolemia. Was the cause of the death due to errors in surgical technique or failure of the anesthetist to adequately monitor and replace lost fluid? A plaintiff's attorney usually will attempt to ascertain multiple causation so that many defendants will be contributing to the damage awards.

Damages

The final element necessary for actionable negligence is damages. This term generally refers to the loss or injury suffered. Damages are usually categorized as special, general, and punitive.

The purpose of compensatory damages is to make an appropriate, and usually counterbalancing, payment to the plaintiff for an actual loss or injury sustained through the act or default of the defendant, thereby "making the plaintiff whole" as much as possible. General damages are those that flow from the wrong complained of and are often known as "pain and suffering." As a result of tort reform legislation seen recently in many states, a cap to general damages has been set by the legislatures. This cap is generally $150,000 to $250,000. Special damages are the actual monetary value of the negligent act and are reflected in such awards as additional money for hospital bills because of anticipated custodial care for life. Punitive or exemplary damages are awarded as punishment to the defendants for acts that the jury considers to be aggravated, willful, or wanton. Punitive damages are awarded or withheld at the discretion of the jury.

Wrongful Death

When a patient dies as the result of negligent acts of the provider, the survivors may collect for wrongful death. A number of states have wrongful death statutes that establish the bases for recovery and the maximum amount of damages that may be awarded.

The issue of recovery for loss of life's pleasures and a wrongful death action were addressed in this Pennsylvania case involving a nurse anesthetist.

> A 5-year-old child, in excellent health, was admitted for a T & A [tonsillectomy and adenoidectomy]. A nurse anesthetist supervised by an anesthesiologist administered the anesthetic. During the procedure, the anesthesiologist was called to an emergency in another OR. When he returned, he noticed the child was cyanotic with no apparent heartbeat. The nurse anesthetist was still administering a full concentration of anesthetic agent and was not using precordial monitoring. Emergency resuscitation restored the patient's heartbeat, but because of the prolonged cardiac arrest, he suffered severe damage and died several weeks later.
>
> The child's father filed suit on behalf of his son's estate for wrongful death. The jury awarded the estate $455,199 and the hospital appealed.
>
> The Pennsylvania Supreme Court ruled on the trial judge's instructions to the jury on the amount of damages. The trial court instructed the jury that it could consider pain and suffering and compensate for loss of future earnings and loss of amenities or pleasures of life. In the higher court's ruling, they said loss of life's pleasures or amenities is one of the elements of recovery for wrongful death and survival.
>
> Willinger v Mercy Catholic Medical Center of Southern Pennsylvania, A2d 1188 (Pa 1978)

Proof of Professional Negligence

Except for certain exceptions, expert testimony is required to establish the appropriate standard of care in professional negligence cases. Both the plaintiff and the defendant rely on the testimony of expert witnesses to prove or to defend their case. Experts may also be used to determine causation and damages. To qualify as an expert witness, a person must possess qualifications and be knowledgeable in the area in question. The federal rules of evidence indicate that an expert is qualified by "knowledge, skill, experience, training, and education."

Possible Exceptions to Expert Witness Requirement

Expert testimony is the primary method for establishing the standard of care for professionals. There are, however, exceptions to this rule, which have a direct application to advanced nursing practice.

Package Inserts and Manufacturer's Instructions

Whether package inserts of drugs or manufacturer's instructions regarding use of equipment should be admissible as evidence of the standard of care is an interesting and a complex question. It is often common practice to use drugs in ways that deviate from the package inserts. The clinician is well aware that package inserts and other drug information protect the manufacturer and can be interpreted as being restrictive in practical situations.

Most courts hold that manufacturer's recommendations are at least admissible as evidence of the standard of care. However, they have seldom, if ever, been considered conclusive. A number of courts have upheld the admissibility of manufacturer's instructions when they are properly validated or refuted by an expert witness. It appears that most courts would not accept a manufacturer's recommendations and package inserts as conclusive evidence of the standard of care. Although the instructions would probably be admitted into evidence, expert witnesses would be called to reinforce the standard of practice.

Medical Literature

The rules of evidence clearly regard the use of textbooks, periodicals, and other literature as hearsay; thus, medical literature is not admissible as direct evidence to prove the statements it contains. The arguments against using this literature for establishing conclusive evidence of the standard of care are many and include the following:

- The author may not be present.
- There is no opportunity for cross-examination.
- The literature may be out of date.

It has been recommended that a more sensible view would be to hold medical literature as admissible under limited circumstances. When a conflict exists between the medical treatise and the standards established by expert witnesses, a good approach would hold both sources admissible as evidence. The jury or the judge could then determine which source was most probative.

Other methods of establishing standard of care include standards and guidelines published by a professional organization, departmental policies, and statutes. Except for nurse anesthetists, there have been few negligence cases against APNs that have appellate court rulings setting legal precedents. It is hoped that the reason is that there are few negligence cases against APNs and not that the law moves at a slow pace.

MALPRACTICE INSURANCE

Along with the independence of advanced practice nursing and the high level of knowledge and skill required, it follows that the responsibility and accountability of advanced practice lead to a greater risk of being sued. For that reason, APNs should be covered for professional negligence through an insurance program.

The employment status of the APN is important in determining whether to purchase an individual policy. Under the laws of agency, the employer is responsible for the acts of its employees and, as such, is responsible to defend and pay damages in a lawsuit occurring under the auspices of that employment. If the APN is self-employed or uncertain of adequate coverage by the employer, it may be advisable that the APN purchase an individual policy. The cost of malpractice insurance depends on the type of practice and its potential for liability claims. Nurse anesthesiology and nurse midwifery are the areas of highest malpractice insurance premiums; however, nurse practitioner malpractice insurance premiums have increased markedly in the past year.

THE PATIENT AND THE APN

We must not lose sight of the patient in all of the discussion of nursing theory, critical learning, and legal standards. Most nurse practitioners select the advanced practice model because they enjoy caring for patients and, in the end, concerns for patients' health and well-being and for delivery of high quality care are the highest priorities. For that reason, the integration of legal and ethical principles into clinical practice is paramount and serves as the focus of this chapter.

Nurses tend to view legal issues from a paternalistic rather than a practical standpoint. Frequently, they want to quote a law to justify a practice, when the law is rarely specific and is open to interpretation, modification, and reversal. It is much more practical for individual APNs to use knowledge of applicable laws, regulations, and standards to determine how to manage their practice, to expect adequate reimbursement, and then to go about doing what they know and love: providing high quality patient care.

PROFESSIONAL ETHICS

The branch of philosophy called ethics, or moral philosophy, deals with questions of human conduct. The word *ethics* is derived from the Greek *ethos,* meaning customs, habitual usages, conduct, and character. Ethics is concerned with defining the moral dimension of life in terms of duties, responsibilities, conscience, justice, and other societal concerns and issues. The stated fact that is nonethical in content is concerned with the "is" of the actions, whereas an ethical judgment concerns the "why" of the actions.[6]

Ethical thinking is shaped by our worldview, which is in turn shaped by all the other dimensions of our existence. Today, the tendency is to separate ethics from traditional moral or religious beliefs. This is probably not entirely possible because every ethical system seems to raise questions about the worldview on which it is based.[7] Even though the world's great religions disagree in many ways, all attempt to point mankind to what lies beyond. Smart[7] stated that perhaps what is needed is "transcendental humanism." He defined this as valuing human welfare and seeing this welfare in the light of an eternal vision—that is, the sense of the beyond allowing one to see anew the sacredness of the person.

To think ethically requires defining the characteristics of an ethical problem. Rational choices are based on factual information but are always somewhat subjective; that is, they involve value judgment and, hence, the potential for value conflict.

This is also a necessary characteristic of an ethical problem. Of necessity, the concept of choice involves freedom, or the ability to make a choice, and responsibility for both right and wrong actions. Choice requires reasoning and decision-making. The unity of knowing and valuing that constitutes an individual is used when human beings make choices, especially when the choices are difficult or perplexing.

Reaching answers to ethical problems will have profound and far-reaching effects on one's perception of:

- The rights of human beings
- Relationships among human beings
- The relationship of human beings to society
- The relationship of human beings to the world

Although difficult, such judgments tend to establish precedent and justification for future activity. The decision may serve as a model for future behavior.

Bioethics is the marriage of ethics and science. It is important for APNs to determine when a decision is a matter of clinical judgment rather than an ethical issue. Ethical reasoning, unlike scientific reasoning, cannot be supported by definitive proof about what is the right or wrong action in a given situation. McManus[6] noted that ethics serves as a guide to the development of a "well-traveled trail" that may lead to better behavior and better actions among people. The APN is often faced with concerns and conflicts among the practice of value-based clinical ethics, business ethics, and social ethics.[8] Different concerns, questions, and conflicts arise in each (Table 13–3). Current Web-based sources for further discussions of nursing ethics are in Table 13–4.

TABLE 13–3. Three Dimensions that Impact the Practice of Value-Based Ethics

Dimensions of the Workplace	Value-Based Questions of Concern to the Specific Dimension
1. Clinical ethics	What judgments about clinical behaviors can be made in light of the relationship of the nurse to the patient? What are the ethical demands and limits of service and staffing? How are these known and agreed upon or established? What are the ethical obligations of the nurses or institution to meet the needs of individuals or families? When are needs ethically not met?
2. Business ethics	What is the obligation of the institution to act in ways that respect the rights, dignity, and values of caretaker and client? What are the duties of the trustees, managers, and other workers as they interact with individuals and social groups?
3. Social ethics	How does the organization meet the needs of its community? How does the organization carry out tasks with providers, payers, regulators, and other entities in health care? How does this affect the larger society?

Adapted from Cofer, MJ: Thoughts on ethics: Value-based ethics in the workplace. VA Nurses Today 8:12, 2000.

TABLE 13–4. Web Sites Devoted to Nursing Ethics	
Source	*Web Site*
ANA Center for Ethics and Human Rights	http://www.nursingworld.org/ethics/
Boston College School of Nursing	http://www.bc.edu/bc_org/avp/son/ethics/ethicsmain.html
Nurse Friendly Site	http://www.nursefriendly.com/nursing/directpatientcare/ethics.htm
Center for Applied and Professional Ethics	http://cape.cmsu.edu/nursing/nursing.asp
Nursing Ethics: An International Journal for Health Care Professionals	http://www.arnoldpublishers.com/Journals/Journpages/09697330.htm
Technology's Dark Side	http://www.curtincalls.com/Ethics/March_2001_ethics.htm

Adapted from Sullivan, BH: Linkages: Web sites devoted to nursing ethics. Wash Nurse 31:38, 2001.

Historical Perspectives

In 1937, C.A. Aikens[9] wrote *Studies in Ethics for Nurses* and included chapters devoted to truth in nursing reports, discretion in speech, obedience, teachability, respect for authority, discipline, and loyalty. Such early works focused on the morality of the individual and on the nurse's duties, obligations, and loyalties.

The American Medical Association (AMA) adopted a Code of Ethics in 1847 when the organization was formed. This was a hallmark event, because before this time there was no regulation of professional behavior. The AMA's initial Code of Ethics dealt with the relationships of physicians to each other, to the patient, and to the public. Revisions followed with continual emphasis on professional conduct. Over time, this activity helped to solidify the idea that medicine was a dignified and honorable calling. Professional codes of ethics generally call for a covenant, or an agreement, between the client and the provider and are considered today as a social contract.[6]

The contrast in ethical development between medicine and nursing has often been remarkable. This is due largely to the fact that nursing has historically been allied to the ideal of treating the person rather than the disease. From this belief, the notion of the superiority of prevention over cure developed. Medicine, on the other hand, has historically emphasized curing as a response to the presence of disease. The APN is often called on to combine the concerns of both perspectives. Complex technological problems, new legal issues, and new economic situations offer a challenging context for ethical thinking and behavior for today's APN.

Ethical Principles

All ethical problems involve moral principles. Such principles are necessary to provide guidance for thought because universal solutions cannot be reached in most ethical dilemmas that can be rotely applied to another problem. Each ethical problem must be examined in the context of the particular circumstances. There are four guiding principles that are important in bioethics:

1. Self-determination
2. Nonmaleficence
3. Beneficence
4. Justice

Self-determination, or autonomy, is a basic social value. An autonomous act is an act of intention that is independent of coercion by others. This moral right was defined by Callahan[9] as follows:

> The right to control one's body and one's treatment and the emphasis given to self-determination, privacy, freedom, and autonomy. The emphasis on not being deceived and being given complete and truthful information all point to an important aspect of a rights-based view, namely the role of an individual patient's will in individual decision making. (p. 19)

Those giving care must acknowledge and respect the autonomy of each client. It may be argued that the only permissible reason to remove a person's social or personal autonomy is to prevent harm to others. Respect for the client's autonomy and the opportunity for professional autonomy in medical practice involve possession of the threshold element of competence, the disclosure of information, and consent without duress. The presence of these three elements imposes an order on conflicting claims and offers finality, which is often sufficiently strong to override the law and prevailing custom.[6]

As a result of the Karen Anne Quinlan case of 1976 and the Nancy Cruzan case of 1989, focus on the autonomous rights of the patient has sharpened. These two cases also focused on the rights of families or surrogates to make choices for an incompetent patient. This enabled the patients' rights to be maintained even when the patients were silent. The Patient Self-Determination Act of 1990 obligated hospitals that accepted payment from federal reimbursement plans to offer education to all patients about advance directives and to provide a means for the individual to execute an advance directive. These events led to the recognition that the decision-making power once accorded only to physicians was now to be shared by the individual patient and any number of other chosen surrogate decision makers.[10]

To be able to make personal health care decisions, patients need to understand all options available to them, the possible consequences of acting on certain options, and the costs and benefits of the possible consequences. Patients must be able to relate these understandings to a personal framework of values and priorities. It must be remembered that disagreeing with the recommendation of the physician or APN is not, singularly, grounds for determining that the patient is incapable of making a decision.[11]

Nonmaleficence is the concern for doing no harm or evil. Generally, the reference is to physical harm, pain, disability, and death, but harm can be defined both broadly and narrowly. Actions that inflict harm may be necessary for ultimate client well-being, but such actions always require moral judgment. Doing something and doing nothing are both actions determined by personal decision. As an example, withdrawal of treatment is often deemed a nonmaleficence decision. If "letting die" seems justifiable, the withdrawal of nutrition and hydration is usually seen as justified. The literature does not support the concept that cessation of artificial feeding and hydration is associated with pain or suffering, although there may be increased stress for caregivers and family. The principle of nonmaleficence requires an interpretation of values and the consideration of risks and benefits as part of a thoughtful and careful action.[6]

Beneficence is the act of promoting or doing good. This principle is action-oriented and requires the provision of benefits and the balance of harms and benefits. Ethical problems arise when benefits are conflicting. The principle of beneficence often appears at odds with the principle of veracity or truthfulness. As a professional, should one ever lie? Many believe that, although truthful alternatives must always be sought, intrinsically a lie may be a right choice if it is necessary to avoid greater evil. Specific criteria have been offered to assist the individual to determine whether a paternalistic lie is justified[12]:

- The lie produces positive benefits for the person lied to that outweigh any evil that might result.
- It is possible to describe the greater good that would occur.
- The individual would have wanted to be lied to.
- All participants would always be willing to allow the violation of truthfulness.

Justice requires weighing issues and responding to the facts that are present. Philosophically, no consensus exists about what constitutes justice. The nurse in advanced practice is responsible for exhibiting just behavior and distributing comparable treatment to each client; therefore, justice is an active process. Retributive justice demands that if a client is harmed, reparation, or a means by which to right the wrong, be applied.

Ethical Theory Bases

Using the basic ethical principles, philosophers have constructed various theories that may form the bases for ethical analysis. Moral theories generally address compliance with rules, consequences of action, or dispositions relative to behavior. These three variants are often classified into normative and nonnormative approaches.

The normative approach explores ethical obligations and duties. This approach allows investigation of what is right and wrong, what we are to be, and what we may value. A concern for reason formed the Socratic roots of ethics in the 5th century BC.[6] At present, all humans live in a global village in which different cultures and worldviews interact. An optimal normative approach would call for tolerance and formation of a society in which there is genuine plurality of beliefs and values in order to breed an ethic of "social personalism." Under this ethic, each person respects the social values of the other because there is genuine respect for that person.

Nonnormative theoretical variants presuppose universally applicable principles of right and wrong and seek systematically to provide justifiable answers to moral questions. One may assess the rightness or wrongness of an act by examining the interests of the actor or by assessing the consequences of the act itself. Deontology, or the act of examining the interests of the actor in performing certain acts, is derived from the Greek *deontais* (duty), which originally meant obedience to rules or binding duties. This sense of duty should consist of rational respect for fulfillment of obligations to other human beings. For example, the commanding duty for the health professional is to respect clients and colleagues and their right to autonomy (self-determination). Immanuel Kant (1724–1804) asserted that respect for persons is the primary test of duty. Kant stated that all persons have equal moral worth and that no rule can be moral unless all people can apply it autonomously to all other human beings. The deontological approach is often applied by health professionals who work with individual clients.[6]

Teleology (utilitarianism) is a consequentialist approach that is paternalistic in application. The root *telos* comes from the Greek for "end of the consequences." All acts are evaluated as positive to the extent to which desirable results are achieved. The right action is that which leads to the best consequence and the greatest good. This is often the ethical foundation applied in the formation of health care policy decisions. A difficulty with this approach is the problem of defining and properly weighing the greatest good as well as deciding who should receive the act.[6]

Ethical Decision-Making and the Clinician

Rapid advances in technology make many demands on the character, education, and abilities of the APN. Applying ethical responsibility in health care does not require the discovery of new moral principles on which to build a new theoretical system, nor does it require the evaluation of new approaches to ethical reasoning. It does encourage professionals to provide a proper foundation for the application of established moral rules. Society and the professions demand that practitioners be knowledgeable in the applied field of health care ethics and the process of ethical decision-making.[6] Ethical issues facing APNs in daily practice include but are by no means limited to informed consent, the right to refuse treatment, the level of competence of incapacitated patients, breaches in confidentiality, dealing with poor prognosis and terminal illness counseling, withholding of information and truth telling, resuscitation/end-of-life decisions, and genetic counseling and privacy concerns.

The emphasis on scientific developments throughout the past several centuries has caused ethics to take a quantitative rather than a qualitative approach. Science has sought to separate itself from concerns about human values and value systems. The changing demands of today's health care environment make it clear that the application of science in medicine is not value-free. The study of values and their effect on human behavior is an area that requires vigorous research.

Providers are bombarded with reams of information each day in clinical practice. Consciously and unconsciously, they make selections from these data and draw conclusions about themselves, their clients, and their lives. All information carries equal weight until value is assigned by the individual. Valued information stimulates further exploration of potential meaning. Dilemmas occur as problems that require ethical decisions. A dilemma is a choice between equally undesirable alternatives. The two essential components of an ethical dilemma are:

1. Existence of a real choice between possible courses of action
2. Placement by decision makers of different values on each possible action or on the outcome of that action

These components are obvious in the dynamics inherent in the current explosion of genetic knowledge. The advances stemming from the National Human Genome Project in the past few years have begun to restructure medical thinking about disease and disease prevention. With the total mapping of the human genome in April, 2003, a new era formally began in which diseases can be categorized based on the amount of genetic and environmental effects responsible for their expression in an individual. APNs, in their roles of patient educator and advocate, will be engaged to an even greater extent in the future in counseling individuals and families about issues surrounding genetic testing, privacy of genetic information, misuse of genetic information, and genetic screening.[13,14]

As an example, genetic screening is a population-based way of identifying people with certain genetic factors associated with a disease or the predisposition to a genetic disease. Newborn screening is carried on in most states to identify infants with genetic disorders that early treatment can prevent or ameliorate the sequelae. While this seems to be in the best interest of all, there are factors to be considered. The validity of the test results is an ongoing concern because false-positive results cause unnecessary concerns for the parents and possible stigmatization of the child, whereas false-negative reports leave the child at significant risk. Criteria for effective newborn screening programs as outlined by Nussbaum et al.[14] include the following:

- Treatment for the disease being screened is available.
- Early treatment of the disease has been shown to reduce or eliminate the severity of the disease.
- Routine oservation and examination of the child will not reveal the disease.
- A rapid and economical laboratory test is available, is highly sensitive, and has reasonable specificity.
- The disease is frequent enough and serious enough in the population to warrant screening costs.
- Health care structures are in place to inform the parents of the findings, confirm the results, and institute the appropriate treatment and counseling.

Phenylketonuria and galactosemia are two heritable diseases that clearly satisfy all the above criteria. Although most parents would readily want their children tested at birth for these diseases, the wishes of parents who dissent must be observed. The APN in the role of advocate would seek, in a nondirective, unbiased way, to make sure that adequate information was available to prospective parents about the nature of the screening, any other genetics tests that might be part of the test battery, any other information that might be obtained about the genetic makeup of the child or other family members, and the parents' right to agree or disagree to screening in accordance with the laws of the state in which they reside.

It is beyond the scope of this chapter to explore fully the social, ethical, and legal ramifications of the constantly increasing genetic knowledge that is now changing and will forever change medical and nursing practice. The APN will need to constantly explore specialty-specific ethical ramifications of genetic discoveries and applications in order to make ethically responsible decisions about care and counseling offered to the individual and family. An excellent source of information is the Ethical, Legal, and Social Implications Human Genome Project. This source may be accessed at http://www.kumc.edu/gec/prof/geneelsi.html. This is a gateway to a number of other on-line ethics sources.

The daily need for adequate ethical decision-making should offer another opportunity for collaboration among APNs, physicians, and other pertinent individuals on the health care team. In a recent editorial, Waldman, a physician, noted that 25 years ago the idea of collaborating with nonphysicians was "akin to conspiring with the enemy."[1] He states that physicians who were able to embrace collaborative practice at the outset were "blessed with the inner strength to not be threatened by professionals with a different approach to women's health" (his specialty). Data from most studies have indicated that collaborative practice has improved access to care and improved patient satisfaction without eroding quality. In order for such skills to be developed, there must be the recognition by physicians that the "sacred trust" of total responsibility for care has shifted from the primary care physician to a more fluid, patient-centered system involving medical specialists, APNs, physician assistants, clinical social workers, therapists, and medical ethicists.[10] The need for excellent collaborative skills between the physician and the APN is of extreme importance when the need for ethical decision-making is paramount in clinical and practice situations.[1]

In their report of a qualitative study, Blake and Guare[15] noted that when practitioners found themselves in ethical dilemmas, their interactions were bound up in adherence to policy, patient's rights, caring, and a shared balance between what they perceived as the ideal action versus the most realistic action. Ethical decisions were also complicated by perceived differences in experience, education, ethnicity, collegialism, authority, and feelings of powerlessness. Most perceived that the ethics of caring had limits that were most often manifest when the application of ethical principles placed them in divergent positions from peers, families, patients, and the power structure within health care organizations.

A survey reported by Smith[16] found that the nurse participants (n = 117) reported that when attempting to resolve ethical dilemmas, the aid of nursing colleagues was sought more often (84 percent) than that of ethics committees, pastors, social workers, journals, or physicians. Ethics committees were chosen as an option in only 28 percent of responses, whereas other frequencies of utilization included journals (33 percent), physicians (38 percent), pastors (48 percent), and social workers (45 percent).

Decision-making models offer the nurse in advanced clinical practice an opportunity for self-examination and self-knowledge. Clinical decisions are most often of mixed character, containing moral dimensions but rarely being solely moral decisions. Ethical decision-making is consistent with critical thinking. Situations must be processed by the identification of ethical dimensions within the context and by the application of principles of moral reasoning. This process offers the greatest assurance that final decisions or courses of action will be the "best." Use of the critical reasoning process produces less chance for mistakes based on ignorance, personal bias, or strong paternalism.[17]

The complex process of ethical decision-making leads to making a decision, acting on it, and justifying the action. In some situations, providers are participants, but at other times they function only to share a point of view. Three levels of decision-making are believed to exist:

1. The immediate level, which is characterized by no time for reflection

2. The intermediate level, in which there is some time for exploration and reflection

3. The deliberate level, in which adequate time exists to gather and examine information and to reach a rational decision after reflection[6]

Iserson[11] provides an interesting algorithm for making decisions about a possible course of action and testing that decision for ethical validity when time is a critical factor. He outlines three tests, which are called the Impartiality Test, the Universalizability Test, and the Interpersonal Justifiability Test. The practitioner applies the Impartiality Test by asking whether he or she would permit the planned action to be performed if he or she was in the patient's place. The Universalizability Test involves asking whether the practitioner would be comfortable with all other practitioners doing the planned action in a similar situation. The Interpersonal Justifiability Test asks whether the practitioner can list or discuss good reasons for the action decision that has been made. If all three of these questions can be answered in the affirmative, there is a reasonable probability that the decision made falls within the scope of ethically acceptable actions.

Dilemma situations have been labeled by some philosophers as incorrigible to moral reasoning. A dilemma may not be solvable, but it is always resolvable. In some cases, lack of available time may limit gathering of sufficient relevant information and consideration of alternative actions. In this situation, the amount of time available has created a dilemma where none would have otherwise existed. Having adequate time for data collection and reflection before a decision is required increases one's responsibility to gather extensive information, to weigh the values of all involved, and to estimate the results of each possible course of action. Providers must guard against a tendency to avoid making a choice when it is necessary to do so. Procrastination used to avoid responsibility should be avoided as well as should hastened judgment that precludes careful reflection. There are levels of immediacy in decision-making. However, the fact that decisions must be made immediately in some situations cannot be used to excuse the lack of thoughtful action in other situations. For example, it is justifiable to give treatment in an emergency situation (i.e., when a person is in immediate danger of death) without the patient's informed consent. However, it is not justifiable to do this in situations in which some time is available. Although often avoided, the deliberate level of decision-making is by far the most common in clinical practice. Making difficult ethical decisions is often avoided because such decisions are personally taxing, require the acceptance of great responsibility, and cannot be accomplished successfully without sensitivity to the human rights and values of others.[11]

Decisions, including ethical decisions, do not occur in a vacuum but are operant within a context that consists of an inner and outer environment. The sum total of an individual's experiences make up the inner environment. The outer environment consists of the actions and reaction of others, time constraints, and material resources. It is improbable that the environmental events that modify the setting of a decision will be repeated, and the operational self brought to the decision-making situation cannot be repeated. In this sense, all decisions are unique but not necessarily unrelated.

Scanlon[18] proposes several models of ethical discernment that can be incorporated into clinical practice settings and may offer practitioners the opportunity to feel more adequately prepared to undertake independent ethical decision-making. These include clinically based educational programs that help the practitioner to explore his or her patient advocacy obligations and assume leadership roles in ethical discernment. Nursing ethics groups may also provide a forum for the acquisition of knowledge and skill development through sample case critiquing and evaluation of ethics practices. Consultation with skilled ethicists and/or participation in multi-disciplinary ethics committees can facilitate communication, mediate conflicts, and alleviate distress related to moral ambiguity. APNs are an important asset to multi-disciplinary ethics teams due to their unique perspective and expertise in direct engagement with the patient. If an APN is available, participation in ethics rounds is to be desired as this allows sharpening of assessment skills and recognition of seemingly nonimportant clinical issues that possess the potential for development into future ethical dilemmas.

Since the early 1970s, a number of decision-making models have been developed for use by health care providers. Most of these models have focused on dilemmas as "triggers" for ethical analysis. An appropriate example, the Thompson and Thompson Decision Model for Nursing,[17] depicts a problem-solving process. The process allows critical review of the operant situation and assessment of all the variables as well as highlighting pertinent ethical issues raised by the situation. Table 13–5 and Table 13–6 provide the model and an analysis of the process of model application. A second example, the Ethical Assessment Framework as outlined by Cassells and Gaul[19] is in Table 13–7. An additional aid to decision-making may be found in the Code of Ethics updated by the American Nurses Association House of Delegates in 2001.[20] The changes in the document reflect the new challenges that are now facing all nurses as a result of technological innovation. Listed in Table 13–8 are the nine general provisions of the Code.

Trends in Ethical Research in Advanced Practice Nursing

The enormous and ongoing changes in the structure of the health care delivery system are greatly affecting practice relationships, producing new concerns for consumers and providers. Often, the resulting complex organizational environments

TABLE 13–5. Thompson and Thompson Decision Model

1. Review the situation and identify:
   a. Health problems
   b. Decisions needed
   c. Key individuals involved

2. Gather information that is available to:
   a. Clarify the situation
   b. Understand the legal implications
   c. Identify the bureaucratic or loyalty issues

3. Identify the ethical issues or concerns in the situation and:
   a. Explore the historical roots
   b. Explore current philosophical/religious positions on each
   c. Identify current societal views on each

4. Examine personal and professional values related to each issue, including:
   a. Personal constraints raised by the issues
   b. Guidance from professional codes or standards
   c. Moral obligations to individuals

5. Identify the moral positions of key individuals by:
   a. Direct questioning
   b. Consideration of advance directives
   c. Consideration of substituted judgments

6. Identify value conflicts, including:
   a. Potential sources of each
   b. Possible strategies for the resolution of each

7. Determine who should make the final decision, considering:
   a. Who owns the problem
   b. Whether the patient can participate in the decision process
   c. Who can speak on behalf of the patient (substituted on basis of best interest judgment) when the patient cannot

8. Identify the range of possible actions and:
   a. Describe the anticipated outcome for each action
   b. Identify the elements of moral justification for each action
   c. Note if the hierarchy of principles or utilitarianism is to be used

9. Decide on a course of action and carry it out:
   a. Knowing the reasons for the choice of action
   b. Sharing the reasons with all involved
   c. Establishing a time frame for a review of the outcomes

10. Evaluate the result of the decision/action and note:
    a. Whether the expected outcomes occurred
    b. If a new decision process is complete
    c. Whether elements of the process can be used in similar situations

produce significant changes in the cultural context of practice and provide the basis for a revised starting point for future research in health care ethics. The communal moral experience that results may be used as a starting point for such research.[21]

Recently, researchers have looked to practice itself as the operant domain for nursing ethics-grounded theory because ethical decision-making applications from formal or utilitarian philosophical frameworks have not always provided adequate answers to ethical dilemmas in practice. For example, a qualitative field study by

TABLE 13–6. Analysis Steps for Utilization of the Thompson and Thompson Decision Model
Step 1: Review the situation. The first step involves identifying significant components of the situation as well as the individuals involved in making the decision. A clear understanding of the situation facilitates each subsequent action.
Step 2: Gather additional information that may influence the situation. Demographic data, socioeconomic status, health status, prognosis, level of understanding, preferences, competence, and family members and/or significant others involved with the situation are examples of additional information that needs to be assessed.
Step 3: Identify the ethical issues. Understanding ethics and ethical principles is essential to identify the issues of the situation accurately. Another key to successful identification of the ethical issues is to gain a historical perspective on the issues.
Step 4: Identify personal and professional values. When a nurse defines his or her personal and professional moral positions as they relate to ethical issues, the nurse is better prepared to understand his or her position in a particular situation. Awareness of professional codes will help to identify professional values.
Step 5: Identify and assess values of key individuals. The moral values of the key people involved in the situation are as important as those of the nurse.
Step 6: Identify value conflicts. Value conflicts can occur within an individual or between the persons in the situation. Understanding why conflicts exist and keeping track of how conflicts have been resolved assist with the final decision.
Step 7: Determine who should decide. Many people are available to assist in making the final decision. The physician, nurse, social worker, patient, and patient's family are all involved in health care ethics. At this point, it must be decided who should be responsible for the decision or action.
Step 8: Identify range of actions, with expected outcomes. A clear list of alternatives helps the nurse recognize possible consequences of a decision and identify a course of action.
Step 9: Decide on the course of action, and carry it out. The person must decide on the course of action.
Step 10: Evaluate results of the decision. The final step involves evaluating the decision made to determine if the outcome was the one anticipated. Evaluation also provides information that assists in future ethical decision-making.

Carpenter[22] revealed that ethical decision-making in the clinical setting appears to be a 10-step process, beginning with an emotional response to an event affecting clinical practice and ending with feelings that affect the nurse's view of self and the profession. Ethical dilemmas in practice appear to have a direct impact on whether a nurse remains in the profession. Value differences between the members of the health care team and clients and the significance of the clinical context in making ethical choices are extremely important

The nursing philosopher Gadow,[23] more than any other, has emphasized the moral position of advocacy in nursing. According to Gadow, the nurse must enter into and experience as far as possible the subjective world of the client to be an advocate through a caring presence with and for the client. Gadow further emphasized that truth-telling in clinical judgment is critical and is the place where both client and nurse must be involved in disclosing information and personal values. The importance of community dynamics in ethical behavior by health care

TABLE 13–7. Ethical Assessment Framework

Steps	Activities
ASSESSMENT 1. Identify the problem 2. Gather relevant facts 3. Identify methods of ethical justification to help resolve the dilemma	Issues, conflicts, and/or uncertainties Medical (objective data), contextual (subjective data), policies, state and federal laws, etc. Consequentialism (consequences), deontology (duty), principalism (principles), care (relationships), casuistry (cases), virtue (character)
4. Consciously clarify values, rights, and duties of patient, self, and significant persons associated with the issue 5. Identify if there are ethical problems 6. Identify guidelines from nursing and professional codes of ethics 7. Identify and use relevant inter-disciplinary resources 8. Identify and prioritize alternative actions/options	Ethics committees, ethics consultants, clergy, literature, administrators, lawyers, colleagues, etc.
PLAN OF ACTION 9. Select a morally justified action/option from the alternatives identified	
IMPLEMENTATION 10. Act upon/support the action/option selected	
EVALUATION 11. Evaluate action/options taken	Perform short-term and long-term follow-up

Adapted from Cassells, JM, and Gaul, AL: An ethical assessment framework for nursing practice. MD Nurse 17:9, 1998.

providers has been used to link caring to public policy.[24] Benner[25] corroborated the idea of community and the importance of a community of practitioners where the "good" can be expressed and lived out. It was noted that the physician's ability to remain technically expert and humane depended, in large part, on the substance of arrangements worked out with other professionals, especially nurses. The community of practice should be the arena in which individual providers can exercise moral and practical reasoning built on values that have been shaped collectively. In this sense, community becomes an experience of shared meaning about thinking and acting, an ongoing event in which moral virtues, values, and principles guide the behavior of all within the community toward responsible decision-making for the good of the whole.[21]

Experiences of moral caring with clients by nurses and physicians in responsible communal interaction create useful patterns of meaning for future application. The patterns of meaning that emerge are informed and influenced by the inner experience of values, virtues, and principles, the cultural context, and the interaction with each individual in the clinical caring context. This approach places the focus of ethical research and practice on the experience of human beings themselves rather

TABLE 13–8. ANA Code of Ethics for Nurses
Nine General Provisions
1. The nurse, in all professional relationships, practices with compassion and respect for the inherent dignity, worth, and uniqueness of every individual, unrestricted by considerations of social or economic status, personal attributes, or the nature of the health problem.
2. The nurse's primary commitment is to the patient, whether an individual, family group, or community.
3. The nurse promotes, advocates for, and strives to protect the health, safety, and rights of the patient.
4. The nurse is responsible and accountable for individual nursing practices and determines the appropriate delegation of tasks consistent with the nurse's obligation to provide optimal patient care.
5. The nurse owes the same duties to self as to others, including the responsibility to preserve integrity and safety, to maintain competence, and to continue personal and professional growth.
6. The nurse participates in establishing, maintaining, and improving health care environments and conditions of employment conducive to the provision of quality health care and consistent with the values of the profession through individual and collective action.
7. The nurse participates in the advancement of the profession through contributions to practice, education, administration, and knowledge development.
8. The nurse collaborates with other health professionals and the public in promoting community, national, and international efforts to meet health needs.
9. The profession of nursing, as represented by associations and their members, is responsible for articulating nursing value, maintaining the integrity of the profession, and shaping social policy.

From http://nursingworld.org/ethics/chcode.htm

than on the problems of technical competence in the treatment of human beings. It has been suggested that a phenomenological-ethical inquiry into the experiences of virtues, values, and principles of the entire community of health care providers would clarify the foundations of choice-making and guide growing understanding of a new ethic of shared responsibility. The process would offer a vision to decision makers who, by virtue of their activity in the practice of clinical ethics, act as co-creators of the communal moral life.[21]

Additional areas of ethical research of importance to APNs include case management in managed care systems,[26,27] research methods and institutional review board (IRB) issues,[28] cloning and human embryonic issues,[29] and the ethical implications of evidence-based medicine.[30]

Ethical Concerns of the APN

Nurses in advanced practice today experience numerous ethical concerns, but the concept of futility as applied in decisions of patient care and the impact of managed care on practice settings are examples indicative of the changing experiential dynamic for clients and providers. Ethics and the law give primacy to patient autonomy, which is defined as the right to be a fully informed participant in all aspects of medical decision-making and the right to refuse unwanted, even recommended and life-saving, medical care. In spite of the power of this concept, it should be remembered that futile treatments are not obligatory. No ethical principle or law has ever required physicians to offer or accede to demands for treatment that are futile. Futility refers to an expectation of success that is either predictably or empirically so unlikely that its exact probability is often incalculable. Futility should be distinguished from hopelessness. Hopelessness is a subjective attitude, whereas futility refers to an objective quality of an action. Hope and hopelessness are related more to desire, faith, denial, and other psychological responses than to the objective probability that some contemplated action will be successful.[31]

The futility of a treatment may be evident in either quantitative or qualitative terms. Futility may refer to the improbability of an event happening as a result of treatment or to the quality of the event that such treatment might produce. The process of determining futility resembles decision analysis, with one important distinction. In decision analysis, the decision to use a procedure is based on considerations of both the probability of success and the quality or utility of the outcome. A very low probability of success may be balanced by very high utility. However, when determining futility, the quantitative and qualitative aspects are treated as independent thresholds or minimum cutoff levels, either of which frees the physician from the obligation to offer a medical treatment.[32,33]

Futility is a substantive concept but may appear illusive when effects on patients are confused with benefits to the patient or when the "symbolic" representation to society of treating handicapped newborns or patients in persistent vegetative states is allowed to take precedence over patient-centered decision-making. Substantive objective application of futility is suggested to be a professional judgment that takes precedence over patient autonomy and permits physicians to withhold or withdraw care deemed to be inappropriate without patient approval. Decisions of this variety are believed to be representative of the ordinary duties of physicians, duties that are applicable when there is medical agreement that the described standard of futility has been met. Appropriate resource allocation arguments for limiting treatment, although currently under intense discussion in corporate and public arenas, are generally looked on unfavorably in the present open system of medical care. This is true because no universally shared and accepted societal value system for appropriate allocation exists and because there are no guarantees that any limit of care that a physician imposes on the client will be equally applied by other physicians under the same circumstances. Because futility is almost always a matter of probability, objective reason asks: what statistical cutoff point should be chosen as the threshold for determining futility? Certainly, no answer has been derived from current discussions. However, there are some general statements of responsibility available, such as the Statement of the Council on Ethical and Judicial Affairs of the AMA, which concludes that physicians are under no obligation to provide futile cardiopulmonary resuscitation. The statement fails to specify any level of statistical certainty at which that judgment is supported. Even a decision on such statistical points would likely have limited usefulness because studies have corroborated the limitations of clinical assessment in correctly estimating both prognosis and diagnosis.[34]

Growing pressure has been placed on all providers to control health care costs by more rigorously controlling medical options. This produces a tension between the value of autonomy, exercised in the form of consent to use or omit various interventions, and the necessity of better control of medical resource expenditures. No consensus exists about what constitutes a just method of balancing the desires of individual patients against the diverse needs of society.

When providers believe that the requested treatment would not be in the patient's best interest, even from the patient's perspective, or that persistent requests by the patient or the patient's surrogate for further interventions are based on faulty reasoning, unrealistic expectations, or psychological factors such as guilt or denial, an obligation exists to make every effort to clarify exactly what the patient seeks to achieve with continued treatment. Adequate and sensitive communication between patient and provider often successfully resolves such problems.[31,32]

Most cases will benefit from sustained attempts to clarify the patient's values and the likelihood of the various relevant outcomes and to improve communication with patients or their surrogates. If this fails, physicians and APNs should carefully consider whether the care requested is consistent with their professional ethics and ideals. If inconsistency is perceived, alternative venues for care should be found, or the conflict should be discussed in a more public forum, such as in the hospital's ethics committees or in the courts. Public scrutiny furthers the debate over the appropriate use of medical resources and fosters the development of consensus through legislation and public-policy development.

Managed care is not a new phenomenon. Zoloth-Dorfman and Rubin[35] noted that in the 19th and early 20th centuries, groups of marginalized individuals created prepaid, capitated managed care plans in response to the problems they experienced in securing adequate health care services. These attempts at prepaid care included immigrant aid societies, trade unions, and company insurance plans. Such plans developed as a response to a medical delivery system not designed to guarantee access to services for those unable to pay a fee at the time of need. The utility of such efforts is evidenced by the continuing success of the Kaiser Permanente system, Group Health of Puget Sound, and other nonprofit health maintenance organizations (HMOs). Managed care plans differ from their historical predecessors by being increasingly structured as for-profit rather than nonprofit corporate entities. Further, development is occurring in a marketplace that is largely unregulated. The older nonprofit managed care model of medicine provided for rationing the provision of health care, incorporating a system of greater accountability, and resource pooling to provide the highest quality of care in the most cost-effective manner.

Managed care plans, particularly those with for-profit corporate structures, have been characterized by providers as threatening to weaken or displace the professional commitment to beneficence and nonmaleficence that form the foundation of the therapeutic relationship and, hence, quality care. The popular press has responded by raising public concern that the incentive structures built into managed care will lead to the sacrifice of quality and safety for profit.[35]

Managed care does generate concern about who will make actual treatment decisions, how decision-making authority will be established, and on which criteria clinical decisions will be made.

Clients who are ill are in an inherently unequal power relationship with providers and health plans. As buyers of health care, they are rarely in a position to effectively evaluate the practice and standards of care promoted by managed care organizations. APNs should assume the role of advocate and educator in these situations. Strong individual moral agency is developed by reflection on personal goals and aspirations as well as by an understanding of the limits of one's personal and professional commitments. To develop true moral agency, the nurse in advanced practice needs to take risks in preventing all plans that call for a gag order on health care providers or that suppress healthy debate on appropriate treatment modalities. Such risk-taking requires courage because of both threatened and real loss of position and status.

APNs must learn to manage information accurately, work in teams effectively, integrate guidelines and clinical judgment, and manage outcomes. Both APNs and consumers need to assume an activist role and seek positions on the boards of directors of large managed care organizations. APNs must develop as expert reviewers of practice guidelines and encourage the release of such guidelines for consumers' review. Areas for future activism include striving to obtain open review of staffing patterns and reasonable compensation for nursing care providers and administrators and to secure the consumer's right to a cost rebate for improved health status or nonutilization of resources. This type of activism, properly carried out, becomes a defining opportunity for professional growth and personal advocacy of the client's right to ethical care.

SUGGESTED EXERCISES

1 A major problem with access to health care exists in a remote rural area. The county commissioners are considering a clinic staffed by a family nurse practitioner (FNP) and a certified nurse midwife (CNM). The county attorney obtained all the necessary permits and documents; however, one of the commissioners still has concern regarding legality of the nurses' practicing without the immediate presence of a physician. You, an FNP, and your spouse, a CNM, have been accepted to fill those positions, pending final approval of the county commissioners. They have asked you to prepare policies and procedures that will adhere to the national standards of such a practice. Prepare a model document that is realistic and practical. Assume that the state allows full prescriptive authority and physician collaboration (off-site).

2 You are an experienced certified registered nurse anesthetist (CRNA) who has been asked to provide anesthesia services for a plastic surgeon in his office. You will be an independent practitioner and will be paid by the patient per case. In your state, CRNAs are not required to follow protocols or standardized procedures, and your standards of practice are determined by the profession. Prepare a document delineating the clinical policies of your practice, including pre-anesthesia evaluation and testing, selection of patients for elective ambulatory surgery, minimum equipment and supplies, and recovery discharge criteria and responsibility.

③ Prepare documents to conduct an annual legal audit of your practice. Include clinical policies, procedures, emergency situations, transfer of patients to another level of care, medical record documentation, and review of state laws and regulations. Also include your plan for keeping current in the clinical components of your practice.

④ Form two groups. One group will represent the ethics committee of a large HMO. The other group comprises those who have survived cancer for more than 5 years. Collaboratively, seek to set down criteria for appropriate withdrawal of medical nutrition and hydration from terminal cancer patients. Provide written rationales for your decisions.

REFERENCES

1. Waldman, R : A guest editorial: Collaborative practice—balancing the future. Obstet Gynecol Surv 57:1, 2002.
2. Balanced Budget Act P.L. 105-33, Sec. 4511(d), 1997.
3. Federal Support for the Preparation of the Clinical Nurse Specialist Workforce through Title VIII. AACN Clin Issues 11:309, 1997.
4. Cady, R: The Advanced Practice Nurse's Legal Handbook, p. 173. Philadelphia, Lippincott Williams & Wilkins, 2003.
5. Hravnak, M: Credentialing and privileging: Insight into the process for acute-care nurse practitioners. AACN Clin 8:1, 1997.
6. McManus, R: Ethical decision making in anesthesia. In Foster, S, and Jordan, L (eds.): Professional Aspects of Nurse Anesthesia Practice. Philadelphia, FA Davis Company, 1994.
7. Smart, N: Worldviews: Cross-Cultural Explorations of Human Beliefs, 2nd ed. Englewood Cliffs, NJ, Prentice-Hall, 1995.
8. Cofer, MJ: Thoughts on ethics. Value-based ethics in the workplace. Virginia Nurses Today 8:12, 2000.
9. Callahan, D: Minimalist ethics. Hastings Cent Rep 11:19, 1981.
10. Chaitin, D, et al.: Physician-patient relationship in the intensive care unit: Erosion of the sacred trust? Crit Care Med 31:S367, 2003.
11. Iserson, KV: Nonstandard advance directives: A pseudoethical dilemma. J Trauma 44:139, 1998.
12. Gert, B, and Culver, C: The justification of paternalism. Ethics 89:199, 1979.
13. Driscoll, KM: The application of genetic knowledge: Ethical and policy implications. AACN Clin Issues 9:588, 1998.
14. Nussbaum, RL, McInnes, RR, and Willard, HF: Thompson and Thompson Genetics in Medicine, 6th ed, pp. 393-395. Philadelphia, WB Saunders Company, 2001.
15. Blake, C, and Guare, RE: Nurses' reflections on ethical decision making: Implications for leaders. J New York State Nurses Assoc 28:13, 1997.
16. Smith, S: MNA ethics survey report. Mississippi RN 59:8, 1997.
17. Thompson, JE, and Thompson, HO: Ethical decision making: Process and models. Neonatal Network 9:69, 1990.
18. Scanlon, C: Models of discernment: Developing ethical competence in nursing practice. MD Nurse 16:3, 1997.
19. Cassells, JM, and Gaul, AL: An ethical assessment framework for nursing practice. MD Nurse 17:9, 1998.
20. Code of Ethics for Nurses, American Nurses Association, 2001. Available at http://nursingworld. org/ethics/chcode.htm
21. Ray, MA: Communal moral experiences as the starting point for research in health care ethics. Nurs Outlook 42:104, 1994.
22. Carpenter, MA: Clinical Psychiatric Nurses' Ethical Decision Making Process. Paper presented at the 1990 Second Annual Health Care Ethics Conference, Baltimore, May, 1990.
23. Gadow, S: Truth-telling revisited: Two approaches to the disclosing dilemma. In Leininger, MM (ed.): Ethical and Moral Dimensions of Care. Detroit, Wayne State University Press, 1990.
24. Schultz, P, and Schultz, R: Nodding's caring and public policy: A linkage and its nursing implications. In Leininger, MM (ed.): Ethical and Moral Dimensions of Care. Detroit, Wayne State University Press, 1990.
25. Benner, P: Experience, narrative, and community. Adv Nurs Sci 14:1, 1991.

26. Donagrandi, MA, and Eddy, M: Ethics of case management: Implications for advanced practice nursing. Clin Nurse Spec 14:240, 2000.
27. Ulrich, CM, Soeken, KL, and Miller, N: Ethical conflict associated with managed care: Views of nurse practitioners. Nurs Res 52:168, 2003.
28. Sutton, LB, Erlen, JA, Glad, JM, and Siminoff, LA: Recruiting vulnerable populations for research: Revisiting the ethical issues. J Prof Nurs 19:106, 2003.
29. Saran, M: The ethics of cloning and human embryo research. Princeton J Bioethics 5:25, 2002.
30. Gupta, M: A critical appraisal of evidence-based medicine: Some ethical considerations. J Eval Clin Pract 9:111, 2003.
31. Frick, S, Uehlinger, DE, and Zuercher-Zenklusen, RM: Medical futility: Predicting outcome of intensive care unit patients by nurses and doctors: A prospective comparative study. Crit Care Med 31:456, 2003.
32. Arnold, RM, and Kellum, J: Moral justifications for surrogate decision making in the intensive care unit: Implications and limitations. Crit Care Med 31(5 suppl):s347–353, 2003.
33. Lelie, A, and Verweij, M: Futility without a dichotomy: Towards an ideal physician-patient relationship. Bioethics 17:21, 2003.
34. Emery, DD, and Schneiderman, LJ: Cost effectiveness analysis in health care. Hastings Cent Rep 19:8, 1989.
35. Zoloth-Dorfman, L, and Rubin, S: The patient as commodity: Managed care and the question of ethics. J Clin Ethics 6:339, 1995.

CHAPTER 14

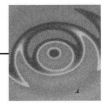

Advanced Practice Nursing and Global Health

CHAPTER 14

Katherine Crabtree, DNSc, FAAN, APRN, BC
Anita Hunter, PhD, RN, CNS, CPNP

Katherine Crabtree, DNSc, FAAN, APRN, BC, received her BSN and MSN from the University of Michigan and her doctorate in nursing science from the University of California, San Francisco. She has been an Adult Nurse Practitioner since 1975 and has taught nurse practitioners since 1977 at Michigan State University; Oregon Health and Science University (OHSU); University of California, San Francisco; and Wayne State University. As Professor of Nursing at OHSU, she also directs the nurse practitioner (NP) training grant funded by Health Resources and Services Administration. She served 4 years as chair of the National Organization of Nurse Practitioner Faculties (NONPF) Education Guidelines and Standards Committee and is now serving on the board of the American College of Nurse Practitioners. She has edited several monographs for NONPF, including *Teaching Clinical Decision-Making* (2000) and *Advanced Nursing Practice: Building Curriculum for Quality Nurse Practitioner Education* (2002). She led the revision of the core competencies for NONPF and codirected the federally funded national validation of NP Competencies for Adult, Family, Gerontological, Pediatric, and Women's' Health Nurse Practitioners.

Anita Hunter, PhD, RN, CNS, CPNP, is a PNP and Associate Professor at the University of San Diego. She is actively involved with international advanced practice, serving in clinical practice, research, and policy-making roles. She has worked as an advanced practice nurse (APN) in Ghana, West Africa, and with APNs in Northern Ireland and South Australia. She has conducted international research in Northern Ireland and Ghana on such subjects as developing cultural competence and adolescent resilience. She has developed short-term cultural immersion clinical experiences for students, developed international NP practice sites, and has been instrumental in the development of standards and scope of practice for the APN in the international arena through her participation in the International Nurse Practitioner/Advanced Practice Nursing Network Policy and Standards Committee. Dr. Hunter is currently Chair of the NONPF International Special Interest Group and past chair of the NONPF Global Advancement Committee.

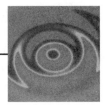

Advanced Practice Nursing and Global Health

CHAPTER OBJECTIVES

At the completion of the chapter, the reader will be able to:

1 Define factors influencing global health.
2 Describe some of the differences in advanced practice nursing in developed and developing nations.
3 Discuss how competencies developed for APNs in the United States have been used internationally.
4 Recognize the ethical and spiritual aspects of developing cultural competence.
5 Identify preparations needed for international nursing assignments, available resources, and opportunities.

GLOBAL HEALTH CHALLENGES

With the world at our doorstep, the World Health Organization (WHO) is calling on APNs to take a leading role in correcting the disparities in health care delivery, filling the deficit of health care providers that currently exists, and addressing the unmet health needs of peoples around the world.[1-3]

Immigration, emigration, and cross-border travel have affected the health and well-being of every nation. Whether escaping from undesirable sociopolitical or physical living conditions or merely seeking a better life, waves of immigrants continue to strain global resources. People fleeing their homelands to escape undesirable conditions are confronted with issues of prejudice, discrimination, and poverty. Nations plagued by civil war and political corruption are doomed to chronic poverty, unstable leadership, and lack of economic development. These conditions adversely affect not only the health of their citizens but also the health of bordering nations and potentially others around the world. HIV is probably the greatest example of inattention to literacy, poverty, hunger, and public health. A disease once localized to Africa has spread throughout the world, decimating families, neighborhoods, and communities.

Increased travel across national borders promotes the transmission of disease. Severe acute respiratory syndrome, which began in China, and HIV/AIDS, which began in Africa, have spread throughout the world. Natural disasters such as flood and famine spread disease and often deplete the resources of developing countries.[4,5]

By assessing and managing old and emerging diseases, APNs can help solve the health problems of immigrants inherent in the transition to a new homeland. Furthermore, APNs counsel and teach individuals how to deal with the health consequences that changes in lifestyle, nutrition, and exercise impose. APNs also can assist individuals, families, and populations as they learn the ways and customs of a new country and teach them how to traverse new health care systems.[6]

When peoples' health and social welfare are not prized, available resources are frequently reallocated to meet other governmental priorities. Ignoring illiteracy, hunger, and poverty and directing resources toward other national goals precludes reaching an optimal level of health for the nation and, ultimately, the world. International communications and media portrayal of conflicting lifestyles, economic discrepancies, racial prejudice, and religious beliefs create a climate of dissatisfaction and distrust, which can turn to hate, frustration, hostility, and sometimes war. Acts of terrorism are increasing. Nations that felt safe and insulated from political unrest and ethnic wars are now required to reallocate resources to protect themselves from these threats, leaving fewer resources to meet the health care mandates presented by society.

While the population of the world's developed nations is aging rapidly, many developing nations report that 60 percent of their population is under the age of 5 years.[7] Because of this drastic demographic change, the question arises: how much of that country's resources should be devoted to saving the past or protecting the future? Clearly, the world is becoming more interrelated and interdependent. World markets, economics, and world resources are becoming more globally accessible.

Decisions made regarding the allocation of national resources and health standards adopted by countries around the world impact each nation's ability to provide health care and protect the health of its citizens. Few nations have the financial resources and trained health professionals to achieve the WHO health goals.

GLOBALIZATION OF ADVANCED PRACTICE NURSING

World interrelatedness and interdependence have had a direct impact not only on global health but nursing and advanced practice nursing as well. The nursing community around the world is striving to emulate practice standards and educational preparation of nurses and APNs in the United States.

To address these challenges directly, the APN community created a nursing network within the International Council of Nursing, the International Nurse Practitioner/Advanced Practice Nursing (INP/APN) Network. The INP/APN is actively working to define advanced practice nursing for the global community and establish policies related to education, standards of practice, and scope of practice for the APN in the international arena. Final definitions and policy decisions must address cultural sensitivity, appropriateness, and competence within the context of ethics, human rights, and nursing practice around the world.

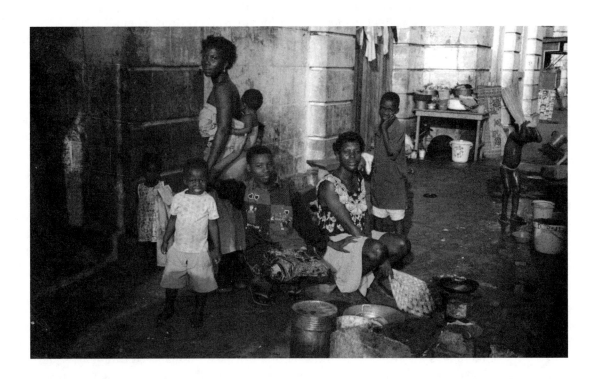

U.S. APN Movement Impacts Nursing Practice Around the Globe

The APN practice in the United States has been in existence since the early 1900s and describes many types of nursing practice. Mary Breckenridge's frontier nursing and Lillian Wald's public health nursing were early examples of advanced practice. The NP role began with Loretta Ford in 1965 with the development of the pediatric NP. Regardless of the population served or care setting, advanced practice nursing in the United States is characterized by complex decision-making, independent functioning, and advanced knowledge and skills obtained through graduate nursing education, either at the master's or the doctoral level.[8]

Four roles requiring special licensure, e.g., clinical nurse specialist, NP, nurse anesthetist, and nurse-midwife, currently describe advanced practice nursing in the United States. These roles are implemented in a variety of settings, including traditional inpatient and outpatient settings and less traditional community-based settings such as Head Start centers, schools, occupational settings, migrant camps, and churches, wherever health care is delivered or health needs identified. These APN roles include delivery of direct care involving the assessment of health, ordering and interpreting diagnostic tests, prescribing medications and performing common medical procedures for the designated patient population as well as consulting, educating, advocating, evaluating care, and applying research. Some APNs specialize in the care of children, adolescents, or elders. Others subspecialize in fields such as lactation, dermatology, and oncology; management of specific diseases, e.g., diabetes mellitus, HIV, or syndromes such as dementia. Some APNs choose to practice in urgent care or long-term care settings exclusively, whereas others move across settings from outpatient to inpatient settings or wherever the patient is located.

The APN role is shaped by the availability of resources, rapidly changing technology, and high consumer expectations for expert care. Care delivery is often provided one on one; at present, care remains predominantly symptom-driven rather than the desired community-based preventive care of populations. APNs are striving to move from an emphasis on disease- or symptom-focused care to health promotion and disease prevention within communities. APNs are politically astute and have the autonomy and the assertiveness to raise questions regarding practice issues, participate in their solution, and change health policies at the local, state, and national levels.[9]

The quality of the care APNs strive for in the United States is compassionate evidence-based care that meets national standards for practice. Regardless of the population or setting, the APN is expected to provide quality care that builds on an expanded knowledge base from the humanities, biopsychosocial, and behavioral sciences. Such advanced clinical knowledge, critical thinking, clinical judgment, and communication skills can be used to address complex problems such as family dysfunction and chronic and life-threatening illnesses. Critical components of the APN role are promoting healthy growth and development from birth to death and helping to resolve psychosocial issues and ethical dilemmas.

Most APN services are reimbursed by private payers and third-party payers. Federal regulations address Medicare reimbursement for APN services. More and more NPs are recognized primary care providers on managed care panels and receive reimbursement for their services from Medicare under their own provider numbers.[10] However, the problems of reimbursement, cost of health care, and health insurance create gaps in access to quality care for the uninsured and working poor. APNs are helping to close this gap, providing indigent care and care to other underserved individuals and families. In such cases, there may be little if any reimbursement. When reimbursement for services rendered is lacking, the neediest people are denied access to health care.

The valued contributions of the APN over the past 30 years have brought recognition and acceptance by the public and the health care system in this country and abroad. The role of the APN has been viewed by the federal government as a cost-effective means of extending care to many citizens who would otherwise go without health services. Federal support of educational programs to prepare NPs has allowed the role to expand and develop models of care emulated around the world. The following are examples of the National Health Service Corps (NHSC) federally funded practice and educational programs:

- Arizona—Combining Native Traditions and Modern Medicine
- California—Building a Healthier Community
- Colorado—Interdisciplinary Approach is a Necessity in Remote Region of Colorado
- Iowa/Illinois—Certified Nurse-Midwives Attentive to Mothers
- Maine—Improving Patient Management of Diabetes
- Minnesota—Rural Community and Good Mental Health
- New York—Improving Oral Health in a New York Community
- North Carolina—Community-Wide Universal Health Care Program
- South Carolina—Providing Mobile Health Care to Underserved Populations
- Washington, DC—Community Spirit Alive and Well in DC

Over the years, the NHSC has helped prepare 22,000 clinicians through such program initiatives as those mentioned above and through educational scholarship programs (http://nhsc.bhpr.hrsa.gov).

Satisfied consumers recognize the value of APN care, and public acceptance has allowed the role to flourish. Many physicians have recognized the value of adding NPs to their practices. However, to maintain this caliber of practice and professional respect, it is important to prepare APNs for tomorrow's practice and not just today's. The National Organization of Nurse Practitioner Faculties (NONPF) has assumed a leadership role in setting the educational standards for APN education in the United States.

EDUCATION COMPETENCIES FOR NP PRACTICE IN THE U.S. AND ABROAD

Framing NP Education Competencies

Based on the work of Patricia Benner[31] and Karen Brykczynski,[36] NONPF developed core competencies for entry-level NP practice regardless of specialty.[11,12]

Benner's original four domains of nursing practice have evolved into seven domains of practice[12]:

- Management of patient health and illness status
- Nurse practitioner–patient relationship
- Teaching/coaching function
- Professional role
- Managing and negotiating the health care delivery system
- Monitoring and ensuring the quality of health care practice
- Cultural and spiritual competence

A national project in 2002, undertaken by NONPF and the American Association of Colleges of Nursing (AACN) with funding by Health Resources and Services Administration, further developed the competencies.[13] The project defined and validated competencies for five primary care NP specialties: adult, family, gerontological, pediatric, and women's health. Together, these five specialties represent more than 80 percent of all primary care NPs (for a complete list of the core and specialty competencies, see the NONPF website www.nonpf.com or AACN website www.aacn.nche.edu). A national panel of NP educators, consumers, and employers of NPs along with representatives from accrediting and credentialing organizations developed the specialty competencies, which were validated by an independent national panel of experts in each of these advanced practice specialties. These national consensus–based competencies have been endorsed by 19 national organizations. These competencies provide educators, employers, and federal funding agencies a guide for the educational programs that prepare NPs in these primary care specialties. The same national validation process is also being used to develop advanced practice competencies for psychiatric–mental health and acute care NPs.

Model for APN Education Abroad

To date, the NONPF core competencies have served as a model for APN education in a number of countries, particularly the United Kingdom[14] and Canada.[15] As the WHO challenge to nurses to care for world populations becomes more pressing, nurses around the world are looking to the United States for help in preparing qualified advanced nursing professionals.

The preparation of APNs for practice in other countries is very different from that required to care for people in the United States. Mentoring nursing colleagues around the world requires an awareness of the rich variety in cultures and environments. Adaptations in teaching methodologies and expected competencies are needed. Most important, adaptations must be culturally relevant to be successful. Individuals sensitive to the beliefs, values, and customs of the people of a particular country can assist others within that culture to design and develop appropriate educational programs to prepare APNs for practice in that culture. In addition, APN consultants must be culturally savvy to help international colleagues achieve the fullest scope of practice possible in their countries and to support their colleagues as they learn to negotiate the political and social structures of their countries.

Impetus for the APN Movement Around the Globe

Certainly, the challenge given by the WHO has served as an important stimulus for the growth of the APN movement abroad. Immigration, emigration, refugees, homelessness, AIDS, starvation, civil war, and natural disasters are just some of the global issues that have attracted worldwide attention. The media have brought us unforgettable pictures of the need for humanitarian aid and health services. World financial, political, religious, and social instabilities complicate national responses to these needs. The APN working with local agencies or international relief efforts can help to revitalize health care systems and affect many of these issues.

The International Council of Nurses (ICN) and INP/APN have endorsed the definition of health care put forward by the WHO:

> Primary health care is essential evidence-based health care practice, brought to the individual, family, and community, at the primary, secondary, and tertiary levels, and is universally accessible, affordable, and able to be a self-sustained practice in that country.[16]

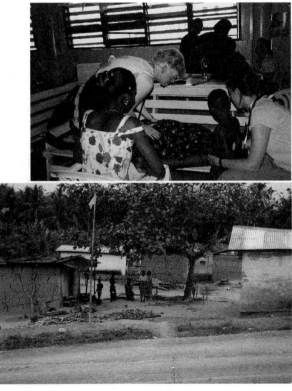

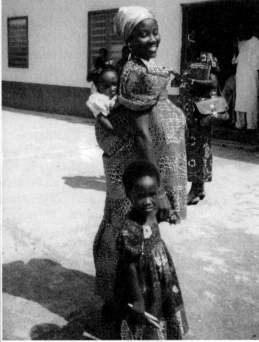

This definition encompasses the work of many nurses around the world, bachelor's- and master's-level nurses, those who perform diagnostic or surgical procedures, midwives, and those who provide acute and public health care.

This definition has framed the work of the ICN, INP/APN, the American Academy of Nurse Practitioners, the Royal College of Nursing (RCN), NONPF, and that of a multitude of other nursing organizations around the world. It defines the practice characteristics and educational preparation needed to become an APN. These organizations, working collaboratively through the INP/APN Network, have defined the NP/APN as a registered nurse who has acquired the expert knowledge base, complex decision-making skills, and clinical competence for expanded practice in primary health care, the characteristics of which would be determined by the context in which he or she is licensed to practice. Given the country in which one practices, an advanced degree, e.g., master's degree, is recommended for entry-level practice in the expanded role.

The characteristics of nurses practicing in the expanded role should include the following:

- Ability to integrate research, education, practice, and management
- Opportunity to practice with a substantial professional autonomy
- Opportunity to have one's own caseload and [provide] case management
- Acquisition of advanced decision-making and diagnostic reasoning skills, advanced health assessment skills, and clinical competence
- Prescribing, referral, and admitting rights
- Legislation that confers and protects the titles of NP/APN/clinical nurse specialist/nurse midwife[17]

Currently, not all nations can provide the education, endorse the scope of practice, or adopt a restricted title for APNs. It is not uncommon for nurses prepared in many developing nations to be expected to practice as APNs yet not be legitimized by the political or medical establishments of those nations.[18]

Acceptable APN practice in developed nations is very different from that in many developing nations. Traditional beliefs about the role of women and the traditional practices of physicians have impaired the forward movement of nursing. Unstable political systems in developing countries also impede long-term planning for health services and education of APNs. Differences in the etiology and treatment of diseases in developing nations also require modification in the APN educational preparation and scope of practice. In the United States and other developed nations, one of the major functions of the APN role is to ameliorate or stabilize the conditions associated with unhealthy lifestyles and to teach adoption of health behaviors for better self-care. In developing nations, the nurse must focus on public health and other environmental factors such as poor air and water quality, inadequate nutrition, and lack of sanitation that give rise to disease or complicate disease responses and treatment. Differences in roles and educational preparation must be recognized in defining APN practice in developed and developing nations. Valuing and recognizing what nurses do in their world where educational and health care resources are limited may give credence to the legitimacy of the nurses' expanded role in these developing nations.

ADVANCED PRACTICE NURSING IN OTHER DEVELOPED NATIONS

Developed and highly industrialized countries outside the United States have recognized the need for advanced nursing roles. The shortage of general practitioners, decreased numbers of physicians, and difficulties providing primary care to inner city, urban, suburban, and rural areas have contributed to a health care crisis not just in the United States but in other developed nations as well.

United Kingdom

Morag White, Chair of the Royal College of Nursing (RCN), NP Association,[19] reported on the effort in the United Kingdom (UK) to develop the NP role to fill these gaps. Specific NP preparatory programs, whose curricula are similar to our master's NP education programs, have been developed in England, Wales, Scotland, and Northern Ireland. In each country, NPs are required to complete an advanced educational program beyond basic nursing training. These programs vary in length and

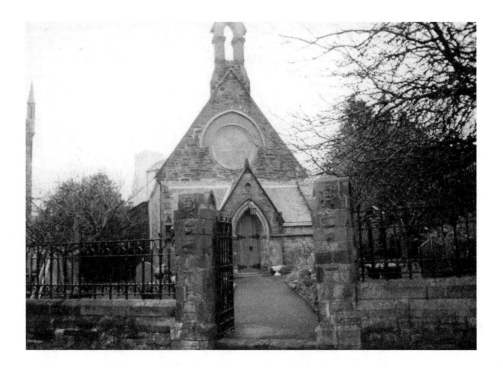

lead to a bachelor's degree, postgraduate diploma, or master's degree.[20] The expanded nurse role in the UK is a broader interpretation of the advanced role than "carrying out tasks that would normally be performed by the doctor."[18] Rather than "pseudo-doctors" performing functions physicians choose to delegate, the nurse is accountable for assessing the needs of the patient and providing holistic, competent care in an increasingly complex environment.

The RCN[14] has published standards describing the role, competencies, and accreditation standards for NP programs in institutions of higher learning. The first cohort of 15 NPs graduated from the RCN NP program in 1992. Development of distance learning programs may provide access to NP education for many more nurses in the UK, just as it has in the United States.

In the UK, NPs are well prepared to become autonomous and/or interdependent practitioners, with full prescribing rights. Regulations restricting the title of NP are under discussion by the new nursing regulatory board, the Nursing and Midwifery Council (NMC). The NMC aims to formally recognize the NP role within the UK and register NPs who hold the required educational qualifications. NPs offer health promotion, diagnosis, and management of acute and chronic illness. They function in community-based clinics; specialist hospital units, e.g., dermatology, cardiology, accident, and emergency; minor injury units; oncology; and in projects working with the homeless and male and female sex workers in inner city areas. NPs lead the minor injury units and are linked to physicians at nearby hospitals by telemedicine if consultation is needed. NPs work as part of a professional team in both primary and secondary care. They are autonomous practitioners with the ability to manage patient care. They treat, review, and discharge patients and make referrals to other professionals in primary or secondary care settings. Although prescribing privileges for NPs are currently under governmental and Department of Health review, it is expected that full prescribing rights will be given to NPs. At the present time, health visitors (community nurses), district nurses (public health nurses), family planning, tissue viability, and asthma and diabetic nurses prescribe from a limited formulary.

In the UK, the NP/APN role is being adapted to fit the national health care system and to meet the unique needs of the people of each country, including the itinerant population known as the "travelers," new refugees, an increasing number of homeless, mentally ill, and elderly persons, and those from rural or underserved areas of the country. Data from a national survey conducted by the University of Central England revealed many of the more than 60 different advanced practice nursing roles identified in the UK are located within hospital settings rather than in community settings.[21] The challenge of differentiating the NP role and defining the scope of practice and role characteristics acceptable to patients, communities, and government remains. Determining which of these multiple roles are viable will also entail evaluation of the financial sustainability of each role; that has yet to be done.

Canada

Because the national health care system in Canada is similar to that in the UK, the NP/APN role is very similar to that in the UK system. The scope of practice varies from Canadian province to province just as it does from state to state in the United

States. In an effort to provide a national umbrella for advanced practice nursing in Canada, the Board of Directors of the Canadian Nurses Association[15] finalized a broad framework to guide development of advanced practice nursing. The framework, which includes core competencies, provides national consistency in key elements in defining advanced nursing practice yet allows provinces to adapt the model to their regional needs and pursue legislation to enact and enable the role. The Registered Nurses Association of British Columbia and the Ministry of Health in Ontario have developed entry level competencies for NPs adapted from the NONPF core competencies.[22]

NPs are registered nurses who have advanced competencies gained through additional education and practice. NPs have advanced knowledge, clinical judgment, and decision-making skills that enable them to offer services beyond those generally provided by registered nurses. These services include assessment, diagnosis, and health care management of common acute and chronic illnesses, including prescribing medications.[22]

Decisions are being made regarding the number and types of NP specialties that will be licensed. For example, some of the issues being discussed are: should mental health nurse practitioners be licensed separately; how should acute care NPs be defined; should gerontological nursing be recognized as a subspecialty of adult nursing or as a separate specialty?

The advanced practice role in Canada also differs depending on whether the population the NP is working with is urban or rural. In the major cities, the clinical nurse specialist/APN works collaboratively with the physician within the hospital in an interdependent relationship. This model is similar to the CNS role in the United States, focusing on patient, educator, and staff development. The APN in the rural community assumes a more autonomous position, working in a position similar to the general practitioner model, with the physician remote from the practice site.

Australia

Elaine Duffy, Monash University School of Rural Health in Australia,[23] attributed the development of the NP role to a shortage of medical practitioners, especially those willing to work in rural, aboriginal health care. The Nurse's Registration Board has been working for more than 8 years to implement the NP role. In the year 2000, the Minister of Health gave full support to the concept. The NP role is tailored after the NP role in the United States and encompasses assessment, diagnosis, treatment, and prescribing authority. Because of the rural nature of their practice, NPs practicing in these areas may have total medical responsibility for the community. Therefore, stringent education and accreditation criteria are being established to ensure public safety and to support the autonomy of the role. Changes are being made in the Nurse's Act, the Poison and Therapeutic Goods Act, and the Pharmacy Act to pave the way for implementation of the NP role in Australia. Issues surrounding education, titling, and licensure are at the center of the debate as the NP role is adopted. The sociopolitical struggle for recognition and protection of the NP title and for full scope of practice are similar to the struggles experienced since 1965 by NPs in the United States.[24]

APN Role in Other Countries

At the 2002 INP/APN and ICN conference in Adelaide, Australia, it was evident that a number of nations, other than the United States, including the Netherlands, Australia, New Zealand, Taiwan, South Africa, and Japan have established some form of the NP, APN, and clinical nurse specialist roles. Thailand, South Korea, the Philippines, and other nations have expressed an interest in understanding these roles and discussing how the NP or APN role could fit within their health system culture. In each of these countries, differences in culture and role relationships influence the type of APN role developed and expected scope of practice.

In the Netherlands, the educational preparation of the APN is beyond the basic nursing level; however, APNs still work side by side with physicians in the hospitals.[1,25] In Taiwan and Japan, an advanced nursing degree has not been mandated. APNs work interdependently with physicians in the hospital. At present these nurses are often seen as handmaidens to physicians. The APNs serve as health educators and provide advanced nursing care under a medical model.[25]

The INP/APN Network has little information about the advanced practice role or concept in South America, the Caribbean Islands, Mexico, the Middle East, southern European countries, Russia, and the Baltic states. Nurses are prepared in those countries in schools of nursing or universities. Although some universities offer advanced degrees, it is unknown whether an advanced practice degree in nursing is available. Nurse graduates either work in the hospital or serve in an advanced practice role similar to the UK district nurse or public health nurses in rural communities. The role of the APN in these nations appears to be similar to the role of nurses in developing nations.

Currently, there is not a formalized certified registered nurse anesthetist role outside the United States. However, a nursing anesthesia preparatory program for developing countries is offered by Health Volunteers Overseas. This nonprofit, volunteer organization founded in 1986 offers more than 50 training programs in 25 developing nations promoting health care in the least developed nations of the world through training and education in 10 specialty areas (http://www.hvousa.org/fact.cfm). The role of the certified nurse midwife is also specific to the United States; however, the midwife, usually a layperson rather than a nurse, is a well-known and well-respected role around the world.

ADVANCED PRACTICE IN DEVELOPING NATIONS

The most underserved and needy populations typically are found in the developing nations where there is an inadequate number of health care providers and fewer APNs. Screening for disease, providing immunizations, improving nutrition and prenatal care, and ensuring clean water and sanitation for healthy communities are often the priorities in developing nations. The need for APNs to serve as health consultants, health educators, and health providers is critical to the health and even survival of the people. Grace Madubuko,[26] Coordinator of Nursing Affairs, West African College of Nursing, recognized the need for APNs to screen and triage

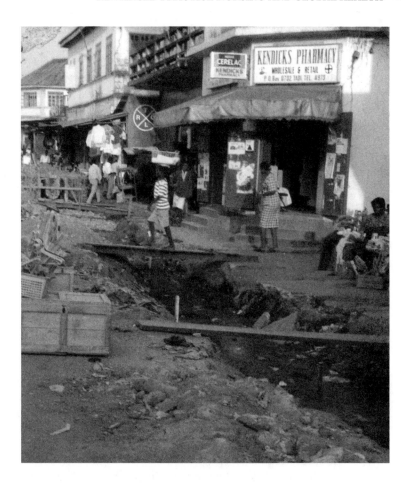

patients, monitor those with chronic illnesses, screen and manage breast and cervical cancer, prevent the spread of HIV/AIDS, reduce maternal/child morbidity and mortality, decrease starvation, and alleviate the health effects of poor sanitation. APNs and other nurses also are needed to help stem communicable diseases and promote prenatal health by providing programs that rely on laypersons trained to carry on the work locally and diffuse knowledge into the community. Nurses also teach others how to avoid transmission of disease, e.g., through adoption of safe sexual behaviors. Collaborative efforts of nursing, medicine, public health, political leaders, and the lay community are needed to achieve the health goals of each developing country.

Some countries sponsor advanced education for their nurses in developed countries such as the United States. These nurses are sent to the United States to be educated so they can return to their country and use their acquired knowledge to improve the health of its citizens. Unfortunately, not all these nurses return to their native countries, creating a "brain drain" of intellectual resources that further depletes the potential leadership and talent available to meet the nation's health goals. Others who do return find their attempts to fully implement new knowledge and change the system frustrated by a lack of resources for quality nursing care, terrain and roads that limit access to health care, illiteracy, and poverty.[26] Basic problems in the systematic dissemination of food and medications to those in need further frustrate the efforts of nurses in countries where resources are scarce and the need is great. At times nurses, because they are the only persons available with professional health knowledge, are sought to perform medical procedures that would otherwise be performed by physicians.

Meeting the need for superb community and public health nursing skills is paramount to reversing the effects of poverty due to war, drought, flood, and famine experienced by many people in third-world nations. The skills needed by APNs in these situations are an intimate knowledge of the community's needs and the ability to obtain and organize resources to meet these needs on a continuing basis. The APN must be trusted by the communities, understand the beliefs and concerns of the people, and be able to communicate complex ideas and concepts simply and clearly. In addition to having extensive clinical knowledge and skills, these APNs must be politically and socially astute to remain trusted members of the community and to survive the changing political landscape.

In Latin America and the Caribbean, because of a lack of physicians, nurses have historically been primary care providers.[27] Using models of public health nursing reminiscent of Lillian Wald's and Mary Breckenridge's practices, they have successfully cared for the people of their countries. Many have been educated as nurse midwives, and some have furthered their education to become family NPs.[27] They create and manage community clinics and home health care agencies to bring health care to rural underserved areas. In addition, these nurses train lay community health assistants and health educators to assist in health screenings, risk identification, and health teaching.[28]

The "village" phenomenon in Africa is similar. Here, lay professionals are often the traditional birth attendants and healers who use herbal therapies and local health practices to help people. Few rehabilitation hospitals, elder-care complexes, or orphanages exist. Access to health care is limited primarily to acute care facilities. People care for one another at home with traditional means. Nurses in several African nations—Ghana, South Africa, Nigeria, and Zimbabwe—have built on these practices by establishing traveling clinics or local clinics to reach out to those in "the bush" who cannot access health care services.[29,30]

Some countries also provide outreach health care services and aid to persons outside their geographical borders. There are many examples of nurses from one country helping people in other countries as part of a "friendly neighbor" program. Two examples illustrate the diversity of assistance that is provided. Nurses in Israel have established an education program to help Ethiopian refugees understand food labeling so they can make informed food choices to meet cultural and health needs.[32] Japan has sponsored the development of a community-based, nongovernmental organization, a hospital for mothers and children, a primary school, and a vocational training school for the impoverished people of the Zia Colony of Pakistan.[33]

ETHICS AND SPIRITUAL AND CULTURAL COMPETENCE IN A GLOBAL ENVIRONMENT

Practicing in an ethical and a culturally and spiritually competent manner is essential, regardless of where an APN practices—developed or developing nation; acute or primary care; city, community, or rural setting. Unfortunately, many wars have been fought in the name of religion to preserve or expand borders and economic resources or to eradicate people of other cultures. Cultural and spiritual tolerance are often lacking in relations among people from different backgrounds within and across national borders. Ethics and spiritual and cultural competence are learned behaviors that arise from values such as respect for human dignity, freedom, and equality. Even in developed nations, civil unrest exists as ethnic minorities compete to meet their needs and preserve their values and communities within an often hostile society. Relations with neighboring countries are strained by economic and environmental policies affecting commerce, natural resources, even imports and exports across borders. In many countries around the world, a nurse of one color, gender, class, ethnic heritage, or religion does not provide care to a patient who is a different color, class, ethnic heritage, or religion without risk to himself/herself and family. Such social divisions make it difficult to meet the needs of people in many countries.

Chase and Hunter[34] discuss cultural and spiritual competence as part of the advanced practice role. Being culturally competent means the APN understands the health and illness perspectives and behaviors of patients, the family health care decision-making processes, treatment expectations, and compliance factors. Cultural and spiritual competence reflects a change in mind-set. Instead of viewing how the patient can fit into the nurse's world because it is assumed the nurse knows best (ethnocentrism), the nurse acquires understanding of the patient's world and examines how to fit into the patient's world. The culturally competent nurse incorporates communication patterns, social organizations, heritage, spirituality, biological variations, beliefs, traditions, and practices that have worked for the patient into the plan of care (ethnorelativism). Ethical practice means respecting the civil rights of people, treating all equally and humanely, advocating on behalf of those in need, valuing life, and facilitating dying with dignity.

Each of these attributes is critical for the APN practicing in a country or community outside of his or her own experience. Without these competencies, efforts to address health and social disparities may be for naught.

OPPORTUNITIES FOR ADVANCED PRACTICE OUTSIDE THE UNITED STATES

Nurses who wish to explore opportunities for advanced practice outside the United States should contact the INP/APN Network within the ICN. This network is composed of APNs from around the world and is a great resource for practice and education issues (http://www.icn.ch/networks_ap.htm).

The need for advanced practitioners is twofold:

1. There is a need for knowledgeable public health nursing consultants who can design and implement community-wide programs. Such programs should include training laypersons to be community health educators who can serve as health educators to the larger community. Training should include teaching about health priorities, maintaining health, preventing diseases, obtaining immunizations, accessing good nutrition, improving sanitation, obtaining prenatal care, and preventing sexually transmitted diseases.

2. There is a need for experienced APNs to help nursing educators around the world develop educational programs to prepare quality APNs who are able to provide health care for the people of their nations.

Several private and public organizations help to place APNs and other nurses overseas. Some religious organizations such as Northwest Medical Teams (http://www.northwestmc.com) recruit health professionals for foreign mission assignments. Some nurses choose short-term assignments of a few weeks or months with, for example, Doctors without Borders (http://www.doctorswithoutborders.org), or Volunteers in Medical Missions (http://www.vimm.org), or Mercy Corps (http://www.mercycorps.org) who dispatch teams of health care providers to disaster areas to provide emergency relief services. Long-term contracts may stipulate a commitment of 2 years or longer.

Nurses are occasionally recruited by foreign governments to set up health care services, organize facilities, and train staff. In the Middle East these nurse consultants may live in a restricted community or compound with other foreign nationals. As guests of the country in which they live, nurses must honor the customs of the country regarding dress and deportment. There may be restrictions on the type of clothing worn for leisure and work. Eating, sleeping, and bathing areas are often segregated by gender. Often, the role of women is more restricted abroad than the role of women in the U.S. culture. Women may not be allowed to travel unescorted, and they may not be allowed to provide physical care to patients of the opposite gender.

Regardless of the country in which a nurse is working, cultural sensitivity and competence are critical. Respect for religious observances, social structure, parenting practices, traditional health and illness beliefs, and marital relations are necessary for a nurse to be successful in any capacity. There are many incentives for engaging in international nursing practice: altruism, respect, providing assistance, and sharing knowledge and resources. However, financial gain is unlikely.

Preparations Needed for International Assignments

Before participating in any international health effort, health providers need to be prepared to work with people in their environment and deal with their health problems. Health problems in the new locale may be unfamiliar. Available therapies may be limited or differ from the treatments the APN has used previously. Protection for the APN includes up-to-date immunizations prior to departure. A list of required immunizations is available through the Centers for Disease Control and

Prevention (CDC) for travel to any country in the world: www.cdc.gov/travel. The CDC also issues health alerts, designating areas where there are known health risks. Protection against disease is important when practicing and living in rural areas or when responding to natural or man-made disasters. Some countries may lack vaccines and prescription medications available in the United States. Universal precautions may not be practiced. Medical supplies may be few. Often, special permits are required on entry to some countries. Travelers may be screened to prevent the spread of disease, such as severe acute respiratory syndrome, before receiving permission to leave an area where there has been an outbreak. Equipment may be older, and low technology may be the norm. Laboratory tests may be unavailable, and treatment may be empirical. Differences in water and food supplies and lack of electricity and refrigeration require adjustment. Temperature extremes and high altitudes may also create health hazards.

Communication and transportation delays are common and expected. Persistence and detailed directions are often needed to locate specific places due to a lack of signage. [35]

Passports and work visas are often required. Obtaining these documents before departure may require additional time and planning. Work restrictions may limit the ability of the nurse to practice abroad due to differences in licensing and educational requirements. Personal safety may be an issue in countries where political unrest is the norm and sentiment against the United States is high.

Reputable organizations require and may provide preparation in the language and culture (beliefs, customs, values, social, political and religious structures) before departure. APNs entering the international arena are responsible for educating themselves about the people and the culture where they will be living and working. Knowledge of priority health problems, their causes, how they are managed, and their long-term outcomes is important preparation for success. Knowledge of personal values, beliefs and prejudices is essential. Having a sense of humor also can be a tremendous advantage with the multitude of adjustments that will most likely be necessary.

PREPARING APNs WITH A GLOBAL PERSPECTIVE

Using the NONPF core competencies[12] as a framework, the following activities could be developed within the curriculum to prepare APNs with a broad global perspective:

I. Professional role learning activities
   A. Debate the strengths and weaknesses of a global perspective on nursing policy, economics, management, and role.
   B. Identify ways to improve access to care for immigrant populations.
   C. Contact nurses or others in an international community via the Internet or at nursing conferences.
   D. Discuss cultures, populations, or communities of interest to identify the socioeconomic and political barriers to furthering their health; explore the

effect of these barriers on health policy development; nursing practice; economic, social, and religious factors within that community.

II. Managing and negotiating health care delivery systems
   A. Incorporate cultural learning activities in core or general graduate courses.
   B. Identify the regional, national, and global context of care for different populations.
   C. Present case studies and problem-oriented scenarios on how to negotiate the U.S. health care delivery system.

III. Monitoring and ensuring the quality of health care practices
   A. Identify political and professional activities needed in an international organization. One example of such an organization is the International Council of Nurses and its INP/APN Network whose goal is to facilitate the development of global standards of practice and education through the sharing of resources and information to help overcome some of the current world health problems.

IV. Demonstrating cultural competence
   A. Identify different cultures, populations, or communities of interest, and use the Internet and literature to plan assessment and intervention strategies.
   B. "Adopt" an international community within a developing nation, identifying health needs of a particular population and planning culturally appropriate interventions for that population.
   C. Assess and plan health-related activities to assist a new immigrant community within the United States.

V. Teaching/coaching function, APN-client relationship, and management of client health/illness status
   A. Identify pathophysiological and pharmacological variations in the presentation and treatment of disease states and responses to medical treatment in given populations.
   B. Explore complementary and alternative health practices of a specific culture, population, or community and their compatibility with modern medical interventions.
   C. Identify health problems of a specific culture, population, or community; using case studies and problem-focused scenarios, identify how to assess and manage these health problems, develop culturally appropriate and manageable interventions to prevent further recurrence, and assist the population in accessing culturally appropriate care.
   D. Participate in short-term domestic and international service-learning and clinical cultural immersion experiences.
   E. Establish faculty practice models for community health and international health. These practice environments would serve as learning centers for nurses, facilitate mentorship, and provide arenas for research and scholarship.

SUMMARY

We live in a global society. As the world grows smaller, APNs are becoming increasingly aware that people around the world are interdependent. Despite differences in skin color, language, dress, and religion, people are more similar than dissimilar. However, the causes of illnesses they face may be very different. Global health needs are rising, resources are diminishing, and emigration of future leaders is occurring in the countries least able to afford such losses. WHO has called on APNs to correct disparities in health care delivery and address the health needs of peoples around the world. APN roles and education programs are being developed, particularly in other developed countries. Advanced practice nursing has a responsibility for the well-being of the world, and APNs are well suited to meet these unmet needs.

SUGGESTED EXERCISES

1. Identify where you would locate information about advanced practice opportunities abroad. Select a country, and obtain information on APNs in that country.

2. Identify immunizations needed if you were planning to spend several months working with an international health care relief organization in rural areas of a South American country such as Nicaragua. Also consider the Ukraine and Japan.

3. Describe personal and professional characteristics you would look for in hiring an APN to develop a new community-based rural health clinic in a developing nation. State why these characteristics are important to the success of the program.

4. Describe the competencies you would expect an APN to possess before seeking a position in international health.

REFERENCES

1. Fawcett-Henesy, A: Disparity versus diversity: Meeting the challenge of Europe's underserved populations. Reflections Nurs Leadership 18, 2001.
2. Jenness, M: Nursing education in Egypt. Int Nurse 12:3, 1999.
3. Uys, L: South Africa. Reflections Nurs Leadership 21, 2001.
4. Douglas, M: The effect of globalization on health care: A double-edged sword. J Transcultural Nurs 11:85, 2000.
5. Diamond, J: Guns, Germs, and Steel: The Fates of Human Societies. New York, W.W. Norton & Company, 1999.
6. Kelleher, D, and Hillier, S: Researching cultural differences in health. London, Rutledge, 1996.
7. Siddiqi, J: World Health and World Politics: The World Health Organization and the U.N. System. Columbia, South Carolina, University of South Carolina Press, 1995.
8. Pulcini, J, and Wagner, M: Perspectives on education and practice issues for nurse practitioners and advanced practice nursing. White paper for the International Nurse Practitioner/Advanced Practice Nursing Network, 2001. Retrieved May 6, 2003, from http://www.icn.ch/networks_ap.htm#reports
9. National Organization of Nurse Practitioner Faculties: Domains and Competencies of Nurse Practitioner Practice. Washington, D.C., Author, 2000.
10. Buppert, C: Nurse Practitioner's Business Practice and Legal Guide. Gaithersburg, MD, Aspen, 1999.

11. National Organization of Nurse Practitioner Faculties: Advanced Nursing Practice: Curriculum Guidelines and Program Standards for Nurse Practitioner Education. Washington, D.C., Author, 1995.
12. National Organization of Nurse Practitioner Faculties: Domains and competencies of nurse practitioner practice. Washington, D.C., Author, 2000.
13. National Organization of Nurse Practitioner Faculties and American Association of Colleges of Nursing: Nurse Practitioner Primary Care Competencies in Specialty Areas: Adult, Family, Gerontological, Pediatric, and Women's Health. Rockville, MD, US DHHS, HRSA, 2002.
14. Royal College of Nursing: Nurse practitioners: An RCN Guide to the Nurse Practitioner Role, Competencies and Programme Accreditation. London, Author, 2002.
15. Canadian Nurses Association: Advanced Nursing Practice: A National Framework. Ottawa, ON, Author, 2000.
16. World Health Organization: Alma-Alta 1978. Primary Health Care. Health for All, Series no. 1. Geneva, Author, 1978.
17. Education Subgroup of the INP/APN: Unpublished statement, 2001.
18. Jones, S, and Davies, K: The Extended Role of the Nurse: The United Kingdom Perspective. Int J Nurs Studies 5:184, 1999.
19. White, M: Nurse Practitioners/Advanced Practice Nursing in the UK. White paper for the International Nurse Practitioner/Advanced Practice Nursing Network, 2001. Retrieved May 6, 2003, from http://www.icn.ch/networks_ap.htm#reports
20. Miller, D: Lecturer in Nursing, University of Ulster, Jordanstown, Newtownabbey, Co., Antrim, Northern Ireland. Personal communication, July 17, 2002.
21. McGee, P, and Castledine, G: Advanced nursing practice in the United Kingdom. Nurse Pract 25:79, 2000.
22. Registered Nurses Association of British Columbia: Competencies Required by Nurse Practitioners in British Columbia. Vancouver, BC, Author, 2002.
23. Duffy, E: Global characteristics of nurse practitioners/advanced practice nurses. White paper of the International Nurse Practitioner/Advanced Practice Nursing Network, 2002.
24. Appel, AL, and Malcolm, P: The struggle for recognition: The nurse practitioner in New South Wales, Australia. Clin Nurse Specialist 13:236, 1999.
25. Chen, C: The Current Issues in Advanced Practice Nursing in Taiwan. White paper of the International Nurse Practitioner/Advanced Practice Nursing Network, 2001. Retrieved May 6, 2003, from http://www.icn.ch/networks_ap.htm#reports
26. Madubuko, G: Nurse Practitioner/Advanced Nursing Practice Development in West Africa. White paper of the International Nurse Practitioner/Advanced Practice Nursing Network, 2001. Retrieved May 6, 2003, from http://www.icn.ch/networks_ap.htm#reports
27. Mc Dowell, HM: International nursing: One nurse's experience. Int Nurs Rev 33:15, 1986.
28. Leininger, M: Transcultural Nursing Concepts. Theories, Research and Practices, 2nd ed. New York, McGraw-Hill, 1996.
29. Avotri, J, and Walters, V: You just look at our work and see if you have any freedom on earth: Ghana women's account of their work and their health. Soc Sci Med 48:1123, 1999.
30. Hunter, A, and McHenry, L: An advanced practice international health initiative: The Ghana Health Mission. Clin Excellence Nurse Pract 5:240, 2001.
31. Benner, PE: From Novice to Expert: Excellence and Power in Clinical Nursing Practice. Menlo Park, CA, Addison-Wesley, 1984.
32. Messias, D: Globalization, nursing, and health. J Nurs Scholarship 9, 2001.
33. Hunter, A, and Pulcini, J: Global Health and Nurse Practitioner Education. National Organization of Nurse Practitioner Faculties 249, 2002.
34. Chase, S, and Hunter, A: Cultural and Spiritual Competence: Curricular Guidelines. National Organization of Nurse Practitioner Faculties, 2002.
35. Ailinger, RL, Zamora, L, Molloy, S, and Benavides, C: Nurse practitioner students in Nicaragua. Clin Excellence Nurse Pract 4:240, 2000.
36. Brykczynski, KA: An interpretive study describing the clinical judgment of nurse practitioners. Scholarly Inquiry Nurs Pract 3:113, 1989.

ADDITIONAL REFERENCES

1. Andrews, M, and Boyle, J: Transcultural Concepts in Nursing Care. Philadelphia, Lippincott, 1998.
2. College of Nurses: Standards of Practice for Registered Nurses in the Extended Class (Primary Health Care Nurse Practitioners). Toronto, ON, Author, 1998.

3. Duffy, E: Evolving role and practice issues: Nurse practitioners in Australia. White paper of the International Nurse Practitioner/Advanced Practice Nursing Network, 2001. Retrieved May 6, 2003, from http://www.icn.ch/networks_ap.htm#reports
4. International Council of Nurses: Definition of nurse practitioners/advanced practice nurse. White paper of the ICN, 2002, at www.icn.ch/networks_ap.htm
5. United States Immigration and Naturalization Service: Statistics, 1999. Retrieved May 6, 2003, from http://www.immigration.gov/graphics/shared/aboutus/statistics/index.htm
6. Wong, F, Chan, S, and Yeung, S: Trends in nursing education in China. J Nurs Scholarship 32:97, 2000.

CHAPTER 15

Advanced Practice Nursing and Health Policy

Eileen T. O'Grady, PhD, RN, NP

Eileen T. O'Grady, PhD, RN, NP, is a certified adult nurse practitioner and serves as policy liaison for the American College of Nurse Practitioners (ACNP), curriculum consultant for the Robert Wood Johnson Foundation's initiative to increase the number of primary care providers, and adjunct assistant professor at the George Washington University School of Medicine and Health Sciences and George Mason University College of Nursing and Health Science. She most recently held positions as a policy analyst at the Center for Health Policy, Research and Ethics at George Mason University and study leader at Abt Associates on the effectiveness of a community nursing organization demonstration project. Prior to that, she was on the faculty of George Washington University Department of Health Care Sciences, where she held a number of roles, including director of the post-MSN nurse practitioner program.

Dr. O'Grady has held several leadership positions with professional nursing associations, most notably as a founder and vice chair of the ACNP. She was a 1999 Policy Fellow in the U.S. Public Health Service Primary Care Policy Fellowship and in 2003 was given the ACNP "Legislative Advocacy Award" for her leadership on nurse practitioner policy issues.

Dr. O'Grady has practiced as a primary care provider for 15 years and has clinical expertise in sports medicine. She has authored numerous articles and chapters on primary care and orthopedics as well as health policy. She has taught nurses and physicians around the United States as well as around the world with the U.S. Peace Corps.

Dr. O'Grady holds an associate of applied science from Marymount University in Arlington, Virginia; a bachelor's of science from George Washington University, a master of public health from George Washington University, a master of science in nursing, and a doctor of philosophy from George Mason University.

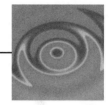

Advanced Practice Nursing and Health Policy

CHAPTER OBJECTIVES

After completing this chapter, the reader will be able to:

1 Analyze the fundamentals of the health policy-making process in the United States.
2 Compare and contrast the major contextual factors and policy triggers that influence health policy-making in the United States.
3 Differentiate the current and emerging health policy issues that impact advanced practice nurses (APNs) and the populations they serve.
4 Summarize the critical elements of political competence.

"Sentiment without action is the ruin of the soul"

—EDWARD ABBEY

Engaging in health policy is central to the advanced practice nursing role; it requires intervening on behalf of the public rather than individuals at the clinical level. APNs witness on a daily basis the consequences of policies that harm patients and populations and that violate human dignity and value. These powerful clinical experiences can become potent influencers in policy formation for the APN who integrates these experiences with two additional skill sets: the ability to analyze the policy process and the ability to engage in politically competent action. The APN movement has made great progress over the last three decades, exerting far-reaching influence on the nation's health delivery system and the nursing profession as a whole. This chapter describes the tensions between cost, quality, and access to health care; the policy process; current APN policy issues; and the skill sets of a "politically competent" APN.

Health policy development is the process by which society makes decisions, selects goals and the best means for reaching them, handles conflicting views about what should be done, and allocates resources to address needs. When influencing health policy, APNs have expertise in using a framework that is directly applicable to the nursing process. APNs are experts in health promotion and disease prevention and have distinguished themselves both in the clinical and policy arenas by their strong belief in the capacity and importance of patients caring for themselves. In order to know how to motivate a patient to change a behavior, for example, one must know where the patient is in the cycle of change. Interventions for patients who do not want to change are very different from those for patients who are determined to change. Knowing what phase a person is in (assessment) helps the APN to customize interventions to effectively promote changed patient behavior. So, too, with the policy-making process. One must identify the phase of the process in order to effectively influence that process.

TENSIONS AMONG HEALTH CARE COSTS, QUALITY, AND ACCESS

A fundamental tension in the 21st century health care system is achieving an appropriate balance between access and quality without excessive increases in costs (Fig. 15–1). The current emphasis on health care quality stems from a large body of research documenting serious quality problems due to poorly developed systems of care.[1] Access to care cyclically becomes a priority as unemployment rates increase, causing the number of uninsured to swell, or census reports are released indicating alarming numbers of uninsured. As systematic quality measures are implemented, health care costs frequently increase, at least initially. Businesses are getting hit with an expense they once thought impossible, paying an average of $8,500 a year per employee.[2] This premium inflation trickles down to employees, who must pay a larger percentage of the premiums or large co-pays out of their

Cost-Quality-Access Tension

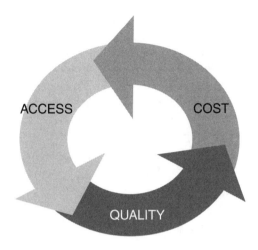

FIGURE 15–1   The tensions between cost, quality, and access.

pocket or choose to go without insurance; this dynamic contributes to increases in the number of uninsured.

Costs

The rapid growth of health maintenance organizations and preferred provider organizations in the 1990s is responsible for the slower growth in health care costs during that decade. Managed care grew because the industry was successful at reducing costs through restricted formularies and choice of providers, preauthorization of some services, and reduced lengths of hospital stay, which shifted care to outpatient sectors. Health care, however, is not delivered in isolation; new technologies such as Web-based spirometry and telehealth can add considerable costs to health care while improving access and quality. The current backlash against managed care is due to the imbalance of cost over quality and access—this overemphasis on cutting health care costs is what led health policy advocates to push Congress to craft the Patients' Bill of Rights. Major legislative activity at the state and federal level continues around benefits packages (defining what services should be covered), resolution of disputes, liability, and patient privacy issues in managed care organizations. Moreover, employer-sponsored health insurance has begun to shift from a defined benefits package to a defined contribution—requiring consumers to become more informed about and actively engaged in purchasing decisions regarding health insurance because they will be contributing more to these costs.

Quality

Today, many people who interact with the health care delivery system are deeply dissatisfied with their experiences. The President's Commission on Consumer Protection and Quality[3] specifies that "the purpose of the health care system must be to continuously reduce the impact of illness, injury and disability and to improve the health and functioning of the people of the United States." Quality is frequently described as having three dimensions: quality of input resources (certification and/or education of providers), quality of the process of services delivery (the use of appropriate procedures for a given condition), and quality of outcome of service use (actual improvement in condition or reduction of harmful effects). Evidence of quality problems include:

- High rates of avoidable errors, resulting in disability or premature death
- Underutilization of services, causing needless complications, higher costs, and loss of productivity for millions of Americans
- Overuse of services, causing unnecessary, costly services that impose risks to patients
- The wide pattern of variation of health care practices, suggesting that health care, for the most part, is not delivered with an evidence base[18]

Access

Access, the third tension in the health care delivery system, is an individual's ability to obtain appropriate health care services. Barriers to access can be:

I. Financial
   A. Insufficient monetary resources

II. Geographic
   A. Distance to providers
   B. Inability to travel to services due to lack of transportation or time or disability

III. Organizational
   A. Lack of available providers

IV. Sociological
   A. Discrimination due to gender, race, ethnic group, sexual preference, age
   B. Language and cultural barriers
   C. Health beliefs

V. Educational
   A. Even the most educated consumers are largely uninformed about the health care delivery system and options available to them once services are required.
   B. Historically, health care services have been delivered in a paternalistic framework, which encourages consumer passivity.

Efforts to improve access often focus on providing/improving health insurance coverage. The Institute of Medicine report on the consequences of uninsurance notes that working-age Americans without health insurance are more likely to:

- Receive too little medical care too late

- Experience more acute sickness and die sooner

- Receive poorer care when they are hospitalized, even for acute situations like motor vehicle crashes[4]

The benefits of having health insurance are even stronger when continuity of coverage is taken into account. Even being uninsured for a relatively short time—1 to 4 months—can be harmful to a person's health. Over the long term, uninsured adults are more likely to die prematurely than people with private insurance coverage. Roughly 42 million Americans are uninsured and, as a result, are at higher risk for poorer health than people who have health insurance.[5] Moreover, the uninsured are much more likely to go without care than are people who have insurance. More than two million Americans lost their health insurance in 2001, the largest one-year increase in the number of uninsured in nearly a decade.[6] In addition to differential access in health care outcomes for the uninsured versus the insured, racial and ethnic disparities exist in all clinical areas, including heart and renal disease, pain management, asthma, and cancer. The causes are multifactorial; the federal government has made the reduction of racial and ethnic health disparities a major priority for research and intervention funding.

THE AMERICAN HEALTH POLICY PROCESS

Health policy–making in the United States is a distinctly incremental process. The key feature of the American health policy process is that no decision is ever final and that all policies are subject to modification. Just as health and heath care are dynamic, the phases of the policy-making process are highly interactive and interdependent. Health policy is very political by nature; political circumstances continually change, and policy decisions are frequently revisited based on those changing circumstances. The distinctly cyclical nature of health policy–making is dependent on the ability of the stakeholders to be strategic and politically competent.

Agenda Setting

There are many health care–related problems in this country that go unaddressed, especially problems that are too costly and too complex to solve readily. If a health care issue is not considered both important and urgent, it will likely never get on the agenda. Other issues, such as the large numbers of uninsured, are difficult to address because there are intense disagreements around possible solutions to expand public and private coverage. These contentious issues often languish at the bottom of the agenda and may receive periodic priority but are put on and taken off the agenda for years. In order for a problem to become a priority for policy makers and to reach the top of the agenda, a confluence of three broad "streams" must occur:

1. Policy triggers (such as those shown in Figure 15–2)
2. Possible solutions to the policy problems
3. Political will[7]

A policy "window" opens when these three flow together, and a policy trigger and solution have the potential to begin the policy-making process. In almost every circumstance, a number of policy solutions emerge and compete with each other. This is where health services research[18] can provide clarity to the solutions being considered. If the policy solutions do not have the real potential to solve the policy problem, the policy issue will not advance in the policy-making process. The crucial third variable is political will, which is the most challenging variable to predict in the policy window stream due to its high level of complexity. Political will is influenced by public opinion, the media, the strength of interest groups and their electioneering skills, executive and legislative branch opinion leaders, and unpredictable election-year pressures (Table 15–1).

The Dance of Legislative Development

Of the thousands of bills introduced in each congressional session, only a small fraction of legislative proposals will ever get to the policy formulation stage and, once there, will follow a highly prescriptive process, or "dance," in order to emerge as a new public law, statute, or amendment to an existing law.[8] The incremental nature of health policy-making and the continuous modifications of existing policies resemble a choreography of steps. An important source for policy ideas is the President's State of the Union Address, which outlines the laws the President believes are necessary for the coming legislative session. Other policy solutions can

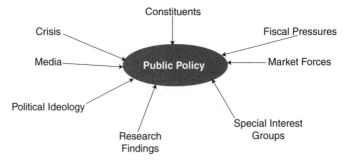

Wakefield's Factors Influencing Public Policy

Constituents

Crisis

Fiscal Pressures

Media

Public Policy

Market Forces

Political Ideology

Research Findings

Special Interest Groups

Source: Mary Wakefield, Director, Center for Rural Health, University of North Dakota.

FIGURE 15–2   Policy triggers.

TABLE 15–1. Factors Influencing Agenda Setting

Influencing Factor	Policy Trigger	Example of Policy Solution/Response
Crisis	Anthrax-laced letters	Millions of dollars are directed at local and national public health efforts.
	Fortune 500 companies engage in criminal accounting activity that causes employees and investors to lose billions of dollars.	Congressional bills are introduced requiring more transparency in accounting procedures.
Media	Drive-through deliveries reported in the lay press	Legislation passed requiring managed care organizations to cover a minimum of 48 hours' stay for normal vaginal deliveries.
Political ideology	The majority party (Democrats vs. Republicans) will have a large impact on health policies.	The Republican leadership opposed the regulations (put into place under a Democratic leadership) that would not require physician supervision of certified registered nurse anesthetists (CRNAs). This change in political context reversed an important decision that has large implications for the patients dependent on CRNAs for anesthesia care, mostly rural Medicare beneficiaries.
Research findings	Biomedical and health services research contributes to the policy process by clarifying problems and identifying solutions. It is estimated that 98,000 people die each year as a result of health care errors.[1]	A number of patient safety bills are introduced in the following legislative session.
Special interest groups	Interest groups with strong grassroots activity and a single clear mission can have a profound impact on the public policy agenda.	The grassroots organization Mothers Against Drunk Driving demonstrates that committed volunteer efforts can influence drunken driving laws, policy, and educational campaigns.
Market forces	In 1999, only 8% of people with employee-sponsored health insurance had traditional indemnity health insurance: 92% of insured people were in some form of managed care. This reflects a sea change in the U.S. health care delivery system, brought on by market forces.	The rapid growth of managed care leads to a number of legislative bills introduced to regulate managed care companies. These managed care reform bills are also known as "Patients' Bill of Rights" legislation and provide a good example of market forces impacting the health policy agenda.

(Table continued on following page)

		Example of Policy
Influencing Factor	**Policy Trigger**	**Solution/Response**
Fiscal pressures	Budget decisions are largely dependent on whether the federal government is in deficit vs. surplus spending.	Downturn of the economy prompts White House Office of Management and Budget Director to tell lawmakers that the federal government cannot afford to pass a $40 billion Medicare provider "giveback" bill because of decreased revenues.
Constituents	Constituents have poignant stories of loved ones with rare diseases; express concern that no private or federal research is being conducted	The Orphan Drug Bill passes into law in 2002 to create incentives for companies to research drugs that do not have commercial viability.
Litigation	Increasingly, interest groups are using litigation to challenge existing policies or obtain specificity to vague legislation.	In September 2002, a federal judge granted class-action status to a lawsuit that claims Wal-Mart's denial of health insurance coverage for birth control is unfair to female employees.

TABLE 15–1. **Factors Influencing Agenda Setting** *(Continued)*

come from "executive communications," often in the form of a letter from a senior member of the executive branch (agency heads, cabinet members, or the President) to members of the legislative branch. Executive communications are often a follow-up to the ideas emphasized in the President's State of the Union Address. One of the most important executive communications is the President's proposed federal budget, transmitted from the White House to Congress. Politically competent interest groups play a pivotal role in developing legislation pertinent to their interests to ensure their concerns and preferences are addressed. Once a bill is introduced by a member of Congress, it is referred to one of the seventeen standing committees in the House and sixteen in the Senate, each with jurisdiction over certain issues.[18] When more than one committee has jurisdiction over a bill, the bill is referred to the appropriate committees and subcommittees sequentially. The majority party controls the appointment of chairpersons to all committees and subcommittees, making political ideology a powerful predictor of both the order and pace with which legislative proposals are considered. Once both legislative bodies approve the legislation, the President signs it, and the legislation is enacted into law. State legislatures follow similar processes, with changes primarily in timing. Individuals should become familiar with the legislative and regulatory processes in the state(s) in which they live and practice.

Policy Implementation: Bringing Laws to Life

The policy-making process now transitions from the Legislative Branch to the Executive Branch of government, starting with the rule-making process. The pertinent federal agency is tasked with "interpreting" the law by adding highly specific rules to the law; for example, when nurse practitioners (NPs) were authorized to receive direct Medicare payment in 1998, the Center for Medicare and Medicaid Services (CMS) defined the education and certification criteria NPs required in order to qualify for a Medicare provider number. Rule-making is also highly procedural, and all proposed and final rules must be published in the Federal Register[18] to ensure that stakeholders and the public have an opportunity to participate in the process. Proposed rules are assigned a comment period, which serves as an invitation to the public and stakeholder community to negotiate, bargain, and provide evidence to support or refute the rules.

Advisory commissions, such as the Medicare Payment Advisory Commission, are established by Congress to "help" the rulemaking process. This is most common in cases when there is widespread disagreement and conflict or when rules will be subject to continual revision, such as the Medicare reimbursement rates.[8] Advisory commissions, which typically comprise members outside the implementing agency, tend to make rules that are much more acceptable to those affected by them. Once the final rules are published, the actual running of the program begins, and most of the responsibility rests with Civil Service employees in the federal government.

Policy Modification: No Policy Decisions are Ever Permanent

Policy decisions are often correct at the time decisions are made, but they can become erroneous with changes in knowledge; demographics; or technological, ethical, or legal events. The need for policy modification occurs when the consequences (intended or unintended) provide feedback into any phase of the process. For example, the de-linking of welfare benefits (such as food stamps) to Medicaid enrollment caused large numbers of children to become uninsured. The unintended consequence of de-linking the two programs led to the creation of the Children's Health Insurance Program (CHIP) to address the growing uninsured rate among children. In fact, modern health policy overwhelmingly comes from modifications of earlier policies. The modification phase should be understood as a continuous interrelated activity in which no decision, including public laws, rules, court decisions, or operational practices, are permanent. Whether the impact of the original policy decision is positive or negative, stakeholders will try to modify the policy for more benefits or retain the existing benefits. Policy changes occur slowly over long periods because the results of the policy are more stable and predictable. Incrementalism also allows time for compromise among the diverse interests and increases the likelihood for consensus and creative solutions.

Unique Structural Characteristics of the United States' Health Policy Arena

The most striking feature of the U.S. constitution is its endurance, the fact that it is still in operation after more than two centuries. The key to this endurance has been its flexibility: the ability of our governmental framework to accommodate tremendous change throughout history. The constitutional framers never imagined political parties, primary elections, the presidential cabinet, or a huge executive bureaucracy; nor could they have envisioned the growth in geography, population, and diversity, the technological advances in travel and communications, and the effects of a civil and two world wars.[9] Yet, the constitutional framework has endured and flourished along with these dramatic changes. The U.S. policy-making system is highly procedural and formal, especially when compared with those of other nations. This formalism stems from the lack of a real power center among the three branches of government and tends to further slow the process and contribute to incrementalism.

Because the majority of health policies are modifications of previous policies or decisions, modifications reflect rather modest changes. Modest policy changes are an intended constitutional construct to keep a power balance within the branches of government and prevent tyranny. Incrementalism in policy development is the United States' preferred political, economic, and social system for change.[10] Increasingly, judicial system input into health policies is playing a more prominent role in clarifying policies, resolving disputes, and setting precedence, which adds another layer of formality and process.

There has been a recent shift in federalism, which forms the boundary of power between the states and the federal government. The shift has been to devolve power to the states. This is often seen in the form of block grants or program waivers to promote the concept of "states as labs." It is also evident that each geographic area of the country requires different or varied approaches to solving health problems. Block grants with broad guidelines allow states to solve health problems unique to their region and population.

Election-year politics in the United States can cause policy makers to make unexpected choices in order to gain the support of an important constituent group at home. Therefore, politically charged issues will often get caught in gridlock until after an election. Table 15–2 summarizes the unique characteristics of the U.S. health policy context.

THE APN HEALTH POLICY AGENDA

The challenges that restrict APNs from expressing or practicing to their full intellectual capacity, such as direct payment, autonomous practice, and the ability to practice in all health care settings, are the foci of many APN organizations' policy agendas. The following are examples of policy issues that demonstrate the ongoing need to monitor regulatory and legislative activity and the interrelationship between legislation and regulations.

Direct Medicare Reimbursement

Skilled Nursing Facilities: Correcting Inconsistencies

Under the current Social Security Act, every skilled nursing facility (SNF) is required by both Medicare and Medicaid to ensure that every resident is provided health care under the supervision of a physician. In the final rules implementing the nursing facility regulations, the CMS, formerly HCFA, made it clear in a preamble that regulations should allow for the effective utilization of NPs, clinical nurse specialists, and physician assistants (PAs), but the statutory language prevented the rule-makers from including these other providers. States have the option to choose

TABLE 15–2. Current Health Policy Contextual Issues Unique to the United States
• Rapidly expanding knowledge base and emphasis on evidence-based practice
• Exploding chronic care needs
• Revolutionary care process in antiquated systems Δ Web based spirometry while the provider is still relying on clinical handwritten data
• Disintermediation Δ Removal of the provider, consumers getting information from other sources
• Managed care domination and backlash
• Work force maldistribution.
• Emergence of New Federalism
• Demographic shift Δ The aging of the U.S. population is the largest ever recorded Δ Shrinking birth rates and growing life expectancy
• Subgovernments emerge, which mingle private and public power to create issue networks
• Election-year politics make for unpredictable decision-making
• Minority of the electorate choosing to vote

Institute for the Future: Health and Health Care 2010. San Francisco, Jossey-Bass Publishers, 2000.

whether a Medicaid recipient's health care can be delivered under the supervision of a clinical nurse specialist, NP, or physician assistant as long as these providers are collaborating with a physician and providing services within their respective scope of practice. The policy that reimburses APNs for Medicaid services is inconsistent with Medicare reimbursement policy.

In addition, the Balanced Budget Act of 1997 authorized NPs to initiate care for rehabilitation services, including physical therapy, occupational therapy and speech therapy, for Medicare beneficiaries. The policy modification to correct this inconsistency that directly impacts access and SNF care quality requires a legislative amendment to the Social Security Act to include " … that the medical care of every resident be provided under the supervision of a physician or APN or Physicians' Assistant."[11] Medicare reimbursement to APNs to initiate (certify) care for Medicare beneficiaries in SNFs will improve the quality of care because of the APN's ability to blend the discipline boundaries of both nursing and medicine. This blending gives APNs the unique cultural and language skills to communicate effectively with nurses, nurses' aids, nursing supervisors, physicians, medical directors, and medial subspecialists.

Home Health Care: A Change is Needed

The Social Security Act stipulates that only physicians can certify and recertify Medicare home health care. However, the 1997 Balanced Budget Act authorized NPs to develop plans of care for Medicare beneficiaries receiving home health care. Rectifying the limitation in APNs' ability to certify and recertify for home care requires a policy modification (amendment) to the Social Security Act or new legislation that would streamline the home health care certification process, which is highly burdensome to home care agencies. Home care and long-term care are two of the fastest-growing sectors of the health care delivery system. APNs could, with this legislative change, play a much more important role in increasing quality of care. APNs are well-grounded in care delivery within the context of the community and the capacity for patients to care for themselves. Current restrictions on APNs to deliver services in these important health care settings must be eliminated.

Professional Autonomy: Restraint of Practice

The CMS rules require nurse anesthetists to practice under physician supervision in order to receive Medicare reimbursement. The rules also allow a state's governor to notify CMS of the state's desire to opt out of the supervision requirement for certified registered nurse anesthetists (CRNAs). Several states have opted out of the physician supervision requirement. For example, in many states like Iowa, 91 of 118 hospitals rely exclusively on nurse anesthetists to provide anesthesia services.[12] CRNAs are the predominant anesthesia providers in rural and other medically underserved areas; without these APNs, many of the facilities serving these areas would be unable to maintain surgical, obstetric, and trauma stabilization services. In addition, rural areas tend to have a high proportion of Medicare beneficiaries. Despite this, physican groups have opposed removal of the supervision requirement at both the federal and state levels, even though removal of the restriction ensures access to care for patients in rural areas and allows facilities to staff their anesthesia departments to best serve their patients. Removal of this major barrier to CRNA practice will require a rule change within CMS, which is not likely to happen until the leadership in the executive branch changes.

Physician Antitrust Legislation: A Threat to APN Practice

In 2000, the House of Representatives passed the Quality Health Care Coalition Act. This legislation evolved from a study in which it was concluded that health plans have greater leverage over quality and coverage of care than do physicians.[13] This bill would have given physicians the ability to force health plans to accept the terms that the physicians negotiate collectively. The ability for physicians to negotiate the terms of their contracts with managed care organizations could significantly disadvantage APN providers in a number of ways. First, legislation of this type has the potential to unfairly block access to more cost-effective providers, thereby raising health care costs. Second, physicians would be given the legal means to limit services provided by APNs. The APN community concluded that there was no amendment or legislative language that could adequately protect APNs from exclusionary practices that would stem from physician antitrust legislation.[11] The Quality Health Care Coalition Act, while not acted on in the Senate, could be reintroduced at any time in either chamber of Congress. APN organizations strongly opposed this or similar legislation. APNs and APN organizations must be constantly vigilant of congressional activity and oppose any antitrust legislation that creates a market barrier to APN practice.

Provider-Neutral Language: Breaking the Physician Monopoly on Health Care

Use of the term *provider* or *health care professional* rather than physician can have enormous impact on scope of practice and reimbursement policies for APNs. Legislative and regulatory recognition is needed to place APNs on par with providers who perform identical services. For example, language in the House and Senate versions of the Patients' Bill of Rights legislation used the term *physician*, which would prohibit APNs from being named as primary care providers or certified nurse midwives as direct obstetric-gynecological access providers. However, using the term *health care professional* enables the rule makers to include providers who are licensed, accredited, or certified under state law to provide health care services within their scopes of practice. APNs continue to advocate for nondiscriminatory language in all legislation and regulations proposed on the federal level. As the number of prescribers and providers who are not physicians increases, provider-neutral language more accurately reflects the current health care work force and diminishes consumer confusion.

APN Workforce: A Dearth of Data

The importance of using good data to make a case for a policy change cannot be overemphasized. However, finding accurate, current data on the APN work force presents a policy challenge. Currently, there is no comprehensive database or practice data, beyond the most rudimentary counts, on all APNs across the nation. This lack of accurate work force data presents a major limitation for moving the APN policy agenda forward. Federal data collected from the Bureau of Labor Statistics, an important source for work force planning data, does not distinguish among different levels of RNs with advanced education, rendering it unusable for APN work force planning. While most states keep track of APNs separately from all RNs, not all do, rendering state nursing licensing data inadequate for national APN work force planning needs. In addition, many APNs hold licenses in more than one state or are certified in more than one practice specialty. Therefore, unless the nurses' state of residence is part of an interstate licensing compact, duplicate licenses and certifications pose another major limitation to creating an accurate APN database.

The quadrennial National Sample Survey of RNs[14], conducted by the Health Resources and Services Administration, is currently the best source of data about the APN work force supply. Since 1977, this national survey, using sampling techniques for the RN population, has estimated and characterized the APN work force size. Because the sampling technique is based on RNs and not on APNs, the sample of APNs in many states is too small for accurate estimates.

The APN community must be able to answer questions frequently asked by policymakers:

1. How many APNs work in areas where there are shortages of health professionals?

2. Do APNs care for a disproportionate share of the uninsured?

3. Do APNs tend to serve in the communities in which they were educated?

4. Are the outcomes, e.g., immunization rates or hospitalization rates, of APN patient populations measurably improved?

Data are needed to inform these important policy questions, and APNs must work to secure meaningful data on the APN work force so that this information can be used in health policy formation. As clinical leaders in nursing, APNs are confronted and affected by policies that seek to address the current nursing shortage. First, students attracted to APN programs come primarily from the basic nursing work force, which is showing a steady decline in growth and will severely limit the future pipeline of APNs. Second, a large proportion of nursing faculty are APNs; therefore, the faculty shortage has significant implications for APN education programs' capacity to accept qualified students. Third, APN support and leadership are needed to promote initiatives that will alleviate the nursing shortage in order to improve patient care and ultimately demonstrate the contribution that nurses make to patient care outcomes.

APN POLITICAL COMPETENCE

Political competence requires the APN to create circumstances that turn ideas into policies. The politically competent APN:

- Participates in the drafting of legislation during the conceptual phase of the process
- Produces and delivers testimony in hearings to inform and refine drafted legislation
- Pays close attention to rule-making
- Provides formal comment on proposed rules

Effective leaders also must understand the strategic consequences of policy decisions (both positive and negative) so that they can gain lead time and position themselves (and organizations or groups) to respond to those decisions thoughtfully. An excellent example of how the luxury of lead time can affect legislation and, ultimately, patient care occurred when the Medicare regulations, being drafted following passage of the 1997 Balanced Budget Act, required NPs to hold a master's degree to be eligible for Medicare reimbursement. Many NP organizations, education programs, and certifying bodies had supported or required graduate preparation as the entry point for NP practice, long before the rules were drafted in anticipation of this rule change. The regulations, however, also reflected the concern about access to health care and included a "grandfathering provision" that allowed NPs without a master's degree to obtain a Medicare provider number (UPIN) for a specified period following implementation of the regulations. This provision allowed NPs who had been practicing for many years to continue to provide care to Medicare patients.

Serving on advisory bodies is another important strategy that APNs can use to exert influence in the health policy arena. The ability to communicate clearly, manage personal feelings, and bring evidence or a strong rationale to support one's positions makes a highly effective advisory board member. However, this also requires the ability to understand those with differing viewpoints while keeping a focus on priorities.

Professional Leadership Skills

As explained above, using data effectively is a powerful tool to make the case for a policy change. Data can play a critical role in explaining why an issue is important. Therefore, understanding how to use and interpret data is critical to influence policy effectively. Wherever possible, data should be incorporated into all communications—when meeting with legislators and other key stakeholders, preparing written material, talking with the media, testifying at a public meeting, or writing letters to policy makers or newspapers.

Use of outside expert opinion, in the event that no data are available, is another important strategy. For example, the American Hospital Association convened a highly diverse commission to examine the hospital and health systems' work force; the commission recommended the use of NPs as hospitalists to fulfill the care manager role in acute care settings.[15] This outside expert recommendation is a powerful tool for any APN negotiating for hospital privileges or working to expand scope of practice laws. There are two basic rules, however, to remember when using data for policy development:

Rule 1: You will depend on data for nearly all aspects of policy development work.
Rule 2: Data alone and especially in their raw form are seldom sufficient to sway anyone over to your side.

When used properly, data help persuade policy makers to think differently about an issue. Effective use of data leads people to a deeper understanding of how an issue is relevant to their lives and helps reframe issues. This reframing is one of the most powerful skills an APN leader can have—the ability to use highly relevant data that alters the way an issue or policy is viewed by those forming the policy. An example of strategic use of data occurred at a CMS Nursing Open Door Policy Meeting. The meeting began with a preview of a newsletter that was to be mailed to all 40 million Medicare beneficiaries. The newsletter described how older adults could make their care safer by asking more questions of their "physician." The one-page newsletter included the term *physician* nine times. The APN leader pointed out that there were nearly 200,000 prescribing providers in the United States who are not physicians: over 101,000 NPs, nearly 10,000 CNMs, 30,000 CRNAs, and over 42,000 PAs. The APN went on to state that using the term *physician* does not accurately reflect the current work force that provides reimbursable care to Medicare beneficiaries and is likely to cause confusion among patients. The CMS official apologized for the oversight and revised the letter to read "health care professional."

APN Professional Organization Fragmentation

One of the greatest lost opportunities for APNs has been the fragmentation of the professional associations representing APN groups. There have been occasions when loose coalitions were formed to jointly support a policy position, but more often the APN movement lacks organizational unity. There are more than six national associations representing NPs, and until the American College of Nurse Practitioners (ACNP) was formed in 1993 there was little opportunity for the NP profession to speak with one voice. Although it is important to acknowledge the uniqueness of each type of APN, political power and influence is lost by this fragmentation. As the APN work force continues to grow in numbers, the APN community will gain strength by flexing the boundaries that distinguish APNs from one another. As the ACNP, whose stated mission is to be fast, friendly, flexible, and funded, moves to increase unity among the NP community, additional emphasis must be placed on the unity of all APNs to garner political resources and strength (Table 15–3).

Proposed APN Political Competencies

Many skills are needed to be influential at the policy level. Most of these skills, however, bridge strong APN skills. APNs have expertise in the assessment, diagnosis, and treatment of the complex responses to human illness and problems.[16] This expertise requires depth, breadth, and synthesis of knowledge of the human re-

TABLE 15–3. National APN Membership Associations	
NP Associations	
American Academy of Nurse Practitioners	www.aanp.org
*American Association of Critical Care Nurses	www.aacn.org
American College of Nurse Practitioners	www.nurse.org/acnp
†*Association of Women's Health, Obstetric, and Neonatal Nurses	www.awhonn.org
*National Association of NPs in Women's Health	www.npwh.org
*National Conference of Gerontological Nurse Practitioners	www.ncgnp.org
*National Organization of Nurse Practitioner Faculties	www.nonpf.org
*National Association of Pediatric Nurse Practitioners	www.napnap.org
*Nurse Practitioner Associates for Continuing Education	www.npace.org
Nurse Midwifery Association	
American College of Nurse Midwives	www.acnm.org
Nurse Anesthetist Association	
American Association of Nurse Anesthetists	www.aana.com
Clinical Nurse Specialist Associations	
†American Association of Critical Care Nurses	www.aacn.org
†Oncology Nursing Society	www.ons.org
National Association of Clinical Nurse Specialists	www.nacns.org

*Denotes national affiliate membership in the American College of NPs. In addition, ACNP has 36 state NP asssociation affiliate members.
†These and a number of other organizations such as the American College Health Association, National Association of Neonatal Nurses, and the National Association of School Nurses have a significant portion of APN membership.

sponse to illness. These same skills that effectively motivate patients to make lifestyle changes can be applied to the policy arena. APNs must hone their interpersonal skills continually and apply them to the policy process. Developing and implementing strategies at the individual and collective professional levels to influence health policy decisions effectively for large numbers of patient populations are critical for high-quality health care, increased access to care, and reduced health care costs.

Interpersonal/Communication Skills

- Identifies and takes action only on select issues about which one feels passionately
- Knows what is wanted out of a situation by establishing rapport versus "being right"
- Works from others' strengths; minimizes weaknesses
- Networks with key stakeholders
- Seeks expertise when needed
- Shares expertise when needed
- Communicates accurately and efficiently
- Manages personal feelings and personal biases
- Uses humor, warmth, and honesty in relationships (using nonthreatening and positive intent)
- Collaborates
- Practices persuasion skills
- Treats patients as colleagues—trusts they can think/act on their own behalf
- Manages personal and professional boundaries
- Creates coalitions
- Avoids role of "shrill" and responds to insults carefully and thoughtfully

Analytic Skills/Policy Knowledge

- Knows policy process as well as stakeholders' views on controversial issues
- Considers the importance of timing before intervening
- Approaches health policy issues with a "solution-finding" attitude to increase access and quality while reducing costs
- Develops and sustains networks within and across professions
- Integrates an understanding of others' perspectives
- Assesses possible policy impacts, both pros and cons
- Assesses possible policy effects on key stakeholders to develop coalitions strategically

- Develops knowledge of individual and organizational patterns or historical positions on critical policy issues
- Identifies power/influence, and develops strategies to increase one's power base
- Crafts coherent arguments in written and oral form
- Uses data effectively to support positions
- Interacts with media effectively
- Demonstrates respect for other health professions and professionals
- Stays active with the APN professional association(s)

Conflict Resolution Skills

- Anticipates, assesses, and responds effectively to the needs of diverse stakeholders
- Employs systems thinking
- Employs strategic thinking ability to conceptualize and articulate a vision
- Takes risks
- Demonstrates active listening by acknowledging and clarifying verbal messages to ensure mutual understanding
- Seeks information to better understand opposing viewpoints
- Diffuses sensitive or difficult situations, and creates a climate for mutual problem-solving

IMPORTANT HEALTH POLICY WEBSITES

Federal Government Sites

Agency for Healthcare Research and Quality	www.ahrq.gov
Congress	http://thomas.loc.gov
Congressional Budget Office	www.cbo.gov
Center for Medicare and Medicaid Services	www.cms.gov
Centers for Disease Control and Prevention	www.cdc.gov
General Accounting Office	www.gao.org
Medicare Payment Advisory Commission	www.medpac.gov
Office of Management and Budget	www.whitehouse.gov/omb
FedStats (statistics from over 100 federal agencies)	www.fedstats.gov

State/Local Health Policy

National Association of State Information Resource Executives	www.nascio.org
National Conference of State Legislatures	www.ncsl.org
National Governors Association	www.nga.org

Foundations

Henry J. Kaiser Foundation	www.kff.org
Robert Wood Johnson Foundation	www.rwjf.org
The Commonwealth Fund	www.cmwf.org

Think Tanks

Academy for Health Services Research and Health Policy	www.academyhealth.org
BCBS Health Issues	www.bcbshealthissues.com
Cato Health Institute	www.cato.org
Center for Studying Health System Change	www.hschange.com
Center on Budget and Policy Priorities	www.cbpp.org
Heritage Foundation	www.heritage.org
National Academy for State Health Policy	www.nashp.org
National Center for Policy Analysis-Health Issues	www.ncpa.org
Urban Institute	www.urban.org

International

Organization for Economic Co-operation and Development	www.oecd.org
World Health Organization	www.who.int

SUGGESTED EXERCISES

1. Describe the APN title recognition laws, prescriptive authority, and reimbursement policies in your state. Does your state appear to be restrictive in comparison with the 49 other states?

2. Craft a three-to-five-page testimony that you would deliver to a legislative body (at the state or federal level) on a health problem that is important to you in your community.

Clearly identify the health policy problem and offer a legislative solution using data to inform your testimony.

3 Identify 10 ways in which you could improve your political competence.

4 Describe a current health policy issue that is important to you. Analyze where the policy issue is in the policy-making process.

REFERENCES

1. Kohn, L, Corrigan, J, and Donaldson, M: To Err is Human: Building a Safer Health System. Washington, DC, National Academy Press, 2000.
2. Kaiser Family Foundation and Health Research and Educational Trust: 2002 Employer Health Benefits Survey. http://www.kff.org/content/2002. Washington, DC, Author, 2002.
3. President's Advisory Commission on Consumer Protection and Quality in the Health Care Industry: Quality First: Better Health Care for all Americans, Final Report. Washington, DC, Author, 1998.
4. Committee on the Consequences of Uninsurance: Care Without Coverage: Too Little Too Late. Washington, DC, National Academy Press, 2002.
5. U.S. Bureau of the Census: Number of Americans With and Without Health Insurance Rises. Press release September 30. http://www.census.gov/Press-Release/www/2002/cb02-127.html. Washington, DC, Author, 2002.
6. Families USA. Going Without Health Insurance: Nearly One in Three Non-Elderly Americans. The Robert Wood Johnson Foundation and Families USA, March 2003. www.familiesUSA.org
7. Kingdon, JW: Agendas, Alternatives, and Public Policies, 2nd ed. New York, HarperCollins College Publishers, 1995.
8. Longest, B: Health Policymaking in the United States, 3rd ed. Washington, DC, AUPHA/HAP, 2002.
9. Pfiffner, JP, ed: Governance and American Politics: Classic and Current Perspectives. Fort Worth, TX, Harcourt Brace and Company, 1995.
10. Lindbloom, C: The science of muddling through. In Etzioni, A (ed.), Readings in Modern Organizations, pp. 154–165. Englewood Cliffs, NJ, Prentice Hall, 1969.
11. American College of Nurse Practitioners: Fact Sheet 2002. www.acnpweb.org.
12. American Association of Nurse Anesthetists: Press release, June 11. http://www.aana.com/press/2002/061102.asp. Washington, DC, Author, 2002.
13. American Medical Association: Competition in Health Insurance: A Comprehensive Study of U.S. Markets. http://www.ama-assn.org/ama/pub/article/5910–5574.html. Chicago, Author, 2001.
14. Spratley, E, et al.: The Registered Nurse Population, Findings from the National Sample Survey of Registered Nurses. Rockville, MD: U.S. Department of Health and Human Services, Health Resources and Service Administration, Bureau of Health Professions, Division of Nursing, 2000
15. American Hospital Association: In Our Hands: How Hospital Leaders Can Build a Thriving Workforce. Chicago, Author, 2002.
16. American Nurses Association: Scope and Standards of Advanced Practice Registered Nursing. Washington, DC, Author, 1996.
17. Academy Health: Glossary of terms. http://www.academyhealth.org/page_resources_glossary_healthcare. Washington, DC, Author, 2002.
18. Field, MJ, Tranquada, RE, and Feasley, JF (eds.): Health Services Research: Workforce and Educational Issues. Washington, DC, National Academy Press, 1995.

CHAPTER 16

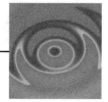

Creating Excellence in Practice

CHAPTER 16

Marla J. Weston, MS, RN
Vicki L. Buchda, MS, RN
Debra Bergstrom, MS, RN, FNP

Marla J. Weston, MS, RN, who is currently a resident of Phoenix, Arizona, received her master's of science in nursing from Arizona State University in Tempe and her bachelor's of science in nursing from Indiana University of Pennsylvania in Indiana, Pennsylvania. Ms. Weston is Executive Director of the Arizona Nurses' Association. Ms. Weston has been a clinical nurse specialist, nurse educator, and nurse executive. She has also served as an adjunct faculty member at Arizona State University and a mentor to advanced practice nurses (APNs) experiencing role transition to their first position and has facilitated the growth and development of experienced APNs. Ms. Weston is affiliated with the American Nurses Association and the American Organization of Nurse Executives. She is a member of Sigma Theta Tau National Honor Society.

Vicki L. Buchda, MS, RN, received her master's of science from Arizona State University in Tempe and her bachelor's of science in nursing from Marian College of Fond du Lac in Wisconsin. She is currently the Director of Patient Care Resources at the Mayo Clinic in Scottsdale, Arizona. In that role she is accountable for professional nursing practice, nursing research, clinical and patient education, case management, nursing quality assurance, nursing informatics, and nursing recruitment and retention at Mayo Clinic and Mayo Clinic Hospital. She has held the positions of clinical nurse specialist, critical care educator, and critical care/telemetry unit director in other facilities and has served as adjunct clinical faculty at Arizona State University. Ms. Buchda is actively involved in several organizations, including the Arizona Organization of Nurse Executives, where she has held a seat on the board of directors for several terms. She is also a member of the American Nurses Association and Sigma Theta Tau International.

Debra Bergstrom, MS, RN, FNP, completed her postgraduate family nurse practitioner certification through Arizona State University in 1995. She received her master's of science in critical care nursing from Arizona State University in 1992 and her bachelor's of science in nursing in 1985 from the University of Texas at El Paso. She served in staff roles in a variety of clinical areas, including postpartum care, cardiovascular intensive care, cardiac care and neurosurgery, and cardiac catheterization laboratory and as an advanced practice nurse in hospital critical care departments. After membership in three group practices of medicine, she now owns and operates Neighborhood Family Practice, P.C.

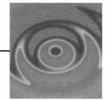

Creating Excellence in Practice

CHAPTER OBJECTIVES

After completing this chapter, the reader will be able to:

1 Incorporate knowledge about concepts of excellence into a personal definition of excellence.

2 Apply principles of excellence to an advanced practice role.

3 Articulate strategies for creating and maintaining excellence.

APNs are expected to exceed the basic standards of nursing practice. Nursing's Social Policy Statement[1] describes APNs as master's-prepared clinicians who:

- Practice within an area of specialization and with greater autonomy than nurses in other roles
- Function at the expanding boundaries of nursing's scope of practice
- Acquire ever-increasing levels of knowledge and skills
- Integrate advanced theoretical concepts and research-based knowledge into clinical practice

Given these already high expectations, how can one distinguish excellence in those engaged in advanced practice?

ATTRIBUTES OF EXCELLENCE

Badness you can get easily, in quantity: the road is smooth, and it lies close by. But in front of excellence the immortal gods have put sweat....

—HESIOD, 700 BC

How does the condition or quality of being excellent arise? Webster defines *excellent* as "superior, very good of its kind, eminently good." Synonyms for excellent include *superior, premium, superb, distinct,* and *admirable.* Two other words expand on this definition. The verb *exceed* is derived from the Latin *ex cedere,* meaning *to go more.* The verb *excel* is from the Latin *ex cellere,* which means *to rise above,* or *project.* The concepts of going beyond and of rising above are inherent in the word excellent. Pinkerton[2] wrote that "Professional excellence implies competence and a striving for high standards in every aspect of life" (p. 280).

Excellence involves an ongoing comparison with a standard or with that which is generally accepted, as well as an unceasing attempt to achieve more and to improve one's performance. Thus, excellence is a dynamic condition that is continually redefined and reinterpreted.

Although the state of excellence is dynamic, excellent organizations and individuals have been repeatedly associated with the following attributes:

- Values
- Vision
- Passion
- Mastery
- Action
- Balance

In this chapter, these attributes establish a framework for exploring excellence in advanced practice nursing. Examples of excellence in organizations and individuals are provided, and strategies for fostering excellence in advanced practice nursing are proposed.

Values

There is no such thing as a minor lapse of integrity.

—TOM PETERS

There is always one true inner voice. Trust it.

—GLORIA STEINEM

A review of the literature on values demonstrates that excellence is characterized by behaviors consistent with certain universally held values as well as with the values of one's profession, the values of one's organization, and one's own personal values. Certain values, such as integrity, honesty, respect for others, and fairness, are held universally and are not based on any particular religion, social philosophy, or ethical system.[3] They are part of all enduring societies. Behaviors consistent with universally held values are necessary for excellence. As Henderson[4] maintained, the personal integrity of the individual [and, we add, organization] is inseparable from the quality of the service given. Integrity requires being honest and authentic with oneself and others as well as taking substantial responsibility for agreements to which one has committed oneself.[5] Behaving with integrity and in a manner consistent with universally held values also creates energy for oneself and others.

When individuals, organizations, or societies fail to act according to universal principles, distrust and fear ensue, power imbalances arise and, ultimately, excellence is inhibited. In present-day America, examples concerning values, or their absence, loom large. Consider the unprecedented corporate betrayals of trust, such as Enron's pension and securities fraud. In contrast, consider the outpouring of patriotism, support, and resources that followed the World Trade Center disaster along with the widespread reassessment of personal and societal values.

Conversely, individuals and organizations that embody universal values promote harmonious relationships and excellence. When Bob Galvin, former chairman of Motorola, was negotiating a lucrative contract with a South American country, he was asked by the country's leaders to write the contract for an extra $1 million, with the understanding that the officials would skim this from the project. Because this request was clearly in violation of the principle of honesty, Motorola turned down the contract and refused further business with the country. Galvin noted that that country's leaders are long deposed, whereas Motorola is still considered an organization of excellence.[5]

However, it has been suggested that there is little economic reason to justify honesty and integrity in business and minimal consequences for failure to tell the truth. In fact, some equate dishonesty with business success.[6] Davidhizar[7] analyzed honesty in nursing practice and found that when nurses were dishonest, they acted this way for reasons including self-protection, protection of other health care providers, and protection of patients. She acknowledged that while paybacks for honesty are few, some important rewards include increased self-respect, peace with oneself, greater trust from others, and a reputation of integrity. Trust and honesty are the cornerstones for relationships between clients and providers and among professional colleagues.

Excellent professionals embody the core values of their professions. Caring, advocacy, accountability, accessibility, and collaboration with other health and community professionals have been articulated as values to which APNs subscribe.[8] In addition, professionals are expected to realize a "higher morality and a greater commitment to the good of others"[9] because of the special nature of the interpersonal relationship entered into with clients. The uniqueness of the relationship is based on the particular vulnerability of clients, which creates an inequality of power in the relationship. The expectation of professionals is that this vulnerability will be the source of trust and obligation, not profit or exploitation.

Excellence, whether in a company or an individual, requires clearly delineating core values. In the early 1980s, after researching attributes of excellent corporations, Peters and Waterman[10] proposed that solid commitment to the values of the organization is linked to the success of a company. Their "one all-purpose bit of advice for management" was to identify, communicate, and base actions on these values. For example, the success of Nordstrom department stores can be traced to clearly profiling, communicating, and enacting the value of "customer above company." The working culture of Nordstrom is filled with anecdotes of salespeople meeting the customer's needs in creative and unconventional ways. One Nordstrom saleswoman went to a rival department store for a customer to purchase a dress that Nordstrom did not carry. She then sold it to the astonished customer for less than the retail price.[11] The saleswoman's behavior was based squarely on her interpretation of the customer-above-company value and was endorsed as such.

Whatever the values ascribed, successful companies are resolutely committed. In their analysis of the successful habits of long-lasting, visionary companies, Collins and Porras[12] identify unchanging core values as a primary attribute of the companies they studied, regardless of what the core values are. Even when these companies are undergoing financial or organizational difficulties, they hold true to their core values. Motorola, for example, strongly values honesty. As a result, discussions in Motorola often involve open disagreement and critique of ideas, even to the point of embarrassing and confronting individuals. Outsiders sometimes describe this as disrespectful or barbaric. Employees of Motorola say anything less is dishonest, and "backroom politics" and "roundabout decision making" is not tolerated.[5]

Peak performance is obtained when the values of the organization, the profession, and the person are aligned.[13] Excellent professionals are knowledgeable about the values of an organization and weigh them in comparison with the core values and traditions of the profession. In situations where the values are aligned, APNs experience a sense of participation and achievement, as well as potential for learning and growth. Koerner[14] found that for APNs, the values and job description were congruent. These values reflected initiative, decision-making, accountability, and internal locus of control behaviors. Most APNs prefer to work in organizations with a participative management style.[15] Involvement in goal-setting and decision-making is associated with increased job satisfaction. Performing interesting and challenging work, assuming responsibility, experiencing achievement, having potential for growth, and receiving recognition as professionals add to their satisfaction.[16]

In the current health care climate, many professional values seem to collide with those of the business environment. If an individual's values are not congruent with those of the organization, several outcomes are possible. Some professionals might continue to perform the job, ignoring the conflict and suppressing personal and/or professional values. Others may be tenacious, continuing to do the job while trying to reconcile the differences. However, excellence in practice is difficult, if not impossible, when professional or universal values are undermined by an individual or an environment.[17] Excellent APNs strive to create or find organizations and practice environments with more compatible value systems, even when the consequences can be considerable, such as making a job change. Initially, for example, the drive for increased efficiency, productivity, and profit can seem diametrically opposed to the APN's core values. To create excellence, the APN must reconcile the desire to provide caring, personalized attention to each client with the demand for ensuring cost-effective outcomes. In right-fit organizations, where individual, professional, and organizational values are aligned, APNs can excel and realize opportunities to improve the quality of care while controlling cost.[18]

At times, ethical predicaments occur when there is no option but to choose between equally unsatisfactory alternatives in which there is no "clearly best" solution. Drucker[19] advised that to obtain excellence, one has to start with what is right rather than with what is acceptable, because compromise is inevitable. In these difficult situations, basing decisions on professional and personal values can lead to excellence. In a study of nurse practitioners, Viens[20] found that strong personal and professional values guided and shaped the resolution of moral dilemmas in clinical practice. Values formed the bases for their rationales, actions, and choices. All the values identified centered on APNs' relationship to the client. Understanding one's motives, acting for the good of the whole and not solely for oneself, caring about the values of the organization, and having concern for others are crucial to the ultimate resolution of the internal battle between the tendency toward self-interest and the obligation to serve.

Vision

If you can dream it, you can do it.

—WALT DISNEY

Reality is something you rise above.

—LIZA MINNELLI

A clear vision of what is possible is necessary for excellence. Creating a new reality occurs by first imagining that possibility. Visions may arise from speculation about the future or by posing these questions: why are things being done in a certain way, what is missing in this situation, what is the desired state? Visions arise from what should be and require rising above "the tyranny of what is." Garfield[13] described the culture at NASA during the Apollo 11 project. The excitement of the mission, the challenge of the task, and the vision of putting a man on the moon all combined to create a culture where otherwise unremarkable people became peak performers.

Making the vision a reality becomes the *raison d'être*. In all excellent organizations, decisions are made, and priorities are set according to the vision. Work that does not support the vision is considered extraneous and consequently aborted.[10] Vision, based on core values, allows a powerful focus toward a future desired state or destination. Organizations and individuals characterized as excellent not only set priorities according to their vision, they also concentrate on the highest priorities; that is, they do first things first.[5,19]

Successful APNs have a vision and know where they want to go. Creating a vision involves knowing what outcomes are desired and can occur on various levels, including personal, clinical, and organizational levels. Having a clear image of the future allows APNs to avoid getting caught in the inefficiency of engaging in activities that may not be vital or productive. On a basic level, creating and maintaining excellence requires the ability to discipline meeting schedules and in-boxes.[21] Moreover, excellent APNs outline long-term agendas, establish priorities, and serve as agents for constructive change. Excellent APNs guard against confusing activity with accomplishment. Bustling activity is not, in and of itself, equated with productivity and organizational imperatives, nor does it necessarily mean that one is moving toward a vision.

Unfortunately, a vision rarely provides a detailed map for a journey, but rather acts as a beacon, providing direction. A prescribed journey with much structure would likely extinguish the opportunities for chance and intuition. As evidenced by hundreds of scientists, including Jonas Salk and Albert Einstein, chance and intuition are very useful in achieving one's vision.[5] The excellent visionary is skillful in integrating reasoning, chance, and intuition.

Garfield[13] described this integrating process as "course correction," an adjustment of the critical pathway whenever cues indicate that desired results are not occurring. Setbacks and mistakes may be valuable signs that it is time to correct course. Course correction employs three skills:

1. Mental agility, which is the ability to change perspective when challenges occur

2. Concentration, which includes stamina, adaptability to changes, and hardiness

3. Learning from mistakes

The ability to correct course enhances the achievement of vision and propels one's movement further in the right direction, despite seeming setbacks.

Passion

People can smell emotional commitment from a mile away.
Remember, passion is contagious.

—TOM PETERS

Commitment to excellence is required for its achievement, and passion is essential to sustain excellence. Peters and Austin[22] described commitment as "hanging in there long after others have gotten bored or given up; it's refusing to leave well enough alone" (p. 415).

Just as consistency between values and behavior produces energy and passion, passion itself also enables energy to create excellence. Passion involves ardently striving for the best, even when repeated efforts seem tedious or appear exceedingly strenuous. Passion motivates via a clear sense of purpose and devotion to high standards.[5] The president of Racing Strollers described her turmoil, speculating about whether she was too demanding when she required that something be done over and over until it was perfect: a seam sewn straighter, a color re-dyed to be purer. She eventually recognized that because she cared so intensely, she was able to see more, to analyze better, and to insist that there be continuous improvement in the product. This ability to recognize the "just-noticeable difference" is a result of passion. She wrote, "Someone has to be slightly crazed, obsessive, and willing to set a high standard"[23] (p. 20).

Passion is not something that can be created artificially. Even the most excellent APNs cannot "motivate" others or themselves to be passionate. When studying companies, Jim Collins[24] and his team recognized that companies that transitioned from good to great *discovered*, rather than manufactured, their passion. Moreover, passion never arises from fear. Rather, passion emerges from an inner force and urge for excellence.

The APN who cares a little more will encourage colleagues to become involved and will facilitate independent thinking and judgment. The APN with passion will not be satisfied with providing less than optimal care and will pursue the latest research, the most up-to-date procedures, and the most effective therapies to produce the best outcomes for patients.

A caution should be noted in the enactment of passion. One may be criticized for being unduly emotional, excessively driven, overly involved, or having unrealistic standards. Many passionate individuals experience a tension between excellence and balance in personal life.[22] Being passionate about creating excellence requires energy, time, and commitment. It may demand late nights and the sacrifice of an occasional weekend. Thus, "the adventure of excellence is not for the faint of heart"[22] (p. 414). Passion requires courage and high self-esteem and should be considered a gift. Yet passion must be disciplined in order to prevent inflexibility and loss of perspective. The APN can compare self-perceptions with those of colleagues to assess the extent to which passion is creating excellence. Colleagues can often assist an APN to channel passion to achieve envisioned outcomes while developing and preserving relationships.

Mastery

People with high levels of personal mastery are continually expanding their ability to create the results in life they truly seek.

—PETER SENGE

Mastery is the ability to channel one's values, vision, and passion via the milieu of expertise to create superlative outcomes. As described by Walsh and Bernhard in Chapter 4, as individuals evolve from novice to expert, they:

- Decrease reliance on abstract principles and increase application of past experience

- Move from viewing situations as comprising equally relevant bits of information to perceiving the whole, in which some parts have greater importance

- Diminish the detached observer orientation in favor of fuller involvement as a performer

Benner[25] described expert nurses (i.e., nurses with a high level of mastery) as having Gestalt, or holistic, understanding. Because of their enormous background of experience, expert nurses perceive patterns of events in an ongoing process of contrasting and comparing scenarios. As a result, experts can sense the wholeness of a situation while recognizing separate components and are able to focus on the nature of the problem without wastefully exploring irrelevant or implausible alternatives.

Masters simultaneously hold an engaging image of a distant vision while dealing with current reality. The ability to translate vision into action, clarify values, use intuition, negotiate, create consensus, implement change, and work with others is essential to progress to the master level. Masters enact these skills because they want to engage others in making a vision a reality.[26] For example, Florence Nightingale demonstrated mastery in nursing not only through technical innovations in care of the sick but also by exerting her influence on powerful individuals to assist her in instituting changes to the practice of nursing. As this example describes, mastery combines expert technical and professional skills with leadership and interpersonal and organizational proficiency.

This combination of leadership and interpersonal and organizational proficiency requires mastering emotional intelligence (EQ). EQ involves monitoring, recognizing, and managing one's own emotions and the emotions of others. Masters develop competence in the four domains of EQ: self-awareness, self-management, social awareness, and relationship management. Masters are skilled at using EQ to create enthusiasm in themselves and others; as a result, performance soars. Masters in EQ recognize, conversely, that when people are anxious or angry, performance suffers. APNs with mastery in EQ can shift among visionary, coaching, affiliative, and demonstrative leadership styles to create a positive emotional reaction from others. They maintain their inner core of integrity, and their passion influences those around them, driving others to higher performance.[27]

Mastery compels a lifelong pursuit of learning. Interestingly, although masters are confident of their competence, they are simultaneously acutely aware of what they do not know. Mastery involves approaching situations with the inquisitiveness of an amateur and a willingness to learn from mistakes. Learning always involves some level of discomfort, risk, and fear of failure. Paradoxically, challenge is one of the greatest human motivators. By definition, as we learn new skills, we are exposed to areas where we are not competent or confident. As one persists in spite of this discomfort, competence builds, fear decreases, and learning becomes exciting. As we repeatedly learn new things, we recognize that the early discomfort and fear make up only a temporary phase that dissolves into the excitement and challenge of learning. Thus, we increase our tolerance for discomfort, ambiguity, and uncertainty associated with learning. Moreover, as the fear decreases, not only does the learning become exciting, it also becomes easier. For example, learning a third language is easier and quicker than learning a second language.[28]

Even with this ongoing learning, the master APN may feel unprepared and inadequate in certain situations. Some believe it is necessary to be perfect at everything they do, lest they be "discovered" as an impostor. Many nurses in advanced practice roles suffer from this "impostor phenomenon."[29] The impostor phenomenon denotes healthy, successful, high-achieving individuals who hide an inner feeling of inadequacy, intellectual phoniness, and a belief that they have fooled everyone. Certain situations, such as starting a new job, moving into a new role, and interacting with authority figures may escalate feelings of being an impostor, including depression, generalized anxiety, lack of self-confidence, frustration, and an overall feeling of ignorance. The risk with the impostor phenomenon is that the APN will settle for the safe and certain to avoid these uncomfortable emotions. Recognizing that many of the feelings associated with the impostor phenomenon may be part of the learning process can help the APN to celebrate achievements and continue to strive for excellence.

Today's rapidly changing health care environment demands that one be able to unlearn old ways of doing things when they no longer apply in order to relearn new methods.[26] Unlearning involves challenging the ways of thinking that worked well in the past but that are no longer appropriate for the future.[30] Home Depot, a warehouse hardware store, is a good example of effective unlearning. Home Depot "forgot" that its customers were male home builders or owners; they learned to provide decorating services and a bridal registry.[31]

Candor concerning one's personal and professional strengths and weaknesses is essential to mastery. Seeking feedback and peer review for self-improvement is one of the most effective avenues for building mastery. APNs who work arduously to get feedback from many sources are more likely to achieve mastery. Peer review provides a forum for sharing information, offering guidance, contributing constructive criticism and direction to other clinical nurses and other advanced practitioners, and getting the same in return. Additional approaches to nurture mastery include ongoing dialogue, education and training, and demonstration of competence by certification. Information obtained from continuing education meetings or conferences as well as from discussions with colleagues are the most frequent sources of practice changes for APNs.[32,33] Masters ensure they have budgeted time for ongoing learning and creative thinking.

Perhaps the most expansive and promising mastery trajectory is that of mentorship. Mentorship is an informal, intense personal relationship in which a senior person offers the wisdom of experience to guide and influence the career of a novice. A mentor is a teacher, coach, taskmaster, confidant, counselor, and friend. Burke in Chapter 9 describes the roles and contributions of mentors in developing excellence in APNs.

Action

We are what we repeatedly do. Excellence, then, is not an act, but a habit.

—ARISTOTLE

I think one's feelings waste themselves in words, they ought all to be distilled into actions and into actions which bring results.

—FLORENCE NIGHTINGALE

Values, vision, passion, and mastery form a foundation for excellence, but action enables it. Action is what gives credibility to the values, vision, passion, and mastery of the APN.

Peters and Waterman[10] described one of eight attributes of America's best-run companies as "a bias for action." These companies are analytic when making decisions but are not plagued by the pursuit of perfection and do not suffer from "paralysis by analysis." Experimentation and a sense of urgency reign in these companies. Standard operating procedure is "Do it, fix it, try it." For example, Bell and Howell proposed the idea of selling movie cameras by direct mail. Realizing that it would take an investment of only $10,000 to try the idea, they decided to act—a decision that ultimately spared them $100,000 worth of time to study the idea.[10]

Excellence in action necessitates reasonable risk-taking. Reasonable risk-taking involves encouraging meritorious attempts while supporting mistakes. For example, knowing that only 1 trial in 10 results in a successful product, excellent companies encourage exploration of all possible trials, rapidly abandoning ideas that show no promise and actively pursuing those that show the potential of success.[10] McDonald's has more experimental menu items, store formats, and pricing plans than its competitors. Although most experimental menu items fail, within 2 years of experimenting with breakfast menus in a few rural franchises breakfast accounted for 35 percent of McDonald's revenues.[10] Risk-taking allows and accepts the potential for failure, minimizes control, and "steps outside of the box." While risk can sometimes be minimized by gaining additional information, time, or control,[34] the optimum direction for action is often unclear. Excellent individuals react to this ambiguity with elegance by making the best decision possible with the information available, then acting on it.

Action may be limited by what Pfeffer and Sutton[35] describe as the "knowing-doing gap." This phenomenon occurs when leaders know what to do and can plot a course to achieve desired results but are not adept at translating ideas into action. Furthermore, the authors found a particular pattern of communication, which they coined "smart talk," to be an inhibitor of organizational action. Smart talk is confident, articulate, and eloquent. At the same time, smart talk is complicated and/or abstract and tends to focus on the negative. Frequently, smart talk only focuses on the problems. As a result, it stops action. The APN can serve as a catalyst for action by asking how the problems can be solved and then working to overcome barriers to produce desired results.

While a bias for action encompasses focusing on results, equally important is focusing on what *not* to do and what to *stop* doing. Many people strive for excellence by creating an ever-expanding list of things to accomplish. The consequence is an endless "doing" that may or may not produce desired outcomes and that frequently results in feelings of being overworked, overwhelmed, and burnt out. Leaders who built great companies made as much use of "stop doing" lists as "to do" lists.[24] Recognizing and discontinuing activities that no longer add value allow for attention and focus on vital activities that produce more significant results, often with less work.

Clearly identifying and measuring contributions assist in creating excellence. Evaluations of APNs' contributions have historically been limited to documenting time spent on various activities, number of patients seen, or amount of revenue generated. For a novice APN, an assessment and documentation of time involvement may assist in learning to effectively prioritize and organize time.[36] However, time documentation alone will not demonstrate the impact of an APN. APNs can focus on results and demonstrate their impact on cost and quality outcomes in any of the following areas[37-39]:

- Reduction of use of costly technology and inpatient care
- Reduction of inpatient lengths of stay
- Improvements in patients' levels of functioning
- Enhanced patient satisfaction
- Improvements in the quality of care provided

Combining process and outcome measurements through research, evaluative studies, or quality-improvement activities will further assist the APN in demonstrating the impact of advanced practice. For example, a clinical nurse specialist developed a comprehensive educational plan for families and children who were newly diagnosed with insulin-dependent diabetes. As an outcome, in a 2-year period, none of the children who participated in the program had been readmitted to the hospital with hypoglycemia or ketoacidosis.[40]

Excellence requires action taken, with a focus on results rather than with concern for who gets credit. Actions carried out in a self-serving manner or directed solely to gain the recognition of others will not result in excellence. Block[41] presented this as the concept of "stewardship": "the willingness to be accountable for the well-being of the larger organization by operating in service, rather than control, of those around us" (p. xx).

Stewardship is based on the value of service: service to clients, the public, colleagues, and the organization. The excellent APN acts as a steward in action. Stewardship and the pursuit of excellence also entail "giving back" to one's profession. As Curtin[42] described: "One of the most effective ways to promote excellence in nursing practice and to disseminate new information is for nurses to offer information, support, guidance, criticism and direction to one another" (p. 28).

Mentoring others is imperative for sustaining excellence in the profession. Serving as a mentor supports the socialization of novices to the profession's values and standards as well as the development of others to take risks, to reach their full potential, and to make substantial contributions to the profession.[43]

Involvement in professional organizations also furnishes APNs with an opportunity to use their knowledge, skills, and talents to create excellence both in practice and in patient care. Involving oneself with professional organizations, both on a community and a national level, not only provides the chance to stimulate the thinking of other nurse colleagues but also stimulates the APN's thinking. In addition, most APNs find that political advocacy is most expedient through professional organizations.[44] Professional organizations monitor health care legislation and provide that information to their members. Professional organizations have the pooled resources of all members to influence political decisions through contributions, lobbying activities, and voting drives. Health care is becoming increasingly shaped by political decisions. Historically, nurses have not been any more active in the political process than other citizens.[45] APNs can be instrumental in working toward political consensus and cohesion with professional groups as well as in using their visibility to influence members of the community on political issues.

Sharing clinical expertise and research results through scholarly presentations and publications provides another way for the excellent APN to give back to the profession. Poster presentations, joint presentations, or authorship with a more experienced colleague; review of an area of clinical literature; or descriptions of innovations in clinical practices provide relatively easy ways to begin presenting and publishing.

Thus, a bias for action, reasonable risk-taking, and involvement enable excellence.

Balance

Balance isn't either/or; it's and.

—STEVEN COVEY, ROGER MERRILL, AND REBECCA MERRILL

Move like a beam of light,
Fly like lightning,
Strike like thunder,
Whirl in circles around a stable center.

—MORIHEI UESHIBA

Balance provides flexibility and stability. Being balanced is similar to having two feet on the ground: A strong wind will cause some sway but not a fall. Being unbalanced is like being tipped so that one foot is off the ground: even a small wind can result in being toppled. Excellence requires that one balance several potentially conflicting areas: logic and emotion, home and work, urgency and importance, production and renewal. Balancing these potential incongruities makes them complementary and creates a stable base or enhances the effectiveness of a person's established base. Creating excellence requires that one be balanced. The challenge to the APN who feels pulled in multiple directions is to develop strategies for maintaining balance. Balance requires actively managing time, carefully selecting renewal activities, and becoming a well-rounded individual.

Effective time management starts with clear values and vision. Balance necessitates that time is spent on activities consistent with the identified values and vision. Balance also entails prioritizing activities and disciplining passion to spend on only selected goals, instead of every goal. It involves resisting getting caught up in the unimportant even though it feels urgent. Saying no to seemingly urgent but lower-priority demands allows time to accomplish the truly important. One of the most effective strategies is to plan your time by first scheduling the most important activities.[46]

Excellence cannot be created in one area of life at the expense of all others. Working to the detriment of health or playing to the detriment of work does not maintain excellence in either category. Balance requires a holistic focus: attention to creating well-rounded, complementary skills and to spending time on renewal activities that reenergize. Corporations are beginning to focus on methods of doing work that supports the "whole person." They are discovering that promoting work-life balance results in synergy and greater gains in both areas of life.[47]

It is unrealistic to expect that the meticulous use of even the best balance strategies will prevent periods of imbalance. Almost anything of excellence requires a short-term burst of intense time and energy. Completing a major project, starting a new job, or finishing graduate school all can require a spurt of concentrated time and attention if excellence is the goal. Short-term periods of imbalance in the use of time do not necessarily result in imbalance in the person. If the period is time-limited, consistent with the overall vision, and accompanied by renewal activities, the individual can remain balanced.

Renewal activities can assist in creating excellence both during times of intense activities and during normal daily existence. Renewal activities restore energy through rest or recreation and can be physical, spiritual, mental, social, and/or emotional.[3] Renewal activities should be selected carefully to reenergize, not merely to become additions to an already lengthy "to do" list. Purposefully selecting renewal activities that complement work activities assists in creating balance and can even enhance productivity. For example, the professional with a mentally demanding job may select renewal activities that are physical. Similarly, taking breaks every 2 hours can improve the efficiency of writing an article. Even stopping to take 10 slow deep breaths in the midst of a hectic day can assist in providing balance.

Balance also includes cultivating and applying synergistic and holistic aspects of the personality. As Henderson[4] stated, "Excellence, to me, suggests the well-rounded, or complete, person." The more complementary skills individuals possess, the more balanced they are. Integrating reason and intuition, combining the technical and the creative, and linking emotion and rationality assist in creating excellence. Finding inner balance means learning to strengthen the inner resources that bring both joy and empowerment to your life.[48]

SUMMARY

How do you create excellence? Tom Watson of IBM would answer that you decide, as of this second, to quit doing less than excellent work.[49] Jim Collins[24] would agree, "Greatness is not a function of circumstance. Greatness, it turns out, is largely a matter of conscious choice" (p. 11). Excellence comes from an inner core: the desire and commitment to be excellent; in other words, valuing excellence, having a vision of excellence, and being passionate about creating and maintaining excellence. APNs must arm themselves with the necessary tools to create excellence, including mastery of clinical, leadership, interpersonal, and organizational skills; the willingness and ability to translate that mastery into action; and the ability to balance conflicting demands to remain centered on achieving excellence.

SUGGESTED EXERCISES

1 Admiral H. G. Rickover[50] stated, "If a profession is to have its proper place in the further development of society, it must be increasingly dissatisfied with things as they are" (p. 12). Identify an area of dissatisfaction within health care or the nursing profession. Using a variety of professional approaches, detail strategies that can be used to create excellence in this area.

2 Develop your own definition of excellence in advanced practice nursing. Identify an APN colleague who embodies excellence as you have defined it. Analyze the attributes of excellence demonstrated by this individual. What strategies did this colleague use to create excellence in advanced practice?

3 Consider whether individuals can be excellent in isolation or whether synergy is required to create excellence. What role have colleagues and mentors played in shaping your vision and achievement of excellence?

4 Evaluate how you are spending your time. Is the way you are spending your time helping or impeding you from achieving your personal and professional goals for excellence? What activities are not adding value and should be added to your "stop doing" list?

REFERENCES

1. American Nurses Association: Nursing's Social Policy Statement. Washington, DC, American Nurses Publishing, 2003.
2. Pinkerton, S: Summary. In Pinkerton, S, and Schroeder, P (eds.): Commitment to Excellence: Developing a Professional Nursing Staff. Rockville, MD, Aspen, 1988.
3. Covey, SR: The Seven Habits of Highly Effective People: Powerful Lessons in Personal Change. New York, Simon and Schuster, 1989.
4. Henderson, V: Excellence in nursing. Am J Nurs 90:76, 1990.
5. Hendricks, G, and Ludeman, K: The Corporate Mystic: A Guidebook for Visionaries with Their Feet on the Ground. New York, Bantam Books, 1996.
6. Bhide, A, and Stevenson, H: Why be honest if honesty doesn't pay? Harvard Business Rev 68:121, 1990.
7. Davidhizar, R: Honesty: The best policy in nursing practice. Today's OR Nurse 14:30, 1992.
8. National Council of State Boards of Nursing: Position Paper on the Licensure of Advanced Practice Nursing. Unpublished material, 1992.
9. Pellegrino, ED: What is a profession? J Allied Health 12:168, 1983.
10. Peters, TJ, and Waterman, RH: In Search of Excellence: Lessons from America's Best-Run Companies. New York, Warner Books, 1982.
11. Spector, R, and McCarthy, PD: The Nordstrom Way: The Inside Story of America's #1 Customer Service Company. New York, John Wiley & Sons, 1995.
12. Collins, JC, and Porras, JI: Built to Last: Successful Habits of Visionary Companies. New York, Harper-Collins, 1997.
13. Garfield, C: Peak Performers: The New Heroes of American Business. New York, William Morrow and Co, 1986.
14. Koerner, JG: Congruency between nurses' values and job requirements: A call for integrity. Holistic Nurse Pract 10:69, 1996.
15. Katims, I: Nursing as aesthetic experience and the notion of practice. Sch Inq Nurs Pract 7:26, 1993.
16. Lucas, MD: Organizational management style and clinical nurse specialists' job satisfaction. Clin Nurse Specialist 2:70, 1988.
17. Koelbel, PW, Fuller, SG, and Misener, TR: Job satisfaction of nurse practitioners: An analysis using Herzberg's theory. Nurs Pract 16:43, 1991.
18. Parr, MBE: The changing role of advanced practice nursing in a managed care environment. AACN Clin Issues 7:300, 1996.
19. Drucker, PF: The Effective Executive. New York, HarperBusiness, 1966.
20. Viens, DC: Moral dilemmas experienced by nurse practitioners. Nurse Pract Forum 5: 209, 1994.

21. Smith, PM: Blazing flashes of the obvious. Executive Excellence 10:4, 1993.
22. Peters, T, and Austin, N: A Passion for Excellence: The Leadership Difference. New York, Random House, 1985.
23. Baechler, M: Loves me, loves me not. Inc 17:19, 1995.
24. Collins, J: Good to Great: Why Some Companies Make the Leap ... And Others Don't. New York, HarperBusiness, 2001.
25. Benner, P: From Novice to Expert: Excellence and Power in Clinical Nursing Practice. Menlo Park, CA, Addison-Wesley, 1984.
26. Senge, PM: The Fifth Discipline: The Art & Practice of the Learning Organization. New York, Doubleday, 1990.
27. Goleman, D, Boyatzis, R, and McKee, A: Primal Leadership Realizing the Power of Emotional Intelligence. Boston, Harvard Business School Publishing, 2002.
28. Harris, J: The Learning Paradox: Gaining Success and Security in a World of Change. Toronto, Canada, Macmillan, 1998.
29. Arena, DM, and Page, NE: The impostor phenomenon in the clinical nurse specialist role. Image J Nurs Scholarship 24:121, 1992.
30. Hamel, G, and Prahalad, CK: Competing for the Future: Breakthrough Strategies for Seizing Control of Your Industry and Creating the Markets of Tomorrow. Boston, Harvard Business School Press, 1994.
31. McGill, ME, and Slocum, JW Jr: Unlearning the organization. Organizational Dynamics 22:67, 1993.
32. Flowers, JS, et al: How obstetric/gynecologic nurse practitioners make practice changes: A national study. J Am Acad Nurse Pract 1:132, 1989.
33. Johnson, TP: Continuing education survey of certified registered nurse anesthetists. AANA J 58:423, 1990.
34. MacCrimmon, KR, and Wehrung, DA: Taking Risks: The Management of Uncertainty. New York, Free Press, 1986.
35. Pfeffer, J, and Sutton, R: The Smart Talk Trap. Harvard Business Rev 77:134, 1999.
36. Hamric, AB: A model for CNS evaluation. In Hamric, AB, and Spross, J: The Clinical Nurse Specialist in Theory and Practice, 2nd ed. Philadelphia, WB Saunders, 1989.
37. Gibson, SJ, et al: CNS-directed case management: Cost and quality in harmony. J Nurs Adm 24:45, 1994.
38. Cronin, CJ, and Maklebust, J: Case-managed care: Capitalizing on the CNS. Nurs Manage 20:38, 1989.
39. Werner, JS, Bumann, RM, and O'Brien, JA: Clinical nurse specialization: An annotated bibliography: Evaluation and impact. Clin Nurse Specialist 3:20, 1989.
40. Peglow, DM, et al: Evaluation of clinical nurse specialist practice. Clin Nurse Specialist 6:28, 1992.
41. Block, P: Stewardship: Choosing Service over Self-Interest. San Francisco, Berrett-Koehler, 1993.
42. Curtin, L: Collegial ethics of a caring profession. Nurs Manage 25:28, 1994.
43. Vance, C: Mentoring for career success and satisfaction. J Adv Nurs 11:3, 1994.
44. Nelson, ML: Client advocacy. In Snyder, M, and Mirr, MP: Advanced Practice Nursing: A Guide to Professional Development. New York, Springer, 1995.
45. Maraldo, PJ: Politics and policy in primary care. In Mezey, MD, and McGivern, DO: Nurses, Nurse Practitioners: Evolution to Advanced Practice. New York, Springer, 1993.
46. Covey, SR, Merrill, AR, and Merrill, RR: First Things First. New York, Simon and Schuster, 1994.
47. Friedman, SD, Christensen, P, and DeGroot, J: Work and life: The end of the zero sum game. Harvard Business Rev 76:119, 1998.
48. Kenny, JW: Women's Stressors, Personality Traits and Inner Balance Strategies. Seattle, Elton-Wolf, 2002.
49. Peters, T: The Pursuit of WOW!: Every Person's Guide to Topsy-Turvy Times. New York, Vintage, 1994.
50. Rickover, HG: Thoughts on Man's Purpose in Life. Paper presented to the Rotary Club of San Diego, 1977.

Index

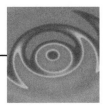

Note: Page numbers followed by the letter f refer to figures; those followed by t refer to tables.